Epidemics

Epidemics

The Impact of Germs and Their Power over Humanity

Joshua S. Loomis

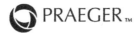 PRAEGER™

An Imprint of ABC-CLIO, LLC

Santa Barbara, California • Denver, Colorado

Library of Congress Cataloging-in-Publication Data

Names: Loomis, Joshua S., author.
Title: Epidemics : the impact of germs and their power over humanity / Joshua
  S. Loomis.
Description: Santa Barbara, California : Praeger, an imprint of ABC-CLIO,
  LLC, [2018] | Includes bibliographical references and index.
Identifiers: LCCN 2017043788 (print) | LCCN 2017045075 (ebook) | ISBN
  9781440861437 (eBook) | ISBN 9781440861420 (print : alk. paper)
Subjects: LCSH: Epidemics—History. | Communicable diseases—Social
  aspects—History.
Classification: LCC RA649 (ebook) | LCC RA649 .L68 2018 (print) | DDC
  614.4—dc23
LC record available at https://lccn.loc.gov/2017043788

ISBN: 978-1-4408-6142-0 (print)
      978-1-4408-6143-7 (ebook)

22 21 20 19 18   1 2 3 4 5

This book is also available as an eBook.

Praeger
An Imprint of ABC-CLIO, LLC

ABC-CLIO, LLC
130 Cremona Drive, P.O. Box 1911
Santa Barbara, California 93116-1911
www.abc-clio.com

This book is printed on acid-free paper ∞

Manufactured in the United States of America

For Kim and Sophia
*This book would never have happened without
your love and support*

Contents

Preface

Infectious agents have been with us as a species for as long as we have been a species. Despite having killed billions of people in every horrific way imaginable, most of us have just a superficial understanding of what infectious diseases are and how they have impacted us. The major reason for this is that few of us have personally experienced the devastating and uncontrolled spread of an epidemic disease in our population. We have thankfully grown up in an era when the vast majority of serious diseases can either be prevented or treated with proper sanitation, antibiotics, or vaccines. As a result, few people spend much time worrying about the possibility of being exposed to dangerous pathogens or having loved ones die from untreatable diseases. While this is an amazing testament to the progress we have made as a species, such advances have unfortunately lulled many into thinking that our technology has made us safe from future threats of new epidemics. It is a dangerous presumption to make, especially considering history is full of examples of unsuspecting populations being wiped out by killer diseases at a time when they thought they were protected in some way. For this reason, it is important that we take a look back at those diseases that have impacted us the most and examine what they have to teach us about who we are and where we are headed as a species.

The central purpose of this book is to look at the human story through the lens of epidemic diseases in order to explain how they have shaped our identity, altered the course of history, and changed how we interact with one another. This journey will take us through several thousand years of human history and traverse dozens of countries and every inhabited continent on Earth. The book will go beyond morbid accounts of disease symptoms and death statistics and tell the interesting and often forgotten stories behind what exactly made these diseases so awful for those who lived through them. The integration of science with history, sociology, religion, and other disciplines will provide the reader with a unique perspective that is not found in most other accounts of epidemic disease. In doing so, it will hopefully create a convincing argument that the history of humans cannot be accurately told without an including a discussion of these diseases.

Selecting which 10 epidemic diseases to include in the book was a difficult decision. The first thing that had to be done was to establish a set of criteria by which all diseases would be judged against. To be included in a book about the most impactful epidemic diseases of all time, it is obvious that a disease had to have killed or maimed a significant number of people. There was no magic number that was needed to make the cut; however, diseases with low morbidity and mortality rates were ruled out because they usually fail to cause any kind of panic. Second, the disease had to have had some historical significance or induced some major change to how we live or behave. This could include epidemics that altered the course of wars, toppled empires, sparked major leaps in technology, and even changed the sequence of the human genome. Finally, the disease had to be broad in its scope, either persisting for long periods of time or affecting people of different cultures in different places. Since smaller outbreaks in defined locations usually do not produce lasting changes on a global scale, they are somewhat less appropriate for this book.

With these limited criteria in hand, I set out to construct a list of the 10 worst epidemics to ever strike our population. There are certain diseases like measles, syphilis, leprosy, and typhoid fever that just missed the cut despite being highly influential in their own right. In fact, nearly any one of these four could have been substituted for polio or yellow fever without losing much in terms of content. However, it was ultimately determined that included diseases were just a bit more impactful and destructive than the others mentioned above. Some of these, like smallpox and plague, were chosen because of the immense effects they had on our ancestors who lived long ago, whereas others, like HIV and polio, were picked because of their role in shaping modern society. In the end, all 10 of the diseases that were selected had an important story to tell us about what it means to be human.

Upon reading the book, it will become readily obvious that it does not present an exhaustive history of every known pathogen. So much amazing scholarship has taken place over the last several decades that each chapter could be expanded into several books of their own. Indeed, there have been many published recently that provide the fine details of just one disease or even a single substory within a broader epidemic. While such books can obviously delve deeper into a topic than what I am able to do with a chapter, they largely fail to reveal big picture relationships that exist between epidemics and humans. For this reason, I chose to broaden the scope of the book and write in it a way that provides the reader with a more holistic understanding of epidemic disease.

CHAPTER ONE

Microbes as Agents of Change

Although they are tens of thousands of times smaller than the human hosts they infect, microscopic germs can produce dramatic and permanent effects on both the individual and populations as a whole. We experience the negative impacts of these parasites throughout our lives—we get the sniffles, wake up with nausea, and suffer through bronchitis. In most cases, we go to the doctor for a week's worth of medication and our immune system eventually defeats the infection. Most of us alive today have never experienced the devastating and uncontrolled spread of a disease in a population and the fear and hopelessness that it produces because we have grown up in the age of antibiotics, vaccines, and modern medicine. However, for most of human history (and still in many parts of the world), pathogens have run amok in our population and caused significant changes to how we interact with one another. Catastrophic epidemics such as the Black Death of the 14th century or the 1918 influenza epidemic almost always produce lasting changes that can be felt hundreds or even thousands of years after the epidemic has ended. The following chapters of this book will review 10 of the most deadly and influential epidemics throughout history and examine their cause, spread, and long-term impacts on humanity.

An epidemic is generally defined as an increased occurrence of a specific disease in a certain location over a given period of time. In some cases, the disease in question is completely absent from a population and is being introduced for the very first time or after a long absence. In this situation, no one in the population will have any natural immunity to the pathogen, and the population as a whole will be very susceptible to its harmful effects. This is the type of epidemic that occurred when Spanish explorers brought small-pox to the New World in 1518 and introduced the disease to native populations. Upon arriving, it spread very rapidly throughout both North and South America and killed tens of millions of people. In contrast, other epidemics arise when a disease is already present in a population at some low, baseline level and experiences a "flare-up" due to some change in the environment. For instance, malaria epidemics often occur following unusually high levels of rainfall and flooding. The excess water causes a temporary increase in the mosquito population, which causes a rise in the number of malaria cases locally (due to the fact that mosquitoes are vectors for malaria).

When an epidemic becomes so widespread that it involves multiple continents, it is generally referred to as a pandemic. For instance, the famous 1918 flu epidemic likely began in the United States and quickly spread to all six inhabited continents, becoming a pandemic in the process. It terrorized the entire world and killed as many as 100 million people in just over one year. After the flu season was over, the disease simply disappeared from the population. A number of epidemic diseases follow this "shock and awe" pattern of wreaking havoc in a population and then leaving after just a short time. However, there are others, like smallpox and plague, that will enter a population, cause great devastation, and then continue to infect people at lower levels for extended periods of time. Some of these long-term epidemic diseases (e.g., chickenpox, measles) become so commonplace that nearly every person in a population is exposed to it at some point in their lives. Semipermanent epidemic diseases like these are said to be endemic. Thus epidemic diseases can turn into pandemics if they spread throughout the world or become endemic if they enter a population and never leave.

The vast majority of epidemics that have arisen throughout our history have been caused by one of three types of germs—viruses, bacteria, or protozoa. To fully understand the diseases they cause and their impact, it is important to quickly review what makes each of them unique.

Viruses

Viruses are by far the smallest of the three types of human pathogens discussed in this book, having an average size that is about 1,000 times smaller than one of the cells in our body. Though remarkably simple, they are responsible for some of the most devastating diseases in human history, including smallpox, flu, measles, yellow fever, and AIDS. Viruses are typically defined by microbiologists as obligate intracellular parasites, which means they require another living thing in order to replicate. Their limitation lies in the fact that they lack the biochemical machinery that is needed to produce more of their own proteins or genetic instructions. Without these building blocks, new virus particles cannot be assembled and the infection essentially stops. Viruses get around this deficiency by entering a host cell and hijacking its machinery for the production of new viruses. Since they are dependent on other living hosts to replicate, viruses are generally not considered to be living entities themselves.

Structurally speaking, viruses are nothing more than a shell of protein (called a capsid) that surrounds the virus's genetic material (called its genome). They are neither made of cells nor do they resemble them in any way. Viruses are like microscopic delivery agents whose goals are to protect its genome and successfully deliver it into the inside of a host cell. Once there, the viral genome provides the necessary instructions for the production of millions of new virus particles by the host cell. The massive presence of virus particles in the cell causes it to become unhealthy, which usually leads to its untimely death. As infected cells start to die off, newly made viruses are released and free to infect the neighboring cells. What follows is the systematic spread of the virus from cell to cell and the gradual destruction of tissue in its wake.

In addition to this viral-mediated cell death, some viruses induce damage in the host by triggering the host to respond too forcefully to the infection. In this case, the virus invades, and the host's inflammatory response is so massive and widespread that it damages the host's own tissue. The virus itself, in these cases, often does nothing directly to induce any kind of tissue damage. For example, in rabies infections, the virus reaches the central nervous system (e.g., brain) and sits relatively innocuously in neuronal cells. When the host detects that rabies virus is present, it mounts a prolonged and potent inflammatory attack in an effort to clear the infection. The gradual buildup of inflammatory chemicals is toxic to neurons and begins to kill them.

Bacteria

Bacteria have caused some of the most feared and devastating epidemics in human history, including bubonic plague, tuberculosis, leprosy, and cholera. Since they are much larger and more structurally and biochemically complex than viruses, bacteria tend to employ a much wider variety of ways of making us sick. First of all, they are not simply shells of protein that cover a genome (like viruses). They are fully living, single-celled creatures that can usually replicate independently of other cells and engage in normal metabolism. Their cells are about 10 times smaller than human cells and are more structurally simplistic. Human cells contain a variety of small, membrane-enclosed structures (called organelles) that work to perform specific functions. For instance, the nucleus stores our DNA, mitochondria help break down sugars, and lysosomes help destroy foreign invaders. Bacterial cells lack all of these internal organelles. Instead, they resemble small, fluid-filled balloons that contain an outer membrane called the plasma membrane. Inside the cell are a single chromosome, water, and small nutrients. Surrounding a bacterial cell membrane is an additional structure called the cell wall. This wall provides an added layer of protection against various types of assaults, including other organisms, toxic chemicals, or our own immune cells.

In terms of causing harm to the host, bacteria follow similar patterns as viruses for the most part. For instance, many types of bacteria cause damage to their human host by directly killing its cells or by triggering the host to have an overactive and damaging inflammatory response. However, some of key differences between viral and bacterial pathogenesis are worth mentioning here. The first is that viruses require the machinery and nutrients found in a host cell in order to replicate themselves. Bacteria, in contrast, are usually much more self-sufficient in how they acquire their own nutrients. In most cases, bacteria will invade the host as a whole but not necessarily reach the inside of individual cells. There are some notable exceptions to this. For instance, some bacteria, like the causative agent of typhus, will only replicate inside of our cells whereas others, like *Mycobacterium tuberculosis*, just prefer to. Therefore, viruses typically kill our cells from the inside out (through nutrient depletion and creating a toxic environment inside) whereas most bacteria do their damage from the outside in.

How bacteria damage and kill cells without entering them is usually accomplished through the production and release of a variety of chemical toxins. The toxins synthesized by bacterial cells can harm the host in a variety of ways including (but not limited to) perforating the cell's plasma membrane, inhibiting vital enzymes, blocking protein production, destroying

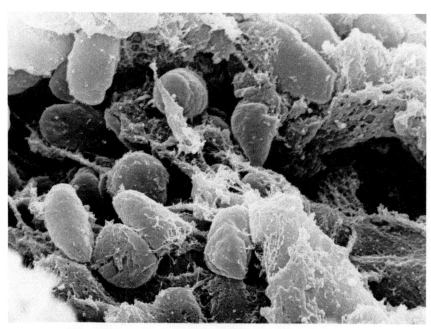

Scanning electron micrograph depicting a mass of *Yersinia pestis bacteria*, the cause of bubonic plague. (Rocky Mountain Laboratories, NIAID, NIH)

proteins that hold our tissues together, disrupting ion flow, blocking the proper transmission of nerve impulses, and sparking massive inflammation. For instance, serious bacterial infections like cholera, botulism, anthrax, and staphylococcus do much of their damage through the production of toxins. The end result in most cases is that host cells die and release their nutrients, which are then quickly picked up by the invading bacterial cells.

Protozoa

Protozoa are single-celled organisms that are amazingly diverse in terms of the environments they can grow in and the types of species they can infect. Of the more than 50,000 species identified, only a small number are known to infect humans and even fewer cause any measurable disease. Some of the more notable human diseases caused by protozoa include malaria, African sleeping sickness, amoebic dysentery, toxoplasmosis, and leishmaniasis. Although, like bacteria, they are composed of single cells, they are actually more similar in size and complexity to human cells. Additionally, they are more genetically related to humans than they are to bacteria.

The mechanisms by which protozoa cause disease are also different from that seen with viruses and bacteria. They usually do not produce extracellular toxins and when they do, the toxins have a much lower potency than what is seen from bacteria. Also, since most reproduce outside of host cells,

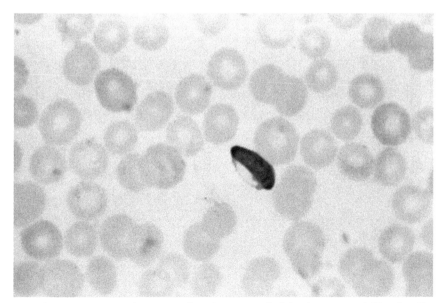

A malaria protozoan (crescent shape) surrounded by human red blood cells. (Centers for Disease Control and Prevention)

they generally do not kill them through nutrient deprivation. Malaria, which directly infects our red blood cells, is a notable exception. Most of the host damage that is seen during a typical protozoal infection is due to the host immune response to the pathogen. Their presence commonly triggers massive inflammation, which throws the host immune system into a tailspin and causes large amounts of tissue damage.

It is clear after reviewing the diversity in the microbial world that our immune system has its work cut out for it. In fact, it is estimated that our immune system fights tens of millions germs every single day. For most of human history (and still in many parts of the world), germs have had the upper hand and have generally run amok in our population. However, with the advent of sanitation, vaccines, antibiotics, and modern diagnostic tools over the last 100 years, we have taken more control over our health and reduced the incidence of epidemics. Although at times it may seem as if we have defeated infectious diseases, our continued fight with HIV, tuberculosis, influenza, malaria, and measles reminds us that the next great epidemic may be right around the corner. As a result, it is vital to look back and learn from our previous fights with these deadly diseases so that we are better prepared for anything we face in the future.

CHAPTER TWO

Plague

There was no one who wept for any death, for all awaited death. And so many died that all believed that it was the end of the world. And no medicine or any other defense availed.

—Agnolo di Tura del Grasso, 14th century, written
after he had buried his five children[1]

Some of the most devastating and influential epidemics in human history have been caused by the deadly disease known as plague. It is a disease that spread over vast areas of land and claimed the lives of 200 million people over the course of about 1,500 years.[2] In doing so, it wiped out as much as one-half of the population of some countries and left many believing that the world was nearing the apocalypse. Of the three major epidemics of plague that have been recorded throughout history, the one that struck Eurasia in the middle of the 14th century was by far the most extensive and historically significant. Termed the Black Death due to the terrifying symptoms it produced, the epidemic spread over the entire continent and killed almost half of the total population. The catastrophic loss of life sent Europe into a political, economic, and cultural tailspin that lasted for decades after the worst of the epidemic had subsided. Amazingly, some of the impacts of the Black Death are still being felt by our population some 650 years later.

The causative agent of plague, Yersinia pestis, is a small bacterium that enters into the human body in one of two ways. The first and probably most well-known route of entry is through the bite of an infected rat flea. When a flea bites a rat or other rodent that is infected with Y. pestis, some of the bacteria move into the gut of the flea as it takes its blood meal and begin to replicate to very high levels. If the infected flea bites a human and takes a blood meal, its stomach becomes so overwhelmed with bacteria and blood that it throws up the contents of its gut onto the person's skin. The person then scratches the area of the bite, which creates microscopic wounds that allow the bacteria to penetrate the skin and invade the body fluids.

Once inside a human, the bacteria quickly get flushed into local lymph nodes, where they have no problem replicating to high levels even in the presence of immune cells. Growth in the lymph nodes produces localized inflammation and tissue death and eventually causes the lymph nodes to swell and turn black (which is common of necrotic tissue). The enlarged, necrotic lymph nodes are called buboes, and the disease state that results is referred to as bubonic plague. Bacteria often then spill into the blood and begin to replicate there, causing inflammation throughout the body. This systemic infection, called septicemic plague, leads to a state of shock, necrotic tissue in the extremities, and mortality rates as high as 90 percent.[3] Having access to the interconnected blood vessel system also allows the bacteria to eventually enter the lungs, which leads a fatal pneumonia called pneumonic plague. Entering the lungs is an important step in the pathogenesis of plague because it allows the bacterium to spread to other human hosts through coughing and subsequent inhalation of infected respiratory droplets. While the flea is typically the vector by which plague gains entry into a new population, it is the pneumonic form of the disease that is believed to cause the high rate of spread and death that is observed in large-scale pandemics like the Black Death.

The Justinian Plague and Its Effect on the Roman Empire

The first major epidemic of plague began during the reign of the Byzantine emperor Justinian I in the year 540 CE. Genetic analysis reveals that it likely originated somewhere in China and then quickly spread throughout the Middle East, northern Africa, Asia, and most of Europe.[4] As was the case with the later Black Death, this first plague left a wake of destruction and panic everywhere it went. Tens of millions perished on three different continents and millions more were left debilitated with high fevers and necrotic buboes. In some cases, whole towns were reported to have been wiped out in just a matter of a few weeks. It remains one of the worst epidemics to ever strike humankind despite occurring before the development of modern modes of transportation or mass urbanization.

One place that was hit particularly hard by the Justinian plague was the capital city of Constantinople. Following the split of the Roman Empire into eastern and western halves in 330 CE, Constantinople quickly became one of the most important cities in Europe.[5] It was a small, densely populated coastal city that served as a major trading port for merchants from Asia, North Africa, and Europe. Ships arrived there daily from all over the world, carrying various types of cargo and occasional stowaway rats. In 541 CE, one such ship traveling from Egypt was unfortunately harboring rats infected with deadly plague bacterium *Yersinia pestis*. Within months of arriving in Constantinople, the disease spread throughout the overcrowded city and began killing unthinkable numbers of people. Accounts from eyewitnesses describe a death rate that approached as many as 10,000 victims a day and left so many dead that survivors were forced to take the roofs off of churches and towers in order to fit the bodies.[6] Although the first and most devastating wave of epidemic eventually passed by 550, the plague continued to torment the population for another 200 years until it finally subsided in 750. In all, the Justinian plague is believed to have killed about 40 percent of the population in Constantinople and between 25 and 100 million people worldwide.

The death of so many in the early part of the epidemic had profound effects on the balance of power in Europe and Asia. In particular, the plague severely weakened the leadership of Constantinople at a time when it was attempting to consolidate its power and regain the lost land of the former Roman Empire. The overexpansion of the empire in the fourth century had led the emperor Constantine to administratively split the land into two halves—one in the west that was ruled by an emperor in Rome and another in the east that was controlled by a co-emperor in Constantinople.[7] While the eastern part of the empire generally experienced expansion and prosperity following the split, the western half began to gradually deteriorate. Several of the Germanic tribes (e.g., Goths and Vandals) began invading large areas of the western kingdom and in the year 476, Rome was officially conquered. With the western half lost, the eastern part of the former Roman Empire (later referred to as the Byzantine Empire) gained much greater autonomy. As a result, the city of Constantinople became the undeniable center of trade, culture, and power in all of Europe. When Justinian I assumed power of Constantinople in 527, one of his primary goals was to raise an army to recapture the land in the west and restore the Roman Empire to its former glory.

Justinian first sent his army to Northern Africa in order to drive out the Vandals that had taken control during the previous century.[8] After winning a series of quick and decisive battles in 534, Justinian moved his Byzantine forces north into Western Europe with the goal of recapturing the Mediterranean from the Goths. It took five years and lots of bloodshed, but Justinian was eventually successful in defeating most of the Gothic armies. With most of the former Roman lands under Byzantine control, it looked as if Justinian was about to usher in a whole new era of the empire. Unfortunately for him, the deadly plague arrived months later in 540 and began killing off massive numbers of his farmers, soldiers, and craftsmen. This significantly depleted his workforce and put enormous strain on his ability to defend the land he just conquered, feed his soldiers, or pay off his debts. Facing a potential catastrophic loss of all that he had just gained, Justinian resorted to hiring foreign mercenaries to repopulate his army.[9] He also began using greater force to collect taxes from his subjects despite the fact that most were fighting to survive the deadly plague. This understandably produced some level of resentment toward Justinian and his perceived waste of resources on unnecessary military conquests.

The Byzantine Empire successfully fought to maintain control of Italy, Spain, and North Africa for the next 25 years; however, soon after Justinian's death in 565, nearly all the land had been taken back by various invaders.[10] Furthermore, subsequent generations would see Persian and Arab empires rise to power and gradually take more of the land of the eastern Byzantine Empire, eventually reducing it to almost nothing. The plague had taken a huge economic, military, and emotional toll on the Byzantine people, and they simply lacked the resources to defend their lands. Within a matter of a few hundred years, the Roman/Byzantine Empire had all but ceased to exist.

No one knows what would have happened to Europe, Asia, and Africa had the plague not hit in the sixth century. It would be overly simplistic speculation to assume that the reunified Roman Empire would have succeeded in maintaining control of its lost land against a constant onslaught by foreign invaders. The western half of the empire collapsed in the fifth century for a variety of reasons (e.g., land decay, food shortages, political infighting), many of which would have still been present a hundred years later. However, it is interesting to think about how a strengthened Rome would have defended itself against the rise of Islam, against the Anglo-Saxon invasion of the British Isles, and against the various Germanic tribes over a long period of time. How would that have changed the long-term history of the world?

The Black Death Begins

The most famous epidemic in human history was the second plague pandemic, the Black Death that started in China in 1334, which reached a peak from 1347 to 1351 and proceeded to kill millions for the next 400 years. Like its predecessor, it is believed to have killed between 75 and 100 million people, wiping out about one-third of Europe and one-fifth of the total population of the world at the time.[11] The pandemic spread in a stepwise fashion, moving between port cities with traders and ships that were sailing throughout Asia, Europe, and Northern Africa. After ravaging China and the Mongolian empire for 10 years, the plague moved south into Crimea and eventually into Constantinople.

As was the case during the sixth-century plague, Constantinople was a busy port city that served as a staging point for the epidemic to sweep westward into Europe and Northern Africa. Once in a new location, rats would jump off the ships, mate with local rats, and transmit the disease to a new population. It is believed to have spread very rapidly between humans through the inhalation of infected respiratory secretions (pneumonic plague) until there were no hosts left to infect. The devastating social impact that such enormous amounts death had on the people is best described by Giovanni Boccaccio, who in the Decameron (1353), wrote, "Citizen avoided citizen, kinsfolk held aloof, or never met or but rarely; in the horror thereof brother was forsaken by brother, nephew by uncle, brother by sister, and oftentimes husband by wife; may, what is more and scarce to be believed, fathers and mothers were found to abandon their own children, untended, unvisited, to their fate, as if they had been strangers."[12] Much as it did 800 years previously, the Black Death produced deleterious effects on all facets of life, forever changing the way people lived, thought, and interacted with one another.

Most historical analyses of the 14th-century Black Death primarily focus on how it affected Europe despite the likelihood that it killed millions in Asia before ever moving westward. Interestingly, there are very few documented accounts of plague activity in Chinese texts from the 14th century and even fewer from Indian sources. Some Chinese medical documents from that time period (the Song-Yuan Dynasty) describe a disease that had characteristic swollen lymph nodes and high fevers and produced a great number of deaths between 1331 and 1353.[13] Also, a census conducted during that time reported that the population of China was nearly cut in half during the second half of the 14th century, with some provinces reporting losses of almost 90 percent of its inhabitants. Since most of Asia at the time was under a constant threat of famine, disease, and war because of the vast Mongol conquests, it is difficult to ascertain whether the sharp drop in population was specifically due to plague or a combination of other factors. It is highly likely that the Black Death did kill millions in western Asia before it moved into Europe; however, the lack of historical records ensures that we will never know exactly how many deaths there were or what its effects were on the population.

One of the few accounts of plague in the Mongol Empire comes from an Italian lawyer named Gabriele de' Mussi who, in 1346, wrote about the Mongol siege of the city of Caffa in Crimea (Ukraine).[14] Caffa was originally founded and used by Italian merchants as an important trading port in the middle of the Mongol Empire. Though relations between the Italians and their hosts were initially civil, their relationship soon deteriorated, and fights between the two led the Mongols to attack the city with an immense army in 1343. When all looked lost for the Italians, de' Mussi writes, "the whole army was affected by a disease which overran the Tartars (Mongols) and killed thousands upon thousands every day."[15] He goes on to describe the disease as having the characteristic symptoms of plague. The new disease absolutely devastated the attackers, which forced the Mongol army to finally concede defeat at Caffa. Upon realizing that their defeat was imminent, "the dying

Tartars . . . ordered corpses to be placed in catapults and lobbed into the city in hopes that the intolerable stench would kill everyone inside. What seemed like mountains of dead were thrown into the city."[16]

This is one of the first instances in recorded history of a live infectious agent being used as a biological weapon. The de' Mussi account and several others go on to describe how successful this strategy was. A large number of Caffa's inhabitants ended up dying of plague in the next several months. Unfortunately, those who managed to escape the city helped spread the disease to Constantinople and Europe. While most historians believe plague would have reached Europe through other trading routes, the fleeing residents of Caffa (and their rats) very likely increased the speed at which the epidemic spread.

This event was a major turning point in the history of warfare that is very often forgotten. The Mongol army's use of an infectious agent to more quickly, thoroughly, and cheaply kill its enemy was brilliant. It provided a model that was followed on and off for next 600 years—kill with a disease first, and once the population is weak, move in with an army. As will be discussed in later chapters, there is some evidence that the Europeans may have used smallpox, measles, and other infectious agents to purposefully decimate the native populations of the Americas and Africa. Similarly, circumstantial evidence suggests that the British destroyed native aboriginal populations of Australia using the same methodology. The Germans are believed to have used anthrax as a weapon in World War I, and the Japanese used typhoid and glanders as weapons in World War II.[17] Thus the use of plague-infected bodies as a weapon, though crude and desperate, proved to be a highly effective strategy that would be mimicked in all future generations.

Decline of European Feudalism and Cause of Revolts

The movement of plague into Europe in 1347 produced such a profound and rapid reduction of population size that the economy of most of the continent changed drastically in a matter of a few years. Europe had been in a recession in the 30 years leading up to the Black Death due to an extensive famine that struck northern Europe in 1315.[18] It left millions of peasants dead from starvation and disease and put an end to the explosive population growth that Europe had experienced for several hundred years prior. Although weather patterns eventually stabilized and harvests continued to improve, the damage from the famine had irrevocably shaken the psyche of the people. It exposed an ugliness in the people that was demonstrated by much higher levels of murder and rape, child abandonment, and even instances of cannibalism. It also strained relationships between feudal lords who managed the land and the peasants who worked it.

Feudalism was a hierarchical system of organizing the population that had been in place throughout Medieval Europe since the ninth century. It was based on relationships that formed as a result of land management. At the top of the feudal system was the king, who owned all the land in a given country. The king would grant portions of the land to nobles/lords, who would pledge their loyalty and protection to the king. Lords would then grant subplots of that land to knights in exchange for military protection. Knights would then hire a large number of serfs/peasants to work the land, who in turn, would pay rent to the knights and receive protection, food, and shelter for their hard work. Much of the money generated from working these self-sufficient manors would be given back to the king in the form of taxes. The bulk of the burden in this system was placed on the backs of peasant laborers, who had little opportunity for upward mobility and improvement to their socioeconomic situation.

The strain on feudalism that was started by the Great Famine of 1315 came to a breaking point during the Black Death.[19] All strata of the feudal society were affected, which left major voids in those managing the land and, more importantly, in the laborers working it. With massive amounts of crops going unharvested and most of the workforce gone, those peasants who survived were now in a position to negotiate greater freedoms and higher pay (as much as five times what they were previously earning). Knights and lords, still having obligations to the king, were forced to comply, and more of the wealth ended up in the hands of the populace.

Local governments in several countries responded to this upward mobility by imposing laws that limited laborer wages and required greater fees from those working the land. The new middle class of laborers were understandably upset by these restrictions, and many responded by revolting against those in power (e.g., English Peasants Revolt of 1381).[20] Labor unrest continued to spread throughout much of Europe, and many laborers moved to towns and cities seeking better opportunities. The economy began to gradually shift away from farming and toward production and trade, which caused feudal lords and knights to lose their power over the lower classes. In the subsequent years, most European nations would shift to a capitalist economic system and feudalism would be gone forever. Although the Black Death was obviously not the sole cause of the end of the feudal system, it was a major factor in precipitating its decline.

God's Wrath, the Church, and Persecutions

Whenever a new disease is discovered in modern times, scientists and doctors quickly mobilize to the affected region, gather patient specimens, and then use an arsenal of diagnostic tools to ascertain the etiological cause of the disease. Once the microbial agent has been identified, infected patients are given appropriate treatments, and the rest of the populace is instructed about to how to prevent any further spread of the disease. The outbreak typically subsides, and the population recovers in a relatively short period of time.

Those living in the 14th century had no such technology available to them when the Black Death began to decimate the population. As a result, their explanations as to the cause of the epidemic were often rooted in superstition and fear rather than reason. They wanted someone or something to blame so that they could rid themselves of whatever was "causing" the epidemic. Some suggested that natural phenomena such as earthquakes or comets had released the plague from the Earth or that the planets were aligned in such a way to cause the disaster. Arguably the most widespread explanation as to why this calamity had struck the people was that it was a punishment from God for the sins of the people. De' Mussi's account of the siege of Caffa by the afflicted Tartar (Mongol) army clearly illustrates this belief when he states, "It was though arrows were raining down from heaven to strike and crush the Tartars' arrogance."[21] The Mongols were attempting to harm Christian Italians, which prompted God to use the Black Death as a weapon to stop them.

Divine retribution against the unrighteous made sense until plague inexplicably turned its wrath on the Christians themselves. People looked to the Church for guidance, and priests provided their flocks with instructions for repentance and protection from the disease. Increased prayer, rituals of piety, placing crosses above doorposts, and visitation to the shrines of saints were prescribed. Some took to more extreme forms of penance to pacify God. Men called flagellants would go from town to town flogging themselves with chains and nail-coated whips until they bled.[22] They would lead public processions in which they punished themselves in an attempt to personally take on God's punishment for the people (much like Christ was thought to have done). Instead of stopping

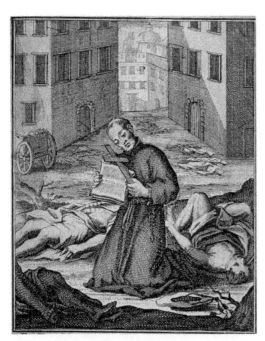

Engraving of a priest giving last rites to plague victims. (National Library of Medicine)

the plague, flagellants are believed to have hastened its spread, as infected fleas moved with them everywhere they went. Thus, despite various acts of appeasement and atonement, God-fearing Christians and their clergy died at unprecedented rates.

Since the clergy often played a significant role in caring for the sick, they typically had very high rates of death from the plague. One contemporary observer wrote that "of the English Austin Friars at Avignon, not one remained . . . at Maguelonne, of 160 friars, 7 only were left . . . at Marseilles, of 150 Franciscans, not one survived to tell the story."[23] If God had not spared even the priests—his elect—what did that mean for the rest of the their flocks? To many, it was as if God had abandoned mankind and nothing could be done to abate His wrath. In the words of poet William Langland, "God is deaf now-a-days and deigneth not hear us, And prayers have no power the Plague to stay."[24] The general response was that people lost trust in the Church and left in record numbers as a result.

The long-term effects on the Catholic Church were equally devastating. First, and probably most significantly, the extensive loss of clergy left a void in quality leadership. In an effort to fill the vacancies as quickly as possible, churches were forced to lower their standards and hire priests with significantly less education, commitment, and training than their predecessors. The result was an increase in abuse and corruption by the clergy. One of the more common abuses, later cited by the reformer Martin Luther in the following century, was related to the selling of indulgences. An indulgence was a form of penance that one performed in order to make up for a sin after it had already been forgiven by God. Normally, penances would involve lengthy prayer, fasting, service to the needy, or giving alms to the poor. However, some corrupt clergy began using these indulgences as a way of extorting large sums of money from their parishioners with the idea that they could either pay now for their sin or risk an eternity in Purgatory. Many in the Church were understandably turned off by this corrupt practice and other abuses seen from the postplague clergy.

The failure of the clergy to save the people from the plague combined with the subsequent corruption have led some historians to suggest that the Black Death indirectly played a role in helping spark the Protestant Reformation. Though the Reformation was initiated due to the complex interplay of a variety of factors, no one can deny the distinct role that the plague played in significantly diminishing the power and perceived infallibility of the Catholic Church prior to Martin Luther issuing his 95 theses.

The Black Death also ushered in a new era of anti-Semitism and Jewish persecution.[25] People were desperate to find someone to blame for their suffering, and the Jews represented a perfect scapegoat. Not only did they have vastly different beliefs and customs than their Christian neighbors, they tended to live together segregated from the rest of the population. When plague unexpectedly arrived in 1347, many Christians began to suspect that the people responsible for the epidemic were the ones who were most different and isolated from everyone else. As the death toll continued to climb among the Christians, that suspicion turned to blame, and the blame eventually morphed into violence.

The persecution began in the spring of 1348 near Narbonne, France, when a group of Jews were rounded up and burned in a bonfire. Shortly thereafter, Jews in Western Europe were openly accused of poisoning wells, lakes, and rivers throughout Europe in an effort to kill the Christians. They were arrested and subjected to various forms of torture in order to force a confession of their crimes. A particularly vivid account of one such "trial" can be found in *The Confession of Agimet the Jew of Geneva* (October 1348):

> Agimet the Jew, who lived at Geneva and was arrested at Châtel, was there put to the torture a little and then he was released from it. And after a long time, having been subjected again to torture a little, he confessed in the presence of a great many trustworthy persons . . . Agimet took this package full of poison and carried it with him to Venice, and when he came there he threw and scattered a portion of it into the well or cistern of fresh water which was there near the German House, in order to poison the people who use the water of that cistern.[26]

So, after being arrested and tortured twice, Agimet "voluntarily" admitted that he was responsible for putting some unknown concoction of venom and poisons into the water supply of Venice. Despite the obvious coercion, news of this and other covert poisonings spread from town to town throughout Europe almost as fast as the plague itself.

The public response to these suspected poisonings was explosive. Jews were rounded up everywhere (often at the behest of the visiting flagellants) and murdered by fire and the sword. Entire populations of Jews in some cities were wiped out in a matter of days. For instance, Christians killed 6,000 Jews in Mainz, Germany, in a single day in August 1349.[27] Similar large-scale massacres were seen throughout Italy, France, Belgium, Switzerland, and most other European countries. During the height of these pogroms, Pope Clement IV tried to stop the mob violence and protect Jews by issuing an edict that declared, "it does not seem credible that the Jews on this occasion are responsible . . . because this nearly universal pestilence, in accordance with God's hidden judgment, has afflicted and continues to afflict the Jews themselves, as well as many other races who had never been known to live alongside them, throughout the various regions of the world."[28] Unfortunately, the Catholic Church was in great political disarray at the time, and there were two popes that claimed to be the true successor of Saint Peter. As a result, attempts by clergy to stop the killings largely fell on deaf ears, and local mobs would continue unimpeded for several decades. No one knows the true death toll of the 14th-century pogroms, but it was conservatively in the tens of thousands.

Failure of Medicine and Its Effects

Medicine in the years preceding the Black Death was more philosophy than practical clinical science. Physicians were trained in medical theory that relied heavily on the ancient teachings of Hippocrates and Galen. Rather than gaining a detailed knowledge of human anatomy and physiology through dissections or examination of clinical data, most curricula were based on 1,000-year-old ideas about disease that were unsupported by any kind of experimental evidence. Physicians learned about how body fluid (humor) imbalances can lead to sickness or how disease was spread by bad, contaminated air called miasma. They often prescribed bleedings, leech treatment, special diets, or fresh air to patients presenting with a variety of symptoms.

When the Black Death arrived in the 14th century, special plague doctors were conscripted to treat those afflicted in their communities and record the number of people who had died of plague. Dressed in elaborate costumes that sometimes included birdlike beaks filled with fragrant flowers (to ward off miasma), plague doctors visited the sick daily and subjected them to the same bloodlettings and leech treatments that had been used for centuries. Unfortunately, no matter what was done, the epidemic only continued to grow worse. The apparent helplessness of the physicians was recorded by a man named Marchione di Coppo Stefani, who wrote, "Almost none of the ill survived past the fourth day. Neither physicians nor medicines were effective. Whether because these illnesses were previously unknown or because physicians had not previously studied them, there seemed to be no cure. There was such a fear that no one seemed to know what to do."[29] Physicians, like the clergy, had few answers for the plague, and people began to lose faith in both.

Despite having no knowledge of the etiology of the plague, some of the treatments and preventative measures recommended did help to a limited extent. For instance, one suggestion was for people to leave cities and seek out "fresh air" in order to avoid the disease-spreading miasma. Although bad-smelling air was obviously not the source of the disease, the idea to flee the city serendipitously allowed some to get away from those who were spreading the pneumonic form of plague. Unfortunately, it was usually only the wealthy who were financially able to uproot their lives and flee to safety. Another somewhat effective measure for slowing the spread of plague involved the quarantining of ships for 40 days in port before allowing them to dock. In doing so, they hoped that the disease would burn itself out on board before potentially infectious sailors were released onto the rest of the population. Interestingly, the Black Death was the first time in history that a quarantine was implemented to slow the spread of a disease (the word quarantine comes from Italian words meaning 40 days).[30] It very likely saved countless lives during the Black Death and many subsequent epidemics from other pathogens.

The failure of physicians and medieval medicine to stop the spread of the Black Death led to drastic changes in the medical profession. For one, the epidemic called attention to the need for better training for physicians and greater regulation of the profession as a whole.[31] The vast majority of medical providers at the time were uneducated, unlicensed, and unregulated. Few attended any type of schooling, and even fewer were given practical experience by trained and experienced professionals. After the plague, many cities began passing ordinances that required medical workers to show some proof of training before they were allowed to practice medicine in a community. Furthermore, medical schools all over Europe began integrating more dissections in their curricula, and several created new, updated medical textbooks. The plague also led to a significant improvement in how practicing physicians shared what they had learned during the course of treating their patients. Many doctors began publishing their experiences in written medical treatises (tractates) that strongly resemble modern-day medical journals.[32] Others gathered information from their colleagues and used it to create practical manuals of prevention, treatment, and surgery. In all, the Black Death helped push medicine out of the Dark Ages and into an era that was based more on reason and evidence than on ancient philosophy.

The Influence of the Black Death on Medieval Art

A popular misconception about the Black Death is that the high mortality rate and utter devastation it produced helped usher in a new period of macabre art that was dominated by images of disease, death, and destruction. While a great number of these plague images certainly do exist, most of the art coming out of Western Europe during and following the peak of the plague (1347–1351) actually show many more images of hope, salvation, and piety. Furthermore, art historians now believe that Medieval Europe had a growing fascination with death and morality in the decades before 1347. Works like Dante's *Divine Comedy* and Buonamico Buffalmacco's fresco *Triumph of Death* clearly demonstrate that people in the early 14th century had begun to express new views of death and the afterlife in their art.[33] Much of this shift has been attributed to changes in Catholic theology (per a papal bull issued by Pope Benedict XII in 1336) that put more emphasis on the soul, afterlife, and Purgatory.[34] Therefore, the Black Death that hit Europe years later would further augment, rather than initiate, a sentiment of mortality that already existed in European culture at the time. Its effects would be significant and long-lasting, as images of both desperation and great hope would permeate European art throughout the Renaissance period.

One of the more common images in plague art is that of victims in various stages of dying as other humans, saints, or angels try to help them. For instance, the *St. Sebastian Intercedes during the Plague in Pavia* by Lieferinxe depicts the martyred St. Sebastian pleading with God on behalf of plague victims, who can be clearly seen suffering in great agony at the bottom of the painting.[35] It is interesting that it shows both the hope that a just God will end the suffering of the people and the great pain and desperation

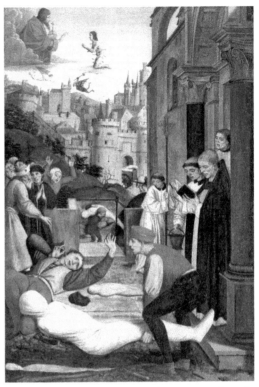

St. Sebastian, pierced with arrows, kneels before God to plead on behalf of humanity, while an angel and a demon battle in the sky. Josse Lieferinxe (French, active 1493–1505) (Artist), 1497–1499 (Renaissance). (The Walters Art Museum)

of those still being affected by the disease. Paintings such as Tintoretto's *Saint Roch Curing the Plague* and the famous illustration of the Black Death from the Toggenburg Bible use very similar imagery whereas others tend to focus more on God's judgment and wrath. The latter type of artwork typically depicts the wrath as arrows falling from heaven onto the people or as an Angel of Death wielding a sword or sickle over the people.

Other common art themes that emerged from the plague era focus on the action of the flagellants and the persecution of the Jews. As mentioned previously, the processions of flagellants and Jewish pogroms were public spectacles that were relatively widespread throughout Western Europe for many years. Both activities involved great suffering and had strong religious undertones, which made them ideal subjects for artwork. One particularly vivid image of flagellants, called *The Procession of the Flagellants*, comes from a medieval manuscript called *Belles Heures*.[36] It shows several masked men violently whipping two men who are lying prostrate on the ground while others carry crosses as part of a procession. In the case of Jewish pogroms, most paintings tended to depict large bonfires engulfing a sea of twisted faces while onlookers throw on more wood or have expressions of satisfaction.

Probably the most enduring metaphor found in plague art is collectively called the Dance of Death (or the Danse Macabre).[37] Most Danse Macabre images depict corpses or skeletons dancing (or moving awkwardly) among members of different social classes in an effort to show that the Black Death did not discriminate. The dancing motions mimic the movements of plague victims near the end of the disease when widespread necrosis and pain cause writhing muscle twitches. A great example of this genre is Bernt Notke's painting from 1466 that was appropriately named *Danse Macabre*. In one section of the painting, death is clearly seen playing music while other images of death joyfully dance and grab hold of the pope and emperor in order to lead them to their ultimate fate. Paintings like this appeared in most Western European countries for several hundred years after the peak of the Black Death, indicating that psychological toll taken by the pandemic lasted well beyond the mid-14th century.

Cause of Human Evolution?

When an epidemic hits a population, there will be individuals in that population who have genetic mutations that make them more naturally resistant to infection. Upon facing exposure to the pathogen, they will be more likely to survive than their normal, nonmutant counterparts. If an epidemic is particularly savage or prolonged (like the Black Death), a great number of people who were susceptible will die, leaving the resistant survivors to repopulate their communities. After many generations of such "weeding out," the new surviving population will have a much higher frequency of individuals with the mutation than did the original, pre-epidemic population. As a result, they will be more genetically prepared if that epidemic were to ever hit again. Therefore, an epidemic can act as a selective pressure that triggers a change in the genetic profile of a population over time; in other words, it can promote human evolution.

There has been much speculation over the past 20 years as to whether or not the 14th-century Black Death had any significant effect on human evolution. This is a difficult question to answer due to the fact that the epidemic occurred nearly 650 years before genetic testing was invented. Therefore, we must rely on a retrospective genetic analysis of bone and tooth fragments from individuals who were known to have died from the Black Death. That DNA, though partially degraded due to time, can be compared with DNA from current populations (the descendants of survivors) to see whether there were any mutations that seemed to increase in frequency after the plague. In other words, comparison of DNA from those who died from plague with those who survived can allow us identify mutations that may have provided some people in the 14th century with a natural resistance to *Yersinia pestis* infection.

Data from these studies strongly suggest that plague helped trigger permanent changes to our immune system.[38] We have a variety of proteins on the surface of our immune cells called Toll-like receptors (TLRs), which function to detect an infection and then initiate an inflammatory reaction. Analysis of genes from different groups who survived the plague revealed that they all shared similar mutations in the TLR genes. These unique TLR sequence changes appear to provide people with an enhanced inflammatory response to *Yersinia pestis* bacteria, which would have given people who had them in the 14th century a better ability fight off the infection than those with normal TLR genes. While those pro-inflammatory mutations were a great help to those who were constantly bombarded with pathogenic bacteria in medieval times, they can cause problems to those living in relatively hygienic conditions in the 21st century. For instance, clinical data suggest that people with these TLR mutations suffer from a higher incidence of autoimmune disorders like Crohn's Disease. Therefore, what helped our ancestors survive one of the worst epidemics in human history was now partially responsible for making our immune systems act inappropriately.

A great deal of investigation has also focused on a mutation in a gene called CCR5 after it was found that the mutation (called CCR5Δ32) is present in about 15–20 percent of Europeans and is almost nonexistent in those of African or eastern Asian descent. This pattern is interesting because the Black Death devastated most of Europe while never reaching into sub-Saharan Africa or eastern Asia. The overlapping geographical pattern of the Black Death and the CCR5Δ32 mutation seems to suggest that the mutation may have provided those in 14th-century Europe with resistance to plague.[39] They would have survived and produced protected (mutant) offspring. The mutation would have then increased in frequency in the population as non-mutants died off at higher rates. Thus, the 15–20 percent of Europeans that have the mutation today may be descendants of those Black Death survivors.

If the theory described above is correct, then animals that have the CCR5Δ32 mutation should theoretically be more resistant to *Yersinia pestis* than normal animals. Unfortunately, results obtained from these studies have been somewhat inconclusive. Experiments seem to suggest that the mutation in rats does provide protection against plague while the mutation in mice does not.[40] As a result of the conflicting findings, whether the Black Death caused the increased prevalence of the CCR5Δ32 mutation among Europeans or whether it was due to some other pathogen such as smallpox is inconclusive. Interestingly and coincidentally, the CCR5Δ32 mutation has been shown to affect the replication of another deadly pathogen, HIV. We know that HIV could not have been the original cause of the unique mutation pattern since it has only significantly affected human populations for about 40 years (about two generations). The relationship between HIV and CCR5Δ32 will be discussed later in the book.

The Final Round of Plague

A discussion of plague and its impacts on mankind would be incomplete without mentioning the third major pandemic, which began in China in the 1850s and killed as many as 12–15 million people over the next 100 years. Unlike its two predecessors, the third pandemic primarily spread throughout Asia rather than Europe, was spread mostly by rats, and had a lower death rate. One reason as to why it did not kill as many as the previous two pandemics had to do with a combination of quarantine and other control measures. Also, microbiology had advanced enough in the 19th century so that the causative agent of plague was discovered in 1894 (by Dr. Alexandre Yersin), a rudimentary vaccine was developed and distributed starting in 1897, and the role of the flea in its transmission was deciphered in 1898.[41] An interesting side note about the vaccine is that the scientist who developed it, Waldemar Haffkine, put such great faith in his own abilities that he first tested the efficacy of the vaccine on himself. When he did not die after being challenged with live plague bacteria, he did another round of testing on prisoners in India. Despite questionable ethics and being only partially protective, the vaccine was successful in drastically slowing the spread of plague in Asia and ultimately limited its impact.

One of the more significant long-term results of the third pandemic was the continued weakening of the relationship between imperial power Great Britain and the people it controlled, most notably those of India and Hong Kong. In an effort to control the spread of plague in India, the British military and regional Special Plague Committees initiated a series of very restrictive control measures on the people.[42] These included the forced quarantining of those suspected of being infected, the seizure and destruction of "contaminated" property, evacuations, and the exclusion of traditional medical practices. As one may imagine, the suffering people, who had already been under oppressive British rule for many decades, did not appreciate the increased restrictions. This led many to respond with protests and violence. One very famous incident that exemplified these growing tensions occurred in 1897. It involved a particularly maligned British officer of one the Indian plague committees named Walter Rand. Three brothers named Damodar Hari, Balkrishna Hari, and Vasudeo Hari Chapekar ambushed Rand's carriage on his way home from Queen Victoria's Diamond Jubilee celebration and brutally killed him and his military escort.[43] They were quickly caught, convicted, and hanged for their crimes. The story was broadcast in the international media and brought attention to the plight of the unstable Indian subcontinent. Although India would not gain its independence for another 50 years, the 19th-century plague epidemic provided a spark of nationalism against imperial Great Britain that would continue to grow as the years went on.

CHAPTER THREE

Smallpox

The smallpox was always present, filling the churchyards with corpses, tormenting with constant fears all whom it had stricken, leaving on those whose lives it spared the hideous traces of its power, turning the babe into a changeling at which the mother shuddered, and making the eyes and cheeks of the bighearted maiden objects of horror to the lover.
—T. B. Macaulay, 1948[1]

Smallpox is one of the greatest scourges that the human race has ever known, killing and disfiguring billions of people over the course of 3,000 years. It killed between 300 and 500 million people in the 20th century alone and may have collectively killed over 1 billion. For those who were fortunate enough to survive smallpox, about one-third were left permanently blinded and three-quarters had pronounced scarring on their faces and extremities.[2] The disease was especially devastating for children younger than the age of five, having mortality rates that approached 95 percent in some places. It was so bad that parents would commonly wait to name their children until after they had survived smallpox. Furthermore, unlike plague, which quickly killed a large number of people and then gradually disappeared over time, smallpox tended to decimate a population during its first exposure and then remain there permanently as an endemic disease, steadily killing about 30 percent of those newly infected, year in and year out. Over time, it would become so common in the population that nearly every person would be exposed to it at some point in their lifetime. This pattern continued from ancient times until the mid-20th century, when a worldwide vaccination effort led to arguably one of the greatest achievements in our history—the total eradication of smallpox from humankind. Smallpox no longer exists in nature, and so for the remainder of this chapter, it will be referred to in the past tense.

The vast majority of smallpox cases (more than 90%) were due to infection with the highly contagious *variola major* virus while a smaller number of less severe smallpox cases were caused by *variola minor*. These viruses were most commonly spread between humans through the direct inhalation of contaminated respiratory secretions and less frequently through skin exposure to contaminated body fluids or inanimate objects. There is some evidence that in rare cases it could also be acquired through eye exposure to infected fluids or spread across the placenta from an infected mother to her fetus. Importantly, human *variola* viruses were never found in any animal vectors nor were they present in the water or soil. Thus smallpox could only be acquired from another infected person.

Once inside the body, variola viruses were internalized by local immune cells called macrophages and moved to the closest lymph nodes. The viruses would then replicate there slowly at first, moving methodically from cell to cell, and then cause a large-scale explosion of infected cells approximately 6–10 days postinfection. This release of virus into the bloodstream, called viremia, allowed the virus to gain access to other tissues and organs. During this time, infected persons would exhibit flu-like symptoms, fever, muscle aches, nausea, and characteristic rashes of the skin and eyes. Most people developed large pustules, predominantly on their face and extremities, whereas others developed a flat, hemorrhagic rash. Further replication and spread of the virus often caused internal hemorrhaging, pneumonia, shock, and death by 16 days postinfection. Since *variola* viruses were effectively removed from the population before the development of modern molecular biological techniques, the mechanisms by which they caused these symptoms or why the infection so often resulted in death is not known.

It is unclear where *variola* viruses came from or when they entered the human population; however, genetics studies suggest that they may have been derived from a poxvirus of small rodents or camels. It is believed that *variola* first entered the human population near the Fertile Crescent when humans began to commonly live among their animals (around 10,000 BCE).[3] The first clear physical evidence of ancient smallpox infections is seen on Egyptian mummies such as that of the Pharaoh Ramses V, who died in 1157 BCE and exhibited characteristic pustules on his face. In addition, ancient tablets written during the Egyptian-Hittite war of 1274 BCE describe a mysterious epidemic that spread from Egyptian prisoners into the Hittite army and remained for another 20 years. While descriptions of this disease suggest that is was smallpox, the historical records were vague enough that it may have been caused by some other infectious agent.

The first few centuries of the Common Era have numerous examples of epidemics that were likely smallpox. For instance, the Antoinine (165–180 CE) and Cyprian Plagues (251–266 CE) that ripped through the Roman

Empire and killed as many as 10 million people were described as causing a rash similar to that seen with smallpox.[4] Similarly, an epidemic that broke out in northern China in 310 CE produced a disease with "seasonal epidemic sores which attack the head, face and trunk. In a short time they spread all over the body. They look like red boils, all containing some white matter. The pustules arise all together, and later dry up about the same time. If the severe cases are not treated immediately many will die. Patients who recover are left with dark purplish scars the color of which takes more than a year to fade."[5] Other even more definitive descriptions of smallpox were recorded in the centuries that followed in Asia, Europe, and the Middle East. It is from these accounts that we first begin to see the long-term impacts of smallpox on our population.

The Downfall of the Roman Empire and Rise of Christianity

As described in chapter 2, the Justinian Plague caused by *Yersinia pestis* helped prevent the reunification of the eastern and western halves of the Roman Empire in the mid-sixth century and ultimately prevented it from regaining its past glory. The empire had been in a state of decline for several hundred years prior to the start of the plague due to a variety of reasons, including political infighting, economic decline, rise of powerful Germanic tribes, and disease. As a result, it is clear that the Justinian plague did not initiate the fall of the Roman Empire but rather helped further weaken what was already deteriorating.

To understand how the Roman Empire began its decline, one must back up about 400 years before the Justinian plague to the year 166 CE. The empire at this point in time had achieved such unprecedented success that it was already being viewed by contemporaries as one of the most powerful, prosperous, and culturally rich empires that the world had ever known. The emperor Marcus Aurelius took over in 161 CE and continued to strengthen the empire, which now included nearly all of Western Europe, northern African, part of the British Isles, and much of the Middle East.[6] Its healthy free-market economy, fueled by a strong entrepreneurial spirit and laws that encouraged trade, created a large middle class and allowed for a relatively high level of economic mobility. The military of the empire was one of the most well-trained and cost-efficient forces ever assembled. An army of just over 350,000 soldiers did such an amazing job of keeping the peace in a far-reaching empire that some historians such as Tacitus complained that they had no great wars to write about. The general peace and prosperity of the time also fostered great advances in art, medicine, law, and science. It was an amazing time to be a citizen of the Roman Empire, and no one could fathom the possibility that this would ever change.

Unfortunately, a relatively minor skirmish that erupted in 162 CE would change everything and trigger a century-long decline that the empire would never recover from. Problems began when a group of people called the Parthians (from modern-day Iran) invaded Roman-controlled Syria and Iraq.[7] This prompted Marcus Aurelius to send in the full force of the Roman army under the command of his brother and co-emperor Lucius Verus. After three years of fighting, the Romans finally captured the Parthian capital city of Seleucia. Roman soldiers sacked the city and others nearby, raided temples, and made off with various forms of treasure. In addition to the plunder, soldiers also returned to Rome with a different kind of "gift" from the Parthian people—a new and especially aggressive epidemic disease. The famous Roman physician Galen described the disease as follows:

> On the ninth day a certain young man was covered over his whole body with an exanthem (rash), as was the case with almost all who survived. Drying drugs were applied to his body . . . On the twelfth day he was able to rise from bed. On those who would survive who had diarrhoea, a black exanthem appeared on the whole body. It was ulcerated in most cases and totally dry. The blackness was due to a remnant of blood that had putrefied in the fever blisters, like some ash which nature had deposited on the skin. Of some of these which had become ulcerated, that part of the surface called the scab fell away and then the remaining part nearby was healthy and after one or two days became scarred over.[8]

The erupting rash that appears at about day nine, hemorrhaging, fever, scabby blisters, and scarring suggest to most historians that Galen was describing an epidemic of hemorrhagic smallpox, though a few have proposed that it may have been caused by typhus or even anthrax.

Once it made it into the empire, the smallpox epidemic spread rapidly along trade routes and killed people indiscriminately in all levels of society. In fact, there is some evidence that it was responsible for the death of both Marcus Aurelius (180 CE) and Lucius Verus (169 CE). Over the next 100 years or so, this smallpox epidemic (called the Antonine or Galenic plague) may have killed as many as 7 million people.[9] Some estimate that it was killing 2,000 people a day in the city of Rome alone.

The death of so many had drastic and long-term impacts on the productivity, safety, and morale of those in the empire.[10] For instance, as the population began to shrink, the military had difficulty finding qualified recruits to defend its borders. As a result, they began having to rely more heavily on paid mercenaries to populate their ranks. Interestingly, many of these mercenary soldiers were actually members of the Germanic tribes who had been launching attacks on the Roman Empire for many years. Such a drastic change in composition of the military produced a gradual weakening of the army and inability to defend its borders. Over time, local Germanic tribes were empowered to form alliances and increase the frequency and ferocity of their attacks on the Western half of the empire. The weakening empire eventually split and the Western half would be permanently lost to these invaders.

Another major impact of losing so many people to smallpox was devastation to the economy.[11] The large cities and the people that inhabited them required an enormous amount of food on a daily basis that came from farms located throughout the empire (most notably in Egypt). The loss of farmers needed to plant, maintain, and harvest crops led to a food shortage and widespread hunger. Furthermore, dead people do not pay taxes, which impacted Rome's ability to fund most of its civil projects and pay its military. The financial situation triggered by the epidemic was so dire that the Marcus Aurelius resorted to auctioning off the imperial jewels in order to pay his debts. The result was a major economic recession, which again weakened the empire and made it easier for other more prosperous and powerful armies to invade and take control.

One of the more interesting by-products of the Antonine smallpox epidemic was the impact that it had on Christianity, a religion that was still in its infancy in the mid-second century and was considered a nuisance to Romans who were still largely polytheistic at the time. Christians, in many ways, lived like outsiders in the empire due to their absolute refusal to worship Roman gods. They would not pray to them, offer sacrifices to them, possess idols of them, or partake in any other rituals that celebrated them. Furthermore, they especially despised the deification of the Roman political leaders and ardently refused to pay homage to Caesar. This general contempt for the emperor and Roman paganism is illustrated in the New Testament book of Revelation. Many theologians believe the apostle John wrote this not as a prophetic description of the end times but rather as an allegorical critique of Rome. He describes Rome as a "great prostitute" and Roman emperors (e.g., Nero) as multiheaded "beasts" who persecuted God's children and was destined for destruction.

The citizens in the very prosperous and nationalistic Roman Empire generally frowned upon any type of critique of their leaders and gods. As a result, when smallpox hit in 166 CE, local authorities were quick to blame the epidemic on Christians and their insults of Roman deities.[12] Similar to how Christians would later persecute Jews during the Black Death in the 14th century, Roman pagans rounded up Christians and murdered many of them in hopes of appeasing their gods and stopping the epidemic. Although popular depictions of this persecution commonly show Christians getting eaten by lions in the Colosseum, most of the time it actually involved unplanned attacks by disorganized local mobs. Such violence continued on and off for many years and even got worse when the empire was hit with yet another deadly epidemic in 251 CE (called the Cyprian plague). The cause of this second epidemic is unclear due to relatively vague eyewitness accounts of the symptoms; however, many have suggested that it was also caused by smallpox.

One may expect that the widespread violence against Christians would have had a deleterious effect on Christianity in the second and third centuries. Counterintuitively, this period is often cited by historians as the time when the religion exploded in popularity and went from being a small, unknown cult to a major force in the Roman Empire. A couple of interesting theories have been proposed to explain this apparent paradox.[13] First, it is well documented that new religions usually arise during times of widespread suffering. People try to make sense of how and why tragedies like epidemic disease or war have befallen them, and when they do not find satisfactory answers in their current religion, they often seek out a new one. They develop a sort of "grass is always greener" mentality and use the hope provided by a new ideology to emotionally deal with the devastation around them. They were worshiping the wrong god, believing the wrong ideas, and performing the wrong rituals before. However, since they have corrected their mistakes, they will be rewarded by being rescued from their suffering.

Early Christianity was an especially attractive alternative to pagan religions due to its propensity to see suffering as a redemptive and purifying tool used by God to draw himself closer to mankind. The epidemics were thus not a punishment being handed down by the Roman gods but were instead something that could be used for good by the Christian God. Also, the belief that Christians continue living in a heavenly paradise after death provided great comfort to those who were dying or watching loved ones die of the disease. The pagan religion of the day provided no such comfort nor did it satisfactorily explain why they were suffering. As a result, large numbers of Romans converted to Christianity in the wake of these two epidemics.

There was also a significant difference between how pagans and Christians acted toward those who were sick. It was noted by both pagan and Christian observers that the Christians were willing to put themselves at risk in order to care for the sick whereas pagans, like the great physician Galen himself, were more likely to flee from the epidemic. The Roman emperor Julian himself wrote that the Christians "support not only their poor, but ours as well; everyone can see that our people lack aid from us."[14] Randy Stark, in his book *The Rise of Christianity*, argues that such uncommon benevolence during these early smallpox epidemics likely played a major role in drawing others into the new religion.[15] As the number of converts continued to grow, Christianity went from being a cult to rivaling paganism as the dominant religion in the empire. In 313 CE, Christianity was officially decriminalized by the emperors Constantine and Licinius in the Edict of

Milan. Just 67 years later, Christianity was declared the official religion of the Roman Empire.

Exploration Creates a Pandemic

After causing numerous epidemics over the course of a millennium, smallpox had become an endemic disease throughout most of Eurasia by the 15th century. Because it was so widespread in the population, people were usually exposed to smallpox at some point during their childhood. Those who were lucky enough to survive this rite of passage enjoyed a lifetime of complete protection against any future infections with the *variola* virus. They could walk among individuals suffering from smallpox and handle contaminated objects without any fear of contracting the disease again. Such immunity would prove to be valuable as Europeans began exploring distant lands and interacting with native populations that had never been exposed to smallpox or had any protection against it.

The age of European exploration began in the 15th century as a direct result of the Ottoman takeover of several key port cities on the Eurasian continent. The first of these, Constantinople, was conquered in spring of 1453 by the Ottoman leader Sultan Mehmed II.

Shortly thereafter, the Ottomans moved eastward and initiated a series of very costly wars with the Republics of Venice and Genoa.[16] In addition to officially putting an end to the Byzantine (Eastern Roman) Empire, the loss of one of the most important port cities in the world and the severe weakening of others produced a massive disruption in trade between Asia and Europe. European monarchs, desperate to find new sources of goods and raw materials that were not under Ottoman control, funded a series of naval expeditions around Africa and into the open Atlantic Ocean in search of foreign lands that could serve as colonies for their expansion.

It was a gamble that ended up paying huge dividends for the Europeans in the centuries that followed. Their settlement of vast areas of land in the Americas, Caribbean, Africa, and Australia gave them access to a near endless supply of valuable natural resources and made them more wealthy and powerful than they had ever been before. Unfortunately, it also put them in contact with millions of indigenous people who were already living in the lands they were trying to colonize. What followed was perhaps one of the worst genocides in all of recorded history. Europeans systematically slaughtered entire civilizations of native peoples using a lethal combination of advanced weaponry and epidemic diseases. Smallpox, in particular, had catastrophic effects on these populations due to the fact that they had no previous exposure to it. Similar to the devastation seen in the early Antonine and Cyprian plagues in Europe, smallpox wiped out as much as 90 percent of the native population in some places and created mass chaos in all levels of society.

Africa

One of the earliest and most influential expeditions out of Europe was that of Portuguese sailors moving down the west coast of Africa in search of a quicker route to India.[17] Through the prompting of Prince Henry the Navigator, Portuguese sailors set sail with a fleet of newly designed, highly maneuverable ships called caravels. They successfully reached mainland Africa in 1434 near the northern coast of the Western Sahara and then proceeded to sail south toward modern-day Senegal, Gambia, and Guinea. By 1480, the Portuguese had explored most of the west coast of Africa, creating semipermanent settlements in several of the countries. Doing so allowed them to trade their goods with local tribes in exchange for slaves, minerals, and gold. The enormous wealth gained from these relationships encouraged Portugal to further explore the southern and eastern coasts of Africa. Upon reaching the southernmost point of Africa, the Cape of Good Hope, in 1488, the Portuguese established a number of trading posts and colonies along the eastern coast of Africa in places like Mozambique, Tanzania, and Kenya. As profits soared and the demand for slaves and gold increased, merchants and caravans moved deeper into the interior of Africa on both coasts.

Although it is clear that the Portuguese had an overall deleterious effect on the African tribes and civilizations it interacted with, the lack of reliable historical records in the 15th and early 16th centuries makes it difficult to decipher the specific impact played by smallpox in the early days of Portuguese colonial rule. For instance, did smallpox and other European diseases like influenza and measles allow the Portuguese to more easily overtake native African populations? We do know that many of the sub-Saharan African populations lived in cities that were equally large, well populated, and complex as those seen in 15th-century Europe. This would have made them well suited for the spread of communicable diseases like smallpox. Also, while there is some limited evidence that smallpox may have intermittently crossed the Sahara Desert sometime after 1100 via Muslim traders, most historians believe that the vast majority of populations south of the Sahara had never been exposed to smallpox at the time the Portuguese arrived.[18] As a "virgin" population, they would have been extremely vulnerable to being hit by a full-scale epidemic. With all this in mind, the only firm evidence that smallpox was active in Africa in the 15th and 16th centuries was that slave ships arriving in the New World were often found to be carrying smallpox.[19] While this clearly indicates that smallpox had to have been present in the cities that the ships departed from, how much it was killing native Africans there or what its impacts were on the native population remain a mystery.

Smallpox had a much more dramatic impact on African populations in the 19th century. Detailed records from various European observers describe widespread smallpox outbreaks in countries like the Sudan, Uganda, Angola, and Mozambique with fatality rates that approached over 80 percent in some cases. For instance, one witness to the 1864 smallpox epidemic in Angola wrote, "the variola epidemic by mid-1864 was on the rampage. It spread inland to the east with many caravans of trade, and spread south along the coast by contact with vessels in the ports . . . The negroes fled in all directions to avoid the epidemic . . . entire populations would migrate from their villages . . . Luanda was on the verge of anarchy as people died in great number."[20] Accounts from coastal towns known for their role in the Atlantic slave trade and slave caravan routes in central Africa describe similar outbreaks. In all, it is very likely that smallpox played a huge role in keeping susceptible African populations sick, weak, enslaved, and unable to mount any kind of resistance against their European colonial rulers.

Although the Portuguese were the first to colonize sub-Saharan Africa and introduce a variety of deadly diseases, other European powers also played a significant role in subjugating the continent with violence and disease. Of significant note to the discussion of smallpox was the colonization of South Africa by the Dutch in 1652. The first outbreak of smallpox in Cape Town occurred in 1713 when a ship arrived from India carrying smallpox-infected linens.[21] While it killed a significant number of the Dutch colonists who had settled there, it was particularly deadly for the susceptible Khoikhoi and Bantu natives living in the area. This epidemic was followed by an even more severe one in 1755 and a third in 1763. The cumulative effect of all three was the near elimination of native peoples from South Africa and relatively easy enslavement of remaining survivors. The Dutch eventually ceded power to the British in 1806, who then recolonized much of the land with their own immigrants and initiate a series of discriminatory laws designed to keep natives in a position of subservience. Although the descendants of this decimated native South African population did eventually escape the grips of slavery, they would continue to face legalized violence and persecution until the official end of apartheid in 1994.

Overall, it is entirely possible that we may be speaking about Africa in much different terms today if not for smallpox and the many other diseases brought in by Europeans during early days of colonial rule. For instance, a healthier African population not decimated by disease may have more effectively defended itself against the invading Europeans and at the very least slow or hinder the takeover of their land. This would have possibly reduced the efficiency by which colonial powers subjugated the native population and used them to steal vast amounts of wealth from Africa. As a result, more of that wealth may have remained on the continent, which would have drastically improved the economic situation of Africa in the centuries that followed.

The Americas

Smallpox first arrived in the New World in late 1518, when a ship from Spain landed on the island of Hispaniola carrying an infected slave or Spaniard.[22] Over the next few months, the disease spread rapidly among African slaves working in the gold mines and then it jumped into native populations all throughout the island. Several eyewitness accounts from 1519–1520 describe the epidemic as a "judgment of heaven" that left the island "desolated of Indians." While these statements were no doubt hyperbolic, the epidemic did kill off as many one-third of the non-European inhabitants of Hispaniola in just over a year.[23] In an effort to continue their lucrative mining activities in the midst of a dwindling workforce, Spanish colonists requested more slaves be brought over from Africa and forcibly relocated the remaining natives into settlement camps for easier control. Since smallpox thrives in crowded environments, doing so only exacerbated the spread of smallpox on the island. By 1519, the epidemic had moved to the nearby islands of Cuba and Puerto Rico, killing as many as 50 percent of their native inhabitants and also putting them at the mercy of the Spanish.[24] For the next several hundred years, Spain extracted millions of dollars' worth of gold from its Caribbean colonies and used its plantations to grow sugar cane, coffee, and ginger.

Although the Spanish were profiting greatly from their successful conquests in the Caribbean, they had their sights set on a much bigger prize— Mexico. In an effort to gain more information about the mainland and the native people inhabiting it, Cuban governor Diego Velázquez commissioned two different expeditions to explore Mexico in 1518.[25] The first was led by Spanish conquistador Francisco Hernández de Córdoba and included just over 100 men and three ships. After sailing through rough seas for about three weeks, de Córdoba's ships made landfall off the coast of the Yucatan Peninsula in early March 1518. The Spanish explorers were met immediately by a large number of Mayan natives who initially appeared to be friendly toward their visitors. However, within a few days, the Spanish were ambushed by the Mayans with spears and rocks and forced to retreat to their ships. In addition to losing several soldiers during the battle, the Spanish were forced back onto ships without fresh drinking water. They sailed around the Yucatan for another few weeks looking for possible water sources and made landfall two additional times. During the course of looking for water near the present-day city of Champotón, the Spanish were attacked by several thousand Mayan warriors and nearly wiped out. Only a fraction of the Spanish force made it safely back to their ships and even fewer returned to Cuba alive. De Córdoba himself died of his wounds just a few days after arriving home.

Although by most measures the Hernández de Córdoba expedition was a total failure, it did succeed in helping Velázquez gather intelligence about the new land and its inhabitants. Several of the survivors reported seeing items made of gold and copper, and one even succeeded in stealing some valuable artifacts from a Mayan temple during their short time on land. This prompted Velázquez to send a second, slightly larger expeditionary force to Mexico in 1518.[26] Led by his nephew Juan de Grijalba, this second group of explorers had much greater success than the first. Not only did they discover the island of Cozumel, they successfully mapped out various rivers and moved into the interior of Mexico. In doing so, they came across representatives of another civilization that lived to the north of the Yucatán Peninsula. The first meeting between the Spanish and the great Aztec Empire was a cordial one that ended with the two groups exchanging gifts. Grijalba returned to Cuba shortly thereafter and reported to his uncle what he had experienced during his exploration of the mainland. Interestingly, Velázquez was not pleased with his nephew upon hearing his report. In particular, he was angry with Grijalba for not seizing the opportunity to establish a formal Spanish colony while he was in Mexico. As a result, Velázquez decided to look for a bolder leader as he began to plan his third expedition to Mexico in 1519.

After much deliberation, Velázquez chose a local politician by the name of Hernán Cortés to lead the next expedition to the mainland.[27] Although Cortés had no previous experience in leading men in any type of exploration or armed conflict, Velázquez initially trusted him and admired his energy and ambition. However, as preparations for the trip began to take form, Velázquez gradually began to suspect that Cortés would double-cross him and claim Mexico for himself. He decided to relieve Cortés of his command and replace him with a man named Luis de Medina. When the papers appointing Medina as the new captain were intercepted and brought to Cortés, he decided to set sail for Mexico immediately. He rallied about 530 men, loaded 11 ships, and set sail for Mexico without the permission of Velázquez or the Spanish crown.

Cortés arrived in Mexico in February 1519 and proceeded to sail his ships north around the tip of the Yucatan Peninsula.[28] He eventually made permanent landfall near the modern-day state of Veracruz in April of that year. After founding a coastal settlement named La Villa Rica de la Vera Cruz and forming an alliance with the local Totonac tribe, Cortés marched his forces (which now included several hundred Totonac warriors) inland toward the Aztec capital of Tenochtitlan. Over the next several months, Cortés saw his army grow as he formed alliances with several large indigenous confederacies who were enemies of the Aztecs. In an effort to appease Cortés and prevent him from initiating any aggressive actions toward his people, Aztec ruler Montezuma II sent Cortés gifts of gold and other treasures on several occasions. Despite Montezuma's best diplomatic efforts, Cortés continued his march to the capital and arrived there in early November 1519 with an army of several thousand Spanish and native soldiers. Knowing that a war was probable, Montezuma tried to diffuse the situation by welcoming Cortés into Tenochtitlan with great pomp and circumstance and with more gifts of gold. However, within two weeks of his arrival (November 14, 1519), Cortés raided the palace and had Montezuma arrested. Cortés forced Montezuma to issue his orders to the empire and made himself the de facto ruler of the Aztecs.

When word of these actions got back to the Cuban governor Velázquez, he sent a large force to Mexico to have Cortés removed and arrested for trea-son.[29] Cortés responded by leading a group of soldiers to fight this new Span-ish contingent led by Pánfilo de Narváez. Though severely outnumbered, Cortés won the battle by mounting a surprise attack against de Narváez's forces at night. Rather than kill the captured Spanish soldiers, Cortés rea-soned with them and convinced them to join his own fighting force. Upon returning to Tenochtitlan, Cortés learned that the Aztecs had violently rebelled against the Spanish leaders that were left in charge in Cortés's absence. The Aztecs won the battle against the Spanish, expelled them from the city, and chased them until the Spanish eventually found safe shelter among the cities of their allies. Though this may seem like a happy ending from the perspective of the Aztecs, it would actually turn out to be the start of the real trouble for their empire.

An African slave who came over from Cuba with de Narváez was actively infected with smallpox. Upon joining forces with Cortés and traveling to Tenochtitlan, the slave inadvertently introduced smallpox to native popula-tions living nearby the capital city. A full-scale smallpox epidemic erupted in October 1520 and ravaged the Aztec population in Tenochtitlan and its sur-rounding cities. This occurred while Cortés was away rebuilding his forces and acquiring supplies in preparation for another attack. A Spanish friar who witnessed the carnage wrote in his book, *History of the Indians of New Spain,*

> At the time that Captain Pánfilo de Narváez landed in this country, there was in one of his ships a negro stricken with smallpox, a disease which had never been seen here. At this time New Spain was extremely full of people, and when the smallpox began to attack the Indians it became so great a pestilence among them throughout the land that in most provinces more than half the population died; in others the proportion was little less. For as the Indians did not know the remedy for the disease and were very much in the habit of bathing frequently, whether well or ill, and continued to do so even when suffering from smallpox, they died in heaps, like bed-bugs and others died of starvation, because, as they were all taken sick at once, they could not care for each other, nor was there anyone to give them bread or anything else. In many places it happened that everyone in a house died, and, as it was impossible to bury the great number of dead, they pulled down the houses over them in order to check the stench that rose from the dead bodies so that their homes became their tombs.[30]

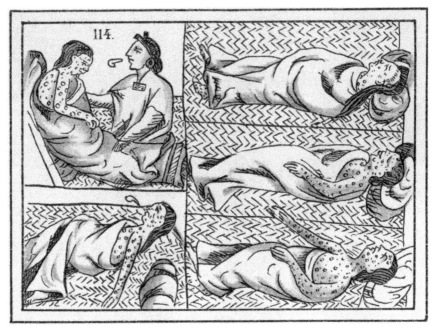

Aztec smallpox victims in the 16th century. From *Historia De Las Cosas de Nueva Espana*, Volume 4, Book 12, Lam. cliii, plate 114. Peabody Museum of Archaeology and Ethnology, Harvard University. (Courtesy of the Peabody Museum of Archaeology and Ethnology, Harvard University, PM# 2004.24.29636)

This graphic account illustrates the utter devastation inflicted on the Aztecs by smallpox and how the large numbers of deaths threw their society into a state of mourning and confusion. The observation that the Spanish aggressors seemed to be largely protected from the disease further demoralized the Aztecs and led them to question their own religious traditions. To make matters worse, the successor to Montezuma was killed by smallpox as were a number of leaders, nobles, farmers, and craftsman.

By the time Cortés returned to the capital in 1521, the once mighty and well-populated Tenochtitlan was a shell of itself. With nearly half of the population dead and another significant portion sick and hungry, Cortés had little problem defeating the Aztecs.[31] On August 13, 1521, the Aztec Empire surrendered and officially became part of the Spanish Empire. In just two years since arriving on the mainland, the Spanish had taken over what some claim was the second largest city in the world. In doing so, they were able to acquire an immense amount of gold. Following the fall of Tenochtitlan, smallpox would continue to ravage the native populations of Mexico for another 100 years. Some conservative estimates claim that from 1500 to 1600, the native population of Mexico declined from 10 million to just over 1 million (a 90% reduction).

While much of this reduction was very likely due to other diseases, war, and famine, smallpox no doubt took the most severe toll physically and emotionally. In addition to experiencing great population loss, the native people of Mexico were forced to watch their culture, language, religion, and overall way of life forever be destroyed by the Spanish and the diseases they brought.

The native people of Central and South America did not fare much better against smallpox. After devastating Mexico, the disease quickly moved south through Central America and made its way into the Inca Empire along the western coast of South America. Just as it had done with the Aztecs, smallpox wreaked havoc on the Inca people, killing 200,000 of them in a relatively short period of time.[32] Included among the fatalities were the Incan emperor and his chosen heir. This left a leadership void in the empire, which sparked a brutal civil war between various successors. At about this time, the Spanish learned of the great wealth in the Inca Empire and launched a new expedition led by Francisco Pizarro. The unrest caused by the war and smallpox allowed Pizarro and his native allies, shortly after their arrival, to overrun the fragmented leadership of the Incas. After some relatively minor skirmishes, the Spanish gained total control of the Inca Empire by August 1533.[33] In the years that followed, smallpox continued to spread rapidly among the Inca people and took the lives of over 60 percent of the local population. Their numbers would further be decimated by successive waves of other diseases including typhus, measles, and influenza. Other countries outside the confines of the Inca Empire would face similar fates. Smallpox brought by Spanish conquistadors would kill much of the native populations in countries like Venezuela, Chile, and Colombia. Furthermore, the Portuguese would go on to colonize Brazil and introduce smallpox there through the importation of infected slaves from Africa.[34] An epidemic in 1560 and several more in the 17th century decimated native populations living in Brazil and gave the Portuguese unquestioned control over the entire region.

Smallpox had similar disastrous effects on the indigenous peoples of the United States and Canada; however, it spread through the continent in a much different way than it had in other New World areas. Unlike the great Aztec and Inca empires, whose people lived in densely populated cities that favored transmission of communicable diseases like smallpox, Native Americans north of Mexico typically lived in smaller, more isolated hunter-gatherer groups. As a result, smallpox was unable to spread and kill as quickly as it had done in the larger New World empires. Instead, it steadily and slowly moved across the continent, jumping from one tribe to another over the course of about two centuries.

Although accurate estimates of death rates among native populations are lacking, eyewitness accounts by European settlers suggest that smallpox wiped out as much as two-thirds of tribes/nations like the Cherokee, Iroquois, Catawba, Omaha, and Sioux.[35] Smallpox was followed by a variety of other

European diseases, widespread malnutrition, and years of war. The end result was the near eradication of native people from North America and the opening up of the entire continent to settlement by Europeans and the United States.

To the colonists, smallpox was seen as a divine gift from God, a "miraculous" tool used against the non-Christian natives who had become a nuisance to them. The Puritan pastor Increase Mather, who was the father of Cotton Mather and a former president of Harvard, once expressed this sentiment when he wrote, "the Indians began to be quarrelsome concerning the bounds of the land they had sold to the English; but God ended the controversy by sending the smallpox amongst the Indians at Saugus, who were before that time exceeding numerous. Whole towns of them were swept away, in some of them not so much as one soul escaping the destruction."[36] Mather was essentially expressing what many in the United States had come to believe during this time; that God wanted "civilized" people to settle all of the land north of Mexico and was willing to use smallpox to execute this plan. When God was not moving fast enough for the colonists, however, there is some evidence that they may have taken matters into their own hands and purposely tried to infect nearby native populations with smallpox.

One of the more famous cases of suspected smallpox biowarfare involved Lord Jeffrey Amherst, who was commanding the British forces in America during Pontiac's War. In July 1763, he wrote to the commander at Fort Pitt in Pennsylvania and proposed, "Could it not be contrived to send smallpox among these disaffected tribes of Indians? We must on this occasion use every stratagem in our power to reduce them."[37] About a week later, he wrote, "You will do well to try to inoculate the Indians by means of blankets, as well as to try every other method that can serve to extirpate this execrable race." No one knows if the recipient of these letters, Colonel Henry Bouquet, carried out the suggested actions; however, a smallpox epidemic did break out among the tribes of the Ohio Valley about this time, resulting in the death of as many as 500,000 natives. Similar genocidal sentiments were made by others during this time as were other accusations of intentional infections of natives with smallpox. While some historians question the veracity of these claims, the fact that high-ranking military leaders made the suggestion and Native Americans were in fact nearly eliminated from the continent suggests that there may be some truth to the accusations.

Oceania

Due to their distance from Europe, the islands of Australia, New Zealand, Papua New Guinea, and Polynesia were not exposed to smallpox until the late 18th century. It was not until the loss of the United States in the Revolutionary War that Great Britain sought out new land to send their malcontents and criminals. After some initial charting of Australia in 1768–1771, Great Britain sent two larger fleets to the island 20 years later with the purpose of establishing a colony. In 1789, just one year after colonization, a major smallpox epidemic erupted, reportedly wiping out about 50 percent of the native Aboriginal people.[38] No one knows for sure how smallpox made its way to the island. Anyone who would have been infected on ships during four-month-long journey from England would have either died or recovered before arriving, thus making it unlikely that it was introduced by an infected traveler. The most likely explanation is that the primary physician who was on board the first fleet was carrying vials of smallpox material that would be used for variolation (an early precursor to immunization) if necessary. It is possible that this material either was accidentally released into the native population or purposely done so. In either case, this epidemic, along with others in 1828 and several in the 1860s, caused a calamitous decline in the Aboriginal population while doing very little to the white invaders.[39] Similar devastations occurred when smallpox first reached New Zealand, Papua New Guinea, and the isolated islands of the Pacific. For instance, smallpox (along with tuberculosis) reduced the population of a once-thriving Easter Island to just 110 people.

By the end of the 18th century, smallpox had spread from Eurasia to every inhabited continent on Earth. Everywhere it went and in every virgin population it entered, smallpox caused great devastation and empowered aggressive imperialistic European nations to seize control of great amounts of land and wealth without much resistance. Despite great diversity in their population demographics, cultural norms, religions, and environment, the histories of indigenous peoples of Africa, South America, North America, and Australia following the arrival of colonists and their smallpox are eerily similar. It is interesting to consider how history may have been different on these continents without the presence of smallpox. Would the Spanish conquistadors have had enough manpower or firepower (in the form of weapons and other diseases) to have overtaken powerful empires like those of the Aztecs and Incas? Would the U.S. military and colonists have been able to settle the vast lands across the North American continent had it not been for the decimation of powerful native tribes/nations like the Iroquois or Cherokee? How would have the power balance in Europe been different had certain countries not been able to extract such great wealth from the Americas and Africa? While no one knows the answers to these questions, it is clear that what would have taken military force and diplomacy many years to accomplish took smallpox a fraction of the time and cost.

Creator of Saints and Deities

One of the clearest indicators of how drastically smallpox affected the human psyche throughout the world is the fact that a number of religions created gods, goddesses, and saints specifically devoted to the disease.[40]

Some of these deities/saints were thought to heal the afflicted or protect the fearful against smallpox while others were believed to purposefully inflict the disease on the wicked. As a result, responses from followers included offering up of prayers and sacrifices, widespread building of temples and shrines, and performing rituals to scare off those deities who were particularly mean or angry.

The earliest religious figure specifically associated with smallpox was a Catholic bishop named Nicaise who lived in France during the 5th century. He had survived a serious case of smallpox prior to being beheaded by either invading Huns or Vandals. His almost miraculous recovery from smallpox saw him become the patron saint of smallpox shortly after his death. Europeans frightened of smallpox and those already suffering from it continued to pray to him for protection and healing for the next 900 years (until bubonic plague became more of an issue). One of the more common prayers to St. Nicaise, believed to have been written for nuns in the 10th century, is as follows: "In the name of our Lord Jesus Christ, may the Lord protect these persons and may the work of these virgins ward off the smallpox. St. Nicaise had the smallpox and he asked the Lord [to preserve] whoever carried his name inscribed. O St. Nicaise! Thou illustrious bishop and martyr, pray for me, a sinner, and defend me by thy intercession from this disease. Amen."[41]

As smallpox spread throughout Asia and eventually to Africa and the New World, a number of new gods and goddesses arose in various polytheistic religions. For instance, the Hindu goddess Sītalā mata became strongly associated with smallpox in the 1700s.[42] She is depicted as a beautiful young woman riding a donkey who could be somewhat hotheaded and unpredictable, inflicting the disease or curing it depending on her mood. As a result, she was equally loved and despised, worshipped and feared all throughout India. Similarly, the Chinese goddess T'ou-Shen Niang-Niang was one of the most popular and feared deities in all three of the major religions of the empire (Buddhism, Taoism, and Confucianism) for hundreds of years. Legend says that T'ou-Shen Niang-Niang particularly liked to give smallpox to attractive children in order to scar them. As a result, children would commonly wear paper masks on their faces in order to scare her off. If the child developed smallpox, a shrine would be set up in the home so that the family could worship the goddess and convince her to heal them. Failure of these actions to protect the child from the devastating effects of the disease would often cause the family to remove the shrine and curse the goddess. In Japan, families would often place a picture of the 12th-century hero Chinsei Hachiro Tametomo in the room of a person suffering from smallpox. Tametomo was captured by his enemies and exiled to the island of Oshima, where he reportedly fought off smallpox demons that were attempting to invade the island.

Many of the tribes of Western Africa built shrines to the god Sopona, who provided people of the world with food and other gifts and punished them

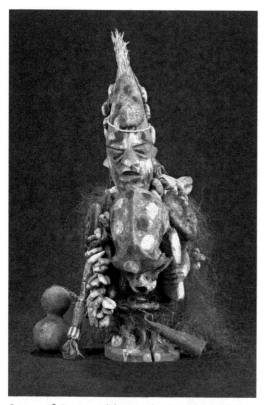

Statue of Sopona (Shapona), the West African god of smallpox. (Centers for Disease Control and Prevention)

with smallpox when they were bad.[43] Local priests called feticheurs would lead worship at these shrines, sometimes charging exorbitant fees for their services and possibly infecting people with smallpox on purpose in order keep business booming. In all, the widespread creation of deities devoted to smallpox not only demonstrates the severity and ubiquitousness of the disease, it also illustrates the primary defense mechanism of people who were completely helpless before the dawn of modern medicine.

From Variolation to Vaccination—A New Hope

One of the more important observations in the history of medicine was that survivors of smallpox were immune to subsequent infections. This fact prompted some individuals to search for methods that could mimic a smallpox infection and induce this immunity without inflicting any serious damage to the recipient. One of the earliest documented attempts at this was done by the Chinese who, in the 15th century, took dried scabs from patients with relatively minor forms of the disease, ground them into a powder, and used a blowpipe to purposely blow them into the nostril of the recipient.[44] In India and Turkey, people took the pus or other materials from smallpox pustules and deliberately introduced them onto the skin of recipients. Very often, small scratches and cuts were made and the pus was carefully dripped into the wound to produce a better inoculation. People in some parts of Africa (e.g., Sudan) would take clothing from those recovering from smallpox and transfer it onto the skin of healthy individuals. The end result of each of these methods of deliberately exposing a person to the smallpox virus was that, as expected, they would develop the disease and become sick. However, since less harmful strains were typically used and people were inoculated through the skin rather than through the more natural route of inhalation, recipients of this treatment would survive about 98 percent of the time and were protected from the disease for the rest of their lives.

Although this technique, which is called variolation, sounds like a godsend and was successful in reducing the incidence and duration of epidemics, it was not without its drawbacks. First, individuals receiving the treatment were fully infectious and could initiate a new epidemic if exposed to a susceptible population. To prevent this, individuals receiving variolation were usually kept in isolation until all symptoms subsided. Second, a death rate of 1–2 percent, though much lower than the 30 percent observed with natural infections, was still a frightening proposition to those considering the treatment.[45] Also, since variolation produced an actual infection, it had the potential to cause the scarring and blindness often observed in survivors of smallpox. Many individuals chose to take their chances and tried to avoid being infected whereas many municipalities utilized quarantining as their preferred means of slowing the spread of smallpox.

By the early part of the 18th century, variolation had become a well-known and still widely controversial prophylactic treatment throughout most of Europe and the United States. Upon witnessing the relative success of variolation in Turkey and the Middle East, several prominent European politicians and physicians (e.g., Charles Maitland, the Suttons, and Ambassador Edward Montague) began advocating its widespread implementation. Several children in the royal families were inoculated as a result. In the United States, Puritan pastor Cotton Mather witnessed the benefits of variolation in the successful treatment of one of his African slaves, Onesimus, and responded by recommending that locals in Boston undergo the procedure as a way to halt the epidemic that was enveloping the city at the time (1720s).[46] These word-of-mouth success stories, combined with data from several scientific tests, allowed variolation to gain much greater acceptance in the medical community and populace by the mid-18th century. For instance, Benjamin Franklin, who lost a son to smallpox, performed a statistical analysis in 1759 to assess the effectiveness of variolation on preventing death from smallpox.[47] He concluded that variolation did in fact drastically reduce mortality rates from smallpox, which led him to enthusiastically recommend its widespread implementation.

One particularly interesting instance in which variolation (and smallpox) played an important role in shaping the course of history was the impact it had on the Continental Army during the American Revolutionary War.[48] Although smallpox had been introduced to North America in the century before the war, it had yet to become endemic in the population as it had in Eurasia centuries before. As a result, most of the colonists who were born and living in North America by the mid-18th century had not been exposed to smallpox as children and were thus susceptible to an epidemic. This was a major concern for the Continental Army, considering that large numbers of susceptible soldiers would soon be living in very close quarters and fighting against an army that had been exposed to smallpox as children. General George Washington and other founding fathers knew this and greatly feared what would happen if a large-scale epidemic were to break out in the army. John Adams revealed such concern in stating that "the smallpox is ten times more terrible than Britons, Canadians, and Indians together."[49]

When an epidemic broke out in British-controlled Boston in 1775, their nightmare was realized as many fled the city and sought refuge behind the American lines.[50] This directly exposed the Continental Army to smallpox and threatened to undo the entire American war effort. Washington responded to the threat by initiating very strict quarantine measures for any soldier showing signs of the disease or anyone who had recently received variolation. His actions were successful, and the Continental Army pushed the British out of Boston without having any major outbreaks. However, the regiment that was marching on Quebec in the north was not so fortunate. Smallpox invaded their camp in the winter of 1775–1776 and wiped out nearly half of them. The following spring, the healthy British, with a fresh supply of reinforcements, pushed the Americans back and destroyed the possibility of adding a portion of Canada to the United States.

The disaster in Canada caused Washington to reconsider his use of quarantine as a means of protecting his army. However, the alternative was equally dangerous. He could inoculate each of his soldiers via variolation and risk either initiating a widespread epidemic in the army or having the British attack when his men were in their two-week recovery. Washington ultimately chose to inoculate every soldier and did so in secret during the winters of 1777 and 1778 (in times when the British were less likely to mount an offensive).[51] This mandated variolation was widely successful in that it allowed Washington to finally forget about smallpox and put all his focus, energy, and resources on fighting the British. Many historians argue that this decision ultimately helped save the war for the Continental Army because a smallpox epidemic among the main fighting force would have likely irrevocably weakened it to the point of defeat.[52]

Although variolation was a huge breakthrough and likely saved millions of lives during its use in the 18th century, it never gained widespread acceptance in the population due to the drawbacks discussed earlier. Knowing that variolation with live smallpox brings with it a 2–3 percent risk of dying, many considered it to be a way more risky option than simply trying to avoid it. Unfortunately, avoidance and quarantine measures failed to adequately contain smallpox for most of history. As a result, it continued to threaten and kill millions worldwide every year.

This all changed at the turn of the 19th century, when a British country doctor named Edward Jenner conducted experiments that forever changed the landscape of preventative medicine. The story begins when Jenner, first working as a teenage apprentice and then later as a physician, spoke with several local milkmaids. When discussing smallpox, they told him that they no longer needed to worry about the disease because they had already contracted and recovered from a relatively mild disease called cowpox. They told him that it was widely known among those who worked around cows that infection with cowpox provided lifelong protection from smallpox. Intrigued by the possibility of developing a harmless and effective alternative to variolation, Jenner decided to conduct a scientific test to determine the validity of these observations. In May 1796, he paid his gardener a modest sum of money for permission to inoculate his healthy eight-year-old son James Phipps with fluid from a cowpox pustule that was taken off the hand of a milkmaid named Sarah Nelmes. James developed minor flu-like symptoms seven to nine days after the treatment but recovered fully within two weeks. In a move that would likely get Jenner arrested if done today, he met with James six weeks later and challenged him with live smallpox. James developed no symptoms and remained immune upon being exposed over 20 more times. Jenner would go on to repeat the experiment with nine other people and all produced the same results.[53]

Despite having his findings rejected by a prominent scientific journal and warned not to continue with his experiments, Jenner published his findings, using his own money, in an article titled "An Inquiry into the Causes and Effects of the Variolae Vaccinae, a Disease Discovered in Some of the Western Counties of England, Particularly Gloucestershire, and Known by the Name of the Cow Pox."[54] The process described by Jenner became known as "vaccination" in honor of the cow that it was derived from (vaca is Latin for "cow"). Physicians in London and elsewhere in England began repeating Jenner's experiments within the year, and before long, the medical community had come to see vaccination as an answer for ending the scourge of smallpox. Thomas Jefferson described these sentiments when he wrote to Jenner, "Medicine has never before produced any single improvement of such utility. . . . You have erased from the calendar of human afflictions one of its greatest. Yours is the comfortable reflection that Mankind can never forget that you have lived; future generations will know by history only that the loathsome smallpox has existed, and by you had been extirpated."[55]

The impact of the Jenner vaccine on the history of smallpox was drastic. By 1800, most European countries had come to embrace vaccination as the best method for preventing smallpox, and the United States and other parts of the world quickly followed. By 1810, some countries and many local municipalities made vaccination mandatory for all citizens. The result was that the number of smallpox deaths gradually declined to the point that it was a rare occurrence in most industrialized countries by the turn of the

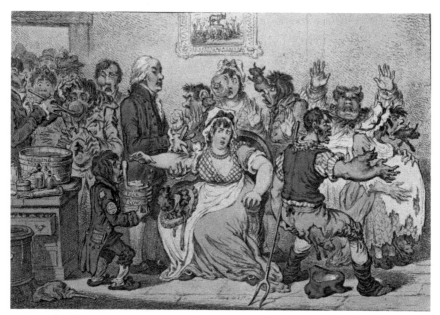

Caricature of vaccination scene at the Smallpox and Inoculation Hospital at St. Pancras, showing Dr. Jenner vaccinating a frightened young woman, and cows emerging from different parts of people's bodies. (Library of Congress)

20th century. However, developing countries in Africa, Latin America, and Asia continued to experience recurring smallpox epidemics due to the prohibitive cost of producing and administering the smallpox vaccine to the populace. In all, the smallpox vaccine not only gave mankind its first weapon for protecting itself against pathogenic microorganisms, it also helped eliminate the fear and power that smallpox held over us for several thousand years.

Jenner's pioneering work in developing the world's first vaccine was also significant for reasons unrelated to smallpox. It provided a proven model by which to attack all infectious disease: find harmless agents that mimic natural infections and purposely inject them into people as a means of priming their immune system for potential exposure to the real thing. The only problem with the cowpox-smallpox model was that most human infectious diseases (e.g., measles, influenza, anthrax, rabies, typhoid, malaria) have no harmless animal version of the disease that provides cross-protection against the human version. As a result, following the success of the smallpox vaccine, it took another 80 years before another vaccine was successfully developed. This next round of vaccine advancement occurred when scientists like Louis Pasteur, Henri Toussaint, and Emile Roux developed ways to artificially weaken dangerous infectious agents (called attenuation), making them both safe and effective as vaccines. Their innovation allowed for the creation of vaccines for diseases like anthrax and rabies in the 1880s and then others like diphtheria, tetanus, and pertussis during the next 50 years. The 1950s and 1960s saw major improvements in biochemical, genetics, and molecular biology techniques, which allowed for the development of the polio, measles, mumps, and rubella vaccines. By the 1980s, vaccine technology had progressed to the point of being able to inject just a select number of purified parts of some infectious agents. For instance, the hepatitis B virus (HBV) vaccine is made up of millions of copies of just one single protein (the HBV surface protein), and the pneumococcus vaccine is composed of just a small number of purified sugars.

What started as an intriguing observation by a country doctor at the end of the 18th century turned into a medical revolution that continues to save an estimated 9–10 million lives every year. Jenner's work was monumental because he showed for the first time that it was possible to stop these epidemic diseases. We were no longer completely at their mercy because we could take an active role in protecting ourselves. In fact, in less than 200 years from when Jenner first injected James Phipps with his vaccine, the world declared that smallpox had been eradicated from the human population.

Eradication and the Cold War

Due to improvements in mass production, distribution, and administration of the smallpox vaccine, the disease had been practically eliminated from most industrialized countries by 1950. For instance, Germany had eradicated smallpox by 1922, France by 1936, and the United States by 1949.[56] These countries had the financial and centralized governmental resources needed to encourage and force, if necessary, its population to receive the vaccine. In contrast, countries like India, Indonesia, Brazil, and most of Africa continued to experience tens of thousands of smallpox cases every year due to a lack of resources and an inability to distribute vaccines to impoverished, isolated, and sparsely populated regions. A similar situation is seen today with diseases like bubonic plague, measles, and polio still arising in poorer countries while being almost unheard of in developed countries. The result of smallpox's persistence in certain regions was that the rest of the world had to continue their very expensive vaccination programs because of the potential of reintroduction due to international travel. If one could eliminate smallpox everywhere, countries could save millions of dollars every year and the problem would be solved once and for all.

In 1958, the Soviet Minister of Health Viktor Zhdanov presented his proposal to the World Health Organization (WHO) Assembly meeting for the creation of a focused and prioritized program for the eradication of smallpox.[57]

Although it was accepted without much disagreement, virtually no new resources were allocated for the program and very little progress was made during the next nine years. The lackluster commitment to smallpox eradication was exemplified by having a total yearly budget of less than $200,000 (U.S.) and only a handful of full-time employees working on it. The reason for this half-hearted effort was due to the WHO devoting a huge amount of its resources to a failing, U.S.-backed malaria eradication program. By 1967, both U.S. and Soviet scientists had come to realize that the malaria program was doomed and more had to be done to eliminate smallpox. As a result, the director general of the WHO drafted a proposal to shift a significant portion of the WHO budget to the smallpox eradication program and it passed the Assembly by a slim margin.[58] With this renewed commitment came a bold goal: to go into the most remote, poor, and violent areas in the world and eradicate smallpox within a decade.

One of the first and most important tasks of the smallpox eradication program was to establish how the United States and Soviet Union would work together and pool their resources to fight a common foe at the height of the Cold War. Following the end of World War II, the Soviet Union sought to expand its influence and spread communism throughout Eastern Europe, Asia, and Latin America, whereas the United States did everything in its power to limit this expansion. The U.S. policy of containment (called the Truman Doctrine) included practical measures such as the massive worldwide buildup of nuclear weapons, economic assistance to weakened countries in war-torn Europe (Marshall Plan), and economic and military assistance to any rebel group or government that was actively fighting communist influences in their country. The Soviet Union, in turn, responded with a nuclear arsenal buildup of its own and provided economic and military assistance to any rebel group or government that was actively promoting communist influences in their country. The end result was a 45-year tense standoff between two superpowers that had the ability to annihilate each other. Although they never fired a single bullet against one another, they were almost always on opposing sides of some of the bloodiest conflicts in the 20th century (e.g., southeast Asia, Somali-Ethiopia, Guatemala). There was a mutual hatred and fear between these two countries that extended through every strata of society and government.

When the revised smallpox eradication program proposal was put forth in 1967, there was a real worry that U.S.-Soviet Union political tension would spread into the WHO and the smallpox program would be doomed as a result. So many vital questions hung over the administration of WHO at this point. Should an American or Soviet scientist be selected to head the program? How much money and vaccines will each country contribute? Is there a risk of these countries amassing smallpox samples for later use as bioweapons? Who will take the credit if the program is successful and the blame if it fails?

When the time came to appoint a director of the program, a well-respected American scientist by the name of Donald Henderson was chosen for the job.[59] The Soviets were initially upset by this choice since they were the ones who first proposed the program and were supplying the majority of the vaccine for it (over 80% of the total). However, Soviet scientists grew to respect Dr. Henderson during the course of the program and many became his lifelong friends. While many of their countrymen were engaged in bitter and sometimes violent conflicts with one another, these scientists, along with many from other countries (most notably Sweden), put politics aside and worked selflessly as a unified team through many financial and logistical problems. They had an insurmountable task of raising nearly $100 million at a time when most excess funds were spent on national defense. They also had to deal with the production, quality testing, and distribution of several billion doses of vaccine to over 30 different countries. Thankfully, their focus, endurance, and hard work paid off. On May 8, 1980, WHO representatives officially declared that smallpox had been eliminated from every human being on Earth. The greatest scourge that our species has known, one that killed hundreds of millions of people in every century, was gone.

As the smallpox eradication program was nearing its completion, several looming issues remained. The first had to do with the fact that labs and hospitals all over the world had thousands of samples of smallpox stored away in their freezers.[60] This obviously posed an enormous threat to the maintenance of eradication since any angry or incompetent lab technician could easily sell smallpox to the highest bidder or accidently release it back into the population. It was therefore vital to identify all lab sources of smallpox and ensure that they were destroyed according to established WHO protocols. Second, once all of those samples had been disposed of, what should be done with the very last tubes of smallpox? Should they be kept somewhere in a secret and secure location in the event of some unforeseen emergency or should they be destroyed? Humans have never purposely caused the extinction of a biological agent before and so this was a major ethical dilemma for both scientists and administrators. In the end, the WHO decided to maintain stocks of smallpox at two facilities, the Centers for Disease Control and Prevention (CDC) in Atlanta, Georgia, and the Research Institute for Viral Preparations in Moscow (these Russian samples were later transferred to the Vector Institute in Koltsovo, Russia).[61] Since that initial decision, the WHO has routinely conducted surveys of virology experts, set deadlines, and held votes to readdress the issue of whether or not to destroy all remaining known smallpox stocks. The deadlines have continually passed without any new action taking place. The most recent reprieve of smallpox took place in 2014, when WHO officials and scientists once again failed to reach a consensus about the future of the last known *variola major* virus stocks. Some believe that research is still needed to gain a better understanding of its pathogenesis and to allow for the production of newer and more effective antiviral drugs. Others think it should be destroyed because its continued existence poses an unnecessary risk to the population.

Their worries may be justified. The sheer abundance of smallpox in the world through the 1960s makes it is highly likely that some countries or smaller groups secretly stockpiled smallpox before the WHO demanded its destruction. There is no way to ensure that WHO investigators found every last vial of the virus in every country in the world prior to 1980. Even more worrisome are the testimonies from defectors (e.g., Ken Alibek) who worked as part of Soviet bioweapons program.[62] They suggest that nearly 20 tons of liquid, weapons-grade smallpox had been produced and stored on several Soviet military bases as late as 1990. Also, there is evidence that Soviet scientists genetically engineered smallpox and fused it with other viruses like Ebola and Venezuelan equine encephalitis virus. These hybrid viruses would be exceptionally more deadly than natural smallpox and could pose a real threat to the health of our species.

When the Soviet Union dissolved in 1991, there were reports that the security at many of these installations was compromised and smallpox and other biowarfare agents may have escaped. One Vector Institute administrator was quoted as saying, "Listen, we didn't account for every ampule of the virus. We had large quantities of it on hand. There were plenty of opportunities for staff members to walk away with an ampule. Although we think we know where our formerly employed scientists are, we can't account for all of them—we don't know where all of them are."[63] What makes this even more alarming is that the modern smallpox vaccine is only protective for about 10–20 years, and most countries stopped vaccinations by the end of the 1970s. There are some vaccines in storage but not nearly enough for 7 billion people. That would mean that nearly the entire population of the world is currently susceptible to infection. Upon receiving conformation of the credibility of these threats from American and British investigators who visited the Russian facilities, Dr. Henderson, who worked so hard to end smallpox, said,

> I feel very sad about this. The eradication never would have succeeded without the Russians. Viktor Zhdanov started it, and they did so much. They were extremely proud of what they had done. I felt the virus was in good hands with the Russians. I never would have suspected. They made twenty tons—twenty tons—of smallpox. For us to have come so far with the disease, and now to have to deal with this human creation, when there are so many other problems in the world. It's a great letdown.[64]

If smallpox were ever to be unleashed again, it would likely kill millions before authorities could mobilize and contain its spread.

Several very important lessons can be learned from the smallpox eradication program. First, due to terrorism and improvements in technology over the past 20 years, it is probably impossible to ever fully eradicate a pathogen from the planet. As long as biological agents continue to be used as weapons and people with enough money can buy scientific equipment on the black market, there will always be a risk that deadly pathogens are being stored away in freezers in some remote part of the world. Secondly, smallpox eradication from a practical sense was an enormous success. Although a risk of reintroduction still does exist, it is important to note that there has not been a case of smallpox anywhere in the world since 1977. That is 40 years without a single death from a virus that was killing 300–400 million people every century. It is an amazing achievement in and of itself, but it also demonstrated that eradication is a possible endpoint. The smallpox eradication program was the fifth such program attempted by the WHO, with the previous four ending in failure. Each failed for a variety of reasons, including ineffective or unstable vaccines/antibiotics/pesticides, lack of funding, lack of regional support, and an inability to identify or contain those who are infected (or vectors). Some in the public health field were beginning to question the feasibility of any large-scale elimination of infectious disease.

The smallpox program was successful while others failed because its vaccine was stable and effective after just one injection and because local health officials were included in decision making and implementation. Thus, it provided a model of success that future eradication programs could look to as they are planned out. Soon after the monumental announcement in 1980, scientists at the WHO began looking for their next target for eradication. Some eradicable diseases include polio, guinea worm disease, measles, mumps, rubella, and lymphatic filariasis. Despite the potential to permanently rid the world of diseases that infect 200 million people every year, neither the WHO nor any other agency or nation has made it a reality. Some have been eliminated regionally and a couple like polio and guinea worm disease are close to being eradicated globally. However, the diseases listed continue to stubbornly hang on in much of the developing world and people are still suffering needlessly as a result.

CHAPTER FOUR

Malaria

If you think you are too small to make a difference, try sleeping in a closed room with a mosquito.

—African proverb

When people are asked what the most deadly animal in the world is, most answers include large, scary-looking animals like sharks, alligators, snakes, lions, and spiders. People are generally shocked to hear that the title belongs to a tiny insect that is less than 2 centimeters in length and weighs only about 2.5 milligrams. The female mosquito, by far, kills more humans than any other animal due to its ability to spread deadly infectious diseases like dengue fever, yellow fever, filariasis, viral encephalitis (e.g., West Nile), and, most importantly, malaria. In fact, well over 90 percent of the deaths attributed to mosquitoes are due primarily to malaria.

Recent estimates from the World Health Organization (WHO) claim that as many as 300 million people contract malaria every single year and about 430,000 die from it, making it one of the leading causes of death in the world.[1] The vast majority of these cases and deaths (more than 90%) occur in sub-Saharan Africa, and most of those killed are children under the age of five; however, malaria is also prevalent in many other warm, tropical areas that receive lots of rainfall and are breeding grounds for mosquitoes. These areas include most of southern Asia (China, India, Southeast Asia), Central America, and the northern portion of South America. Although it does not have the high mortality rates that are seen with plague or smallpox epidemics, malaria is nearly ubiquitous in impoverished tropical areas and causes a debilitating illness that drastically limits the productivity, economic development, and growth of individuals and entire populations. It causes a significant reduction in one's ability to work and go to school and puts a huge financial burden on families that are forced to spend their limited resources on medical care. Many public health experts believe that malaria represents one of the greatest hurdles in allowing developing countries to escape the endless cycle of poverty.[2]

Malaria is caused by infection with one of four species of the parasite *Plasmodium* (*P. falciparum, P. malariae, P. ovale,* and *P. vivax*). *Plasmodium* is not a type of bacterium or virus but rather a unicellular protozoan that has a complex cellular structure (like that of humans) and a life cycle that involves both its mosquito vector and human host. About 30–40 different species of mosquitoes, all belonging to the genus *Anopheles*, naturally serve as vectors for *Plasmodium* parasites.

After a mosquito bites an infected person and takes in a blood meal, the parasite undergoes a type of sexual reproduction in the gut of the mosquito and proceeds to invade the cells that line its gut.[3] After further replication in those cells, new parasite production causes gut cells to burst, releasing the parasite sporozoites. The sporozoites spread to the salivary glands of the mosquito and wait for it to bite another human. Upon landing on a new host, the mosquito inserts its mandibles and the maxillae into the skin and promptly injects its saliva, which has potent anticlotting and pro-inflammatory properties (allowing blood to flow freely). *Plasmodium* sporozoites found in the mosquito saliva enter into the bloodstream of the new host and quickly migrate to the liver, where they invade host hepatocytes.

In many cases, the sporozoites will sit dormant inside the hepatocytes for several days, weeks, or even months before proceeding to the next stage of its life cycle.[4] This asymptomatic incubation period varies for each of the four *Plasmodium* species that cause malaria. Once it becomes activated, it undergoes reproduction inside of the liver cell, causing it to burst and release parasite cells that are now called merozoites. These merozoites move into the blood of the host and invade red blood cells (RBCs) there. Once inside RBCs, the parasite drastically increases its size, ingests host hemoglobin, and undergoes several rounds of reproduction. The infected RBCs eventually pop, releasing a large number of new merozoites that are capable of infecting even more RBCs. This cycle of infection, growth, reproduction, and release from RBCs will repeat about every 2–3 days (depending on the *Plasmodium* species) until the patient dies or is treated.

The large-scale destruction of RBCs every couple of days causes the majority of symptoms that are characteristic of malaria infection.[5] Most malaria patients experience generic flu-like symptoms including high fever, muscle ache, fatigue, chills, headache, nausea, and uncontrollable shivering. However, malaria uniquely produces these symptoms in a repeated, cyclical fashion (i.e., it is paroxysmal); patients feel awful, apparently recover, and then feel awful again every 2–3 days. Some patients infected with *P. falciparum* may experience more severe complications such as anemia, respiratory distress, renal failure, miscarriage, and a variety of central nervous system problems (e.g., convulsions, seizures, and coma). Without proper treatment, patients can remain debilitated with these symptoms for up to six months. Furthermore, even after recovering, patients can have frequent recurrences (due to dormant infections in the liver) for 50 more years. For instance, a significant number of U.S. soldiers who contracted malaria while serving in Vietnam in the late 1960s have reported continual "flare-ups" of malaria nearly 40 years after being treated in military hospitals.

Unfortunately, *Plasmodium* infection does not provide a person with full immunity, which allows for recurrences and brand-new malaria infections. In fact, it is common for people living in locations where malaria is endemic (e.g., Africa) to be reinfected with malaria on an almost yearly basis. The relatively poor immune response toward malaria has also made the development of an effective vaccine very difficult and ultimately helped doom all attempts at full eradication.

The origin and spread of malaria around the world has been one of the more interesting and hotly debated topics in epidemiology in recent years. Although many people tend to associate mosquitoes (and malaria) with hot, humid environments like that found in the jungles of Africa or South America, the *Anopheles* genus has species that are capable of thriving in temperate and even cold climates. For this reason, malaria has been able to spread to all corners of the globe, including regions that are close to the Arctic Circle.

Recent genetic studies strongly suggest that most, if not all four, of the *Plasmodium* species that cause human malaria originated somewhere in sub-Saharan Africa about 100 million years ago as parasites of Old World primates.[6] The jump to humans probably took place very shortly after the appearance of early hominids; however, the low-density hunter-gatherer lifestyle of these early humans did not allow for widespread distribution or spread of the disease. In other words, small groups tended to live far apart from one another, making it unlikely that one would be bitten by a mosquito that had recently bitten another infected person. This changed with the advent of the agricultural (Neolithic) revolution in the Fertile Crescent about 10,000 years ago.[7] People not only began living in fixed locations in much higher population densities, they also significantly changed the land around them, which fostered the reproduction and spread of insect vectors. As agriculture techniques gradually made their way into sub-Saharan Africa, the *Anopheles* mosquitoes living there experienced an explosive population growth. This allowed for the spread of *Plasmodium* parasites beyond the confines of Africa. For instance, paroxysmal fevers characteristic of malaria were reported in a Chinese medical text from around 4,700 BCE, and subsequent references to malaria were made in Egyptian, Sumerian, and Indian texts from about 3,500 BCE.

Malaria had stretched across the Eurasian continent very early in human history, but it likely did not make it to the New World until European explorers and African slaves brought it there in the 16th century.[8] Some have argued that *P. malariae* and *P. vivax* (and thus malaria) were present in the Americas long before the arrival of Europeans due to the fact that they are genetically similar to parasites of New World monkeys. The hypothesis was that the human-tropic *Plasmodium* species evolved from New World monkeys just as they had done separately in Africa previously. However, genetic analyses of Native Americans reveal that they lack genetic markers that are characteristic of populations that have been exposed to malaria for long periods of time (hundreds or thousands of years).[9] The lack of these "malaria" markers indicates that it is likely that Americans had only recently been exposed to malaria and that it was the Europeans who transmitted *Plasmodium* to both the Native Americans and the New World monkeys upon arriving there.

Despite not killing people as efficiently, indiscriminately, or gruesomely as some of the other pathogens discussed in this book, malaria has undeniably had as significant and long-term impacts on our history, development, and genome as any pathogen in the world. Much of its destructive potential lies in its ability to repeatedly infect and incapacitate a person for long periods of time. It has paralyzed armies, altered major public works projects, blocked colonization, and helped keep an entire continent in a state of poverty. Furthermore, it has caused more permanent changes to the human genome than any other pathogen in human history. In fact, several deadly genetic diseases, such as sickle-cell anemia and thalassemia, exist today because of our species' long-term exposure to malaria.

Ancient Killer

References to a fever-causing disease similar to modern-day malaria can be found in 5,000-year-old texts from China, Sumeria, and India. The first irrefutable clinical description of malaria comes from the famous Greek physician Hippocrates in his work *On Airs, Waters, and Places* around the year 400 BCE.[10] He clearly described the paroxysmal fevers that are characteristic of malaria and the times of year when they were mostly likely to occur. Other ancient writers also described malaria as a fever that was associated with wet environments such as marshes and swamps, and some like the Roman writer Marcus Terentius Varro even suggested that tiny insects associated with these wet environments may play a role in the disease transmission.[11] Despite providing a pretty accurate clinical presentation of malaria and astutely identifying environmental factors that contribute to it, ancient writers had no idea as to the true etiology of the disease. The prevailing theory at the time was that a person contracts "marsh fevers" by breathing in poisonous vapors given off from the smelly swamps. This miasmatic (diseased air) theory of disease transmission remained the most accepted cause of malaria for several thousand years. Interestingly, that theory ultimately gave rise to the name malaria, which literally means "bad air" in medieval Italian.

While the historical record clearly indicates that malaria was common in ancient empires such as those of the Romans, Greeks, Chinese, and Mongols, the precise impact it had on those civilizations remains poorly defined. This is due to a lack of widespread record keeping by some of these civilizations and a general inability to effectively distinguish the fevers caused by malaria from those caused by other diseases like typhoid. Despite these limitations, some surviving records do indicate that malaria did in fact play a significant role in shaping the history of the ancient world. For instance, the Roman Empire, which was centered in the relatively marshy Italian Peninsula, continuously had to deal with malaria outbreaks that would kill many and send others fleeing to higher and dryer ground.[12] Part of this was due to the Roman aqueduct system that constantly brought in large supplies of fresh water into the fountains and baths of major Roman cities, creating areas of standing water for mosquitoes to breed in. Similarly, the clearing of land for agriculture led to larger areas of standing water in the region, and the Tiber River, which runs alongside the city of Rome, would flood annually, turning large portions of the city into uninhabitable swampland.

Realizing that excessive stagnant water was having a deleterious effect on the health of the city's inhabitants, Roman officials ordered that a giant underground sewer system be developed in order to drain flood and waste water away from Rome. This sewer, called the Cloaca Maxima, was one of the most revolutionary and advanced public works projects in the world at the time.[13] Almost immediately upon being completed, the city began to dry out, and the number and severity of malaria outbreaks began to diminish. Although malaria would never completely be eliminated, people started enjoying greater periods of good health, and the population of the city gradually increased. In contrast, other densely populated regions of ancient Italy that lacked such a sewage system (e.g., Ostia Antica and the Pontine Marshes) continued to struggle with malaria to the point that several cities were abandoned due to the inherent danger of living there.[14] Thus, the Cloaca Maxima at the very least helped keep malaria in check in Rome and allowed it to prosper more than it would have otherwise. Taking it a step further, it is possible that Rome, like several of its neighbors, may have remained permanently incapacitated by malaria if not for the Cloaca Maxima, and the whole history of the Roman Empire could have been drastically different as a result.

Years later, the city of Rome would face a very different enemy that again threatened its very existence. Attila the Hun, known as the "Scourge of God" by the Romans, rose to power in the year 434 CE and commanded an army that systematically plundered and destroyed cities all across eastern Europe, Gaul (modern-day France, Belgium, Switzerland, and Luxembourg), and northern Italy. By 452, he had reached central Italy and focused his attention on the crown jewel of the Roman Empire. When Pope Leo I heard that the Hun army was approaching Rome, he personally led a party to meet with Attila and discuss terms for a peace treaty.[15] The meeting that followed remains one of the more interesting and mysterious diplomatic discussions in history. Rather than moving forward with his attack plans as he had done so many times before, Attila inexplicably packed up his supplies and ordered his army to leave Italy. What the pope said or did to convince Attila remains unknown. Some scholars believe the pope gave Attila a massive amount of money to leave Rome alone while others say he threatened him with military force. Recently, some scholars have suggested that Attila may have seen the devastation that malaria inflicted upon his susceptible army in their time in Italy and feared that a long-term invasion of Italy would result in the loss of his entire fighting force. Could the pope have warned Attila that God would punish his army with this invisible enemy if they invaded Rome? It certainly is a viable theory considering that malaria would have been widespread in central Italy at the time, and most of his army would have likely been vulnerable to the types of *Plasmodium* species found in the Mediterranean.

Several other ancient armies and leaders faced similar crises. For instance, many scholars believe that malaria took the life of Macedonian commander Alexander the Great during the height of his empire (323 BCE). Ancient sources describe Alexander in the weeks preceding his death as having a high fever, weakness, and pain, all of which are characteristic of malaria and a few other infectious diseases that were endemic to Asia at the time.[16] While no one will ever really know if malaria was the true cause of Alexander's death, the effects of his death were clear and dramatic. In just 20 years, the entire empire that Alexander had built was destroyed and taken over by other powers. A similar fate has also been suggested for the famous 13th-century Mongolian emperor Genghis Khan, who assembled the largest empire in the history of the world.[17] Even though he was infected with malaria for several months before dying, it is not known whether that was the cause of his death or whether it was something else.

White Man's Grave and the Scramble for Africa

An examination of the history of European invasion of distant lands in the 15th century and later reveals a very striking feature—the vast majority of the African continent remained uncolonized up until the late 19th century. In fact, as of 1870, only about 10 percent of the land mass of Africa was under European control (most of this represented coastal cities used in the slave trade).[18] In contrast, nearly all of North and South America, Australia, and significant portions of Asia (e.g., India and Indonesia) were controlled by the French, British, Portuguese, and Spanish by the early 1800s. This hands-off approach toward Africa makes little sense considering the continent had been discovered by traders and explorers many centuries before; the inhabitants of Africa were just as susceptible to European diseases as natives found on the other continents; and Africa harbored an enormous abundance of raw materials and inherent wealth. Thus, there is no logical reason why Europeans would have purposely refrained from taking control of the African land mass and its inhabitants when there was so much to gain by doing so.

The fact is European explorers had attempted to venture deeper into the African continent since arriving there in the late 15th century. One of the major factors that prevented them from doing so to any large extent was the ongoing and widespread presence of a variety of deadly diseases, including yellow fever, sleeping sickness, dysentery, and most importantly, malaria. Unlike native Africans, who often have some genetic resistance to malaria (see later in this chapter), invading white Europeans were almost completely susceptible to the disease. West Africa in particular is an extremely favorable breeding ground for the *Anopheles gambiae* and *Anopheles funestus* species of mosquitoes, which efficiently transmit the deadliest form of malaria caused by *P. falciparum*. The mosquitoes and malarial parasites were so common that a person living in West Africa could be expected to be bitten by infected mosquitoes about 100 times every single year. What this translated to was mortality rates that approached 50–70 percent for Europeans who entered sub-Saharan Africa.[19]

The death rate from malaria and other diseases was so high that Europeans dubbed Africa as "The White Man's Grave." Such high death rates eliminated any possibility of a large-scale invasion by European military forces or civilians and made exploration difficult. In fact, the bulk of Africa's interior was not even mapped to any great extent until the middle of the 19th century. The burden of African diseases like malaria was so great that it was still more profitable and advantageous to colonize less dangerous areas. In a sense, malaria (and yellow fever), despite killing large numbers of native Africans every year, helped protect the continent of Africa and its people from aggressive European imperialism for about 300 years. That protection ended abruptly in the latter part of the 19th century due in large part to the mass production and distribution of a single lifesaving drug called quinine.

Quinine is a natural alkaloid compound produced in the bark of the cinchona (quina quina) tree, a tall evergreen that was originally found only high in the Andes Mountains. A local tribe called the Quechua had accidentally discovered beneficial effects of cinchona bark in the treatment of malaria and other fever diseases as early as the mid-1500s.[20] They would dry the red bark, grind it into a powder, and mix it with sweetened water (masking its bitter taste) to create a medicinal tonic. During this time, a number of Jesuit (Catholic) priests traveled to South America and set up missions there in an attempt to convert local tribes and learn from their customs and herbal remedies. Several of these priests had observed and documented the successful use of the bark tonic in treating malaria. The first such reference of the use of cinchona bark is found in a book by an Augustine monk named Antonio de la Calancha who, in 1633, wrote, "A tree grows which they call 'the fever tree' in the country of Loxa, whose bark, of the color of cinnamon, made into powder amounting to the weight of two small silver coins and given as a beverage, cures the fevers and tertiana; it has produced miraculous results in Lima."[21]

How the bark made its way to Europe and when that occurred is a topic still greatly debated among scholars. Some sources claim that a Jesuit apothecary/pharmacist named Agostino Salumbrino shipped a sample of the bark to Rome in the early 1630s; others claim that a Jesuit missionary named Bernabé de Cobo obtained a sample of the bark while traveling through Peru and hand-delivered it to Spain and then Rome in 1632.[22] A third explanation, first suggested by medic Sebastiano Bado in his 1663 work *Anastasis corticis Peruviae seu china china defensio*, holds that the wife of the Count of Chinchón, the Spanish viceroy of Peru, was gravely ill with malaria until being cured by the miraculous bark.[23] She is then said to have brought the bark back to Europe upon her return to Spain in 1638. However, the discovery of Count Chinchón's diary in 1930 seems to suggest that this latter story was more myth than fact. Most evidence points to the bark being brought to Europe via Jesuit missionaries in the 1630s.

After arriving in Europe, this new miracle treatment, called "Jesuit bark," "Peruvian bark," or "fever bark," sparked a controversial medical revolution that had wide-ranging and long-term effects throughout the world. One of the early European advocates of the bark was a Catholic cardinal named Juan de Lugo who, with the help of Pope Innocent X's personal physician, used it to treat a number of local Romans suffering from malaria. Their results were so encouraging that recommendations for dosage and administration were later published in the *Schedula Romana*, an instruction book issued by the pharmacy of the Collegio Romano in 1649.[24] De Lugo was so convinced of the bark's ability to treat malaria that he personally began distributing it to the poor from his palace and to local Roman hospitals. He also recommended that it be distributed from Catholic missions throughout Europe, which drastically increased demand for the bark.

In contrast to its growing acceptance in the Catholic world, Protestant-dominated countries (e.g., England) and their physicians tended to view the "Jesuit bark" with a bit more skepticism. Many Protestants at the time had a deep mistrust of anything supported by the Catholic Church, which caused them to view the bitter-tasting bark powder as a potential plot by the pope to harm them.[25] Furthermore, many of the classically trained physicians from Protestant countries still largely followed Galenic medical practices that called for bloodletting and purging in cases of malaria (in order to balance the body humors). Suggesting that Galen and 1,400 years of medical teaching were wrong and the Catholics were right was tantamount to sacrilege. The mistrust gradually began to subside; Jesuit bark gained more widespread acceptance as a long litany of Protestant aristocrats, including King Charles II of England and the son of King Louis XIV of France, were treated successfully with the bark. In all, it took well over a century from the time it was first recognized as a potential malaria treatment for the bark to be universally accepted throughout Europe.

By the beginning of the 19th century, demand for the bark was at an all-time high due to the continued presence of malaria in major urban centers and an increased presence of Europeans in tropical environments abroad. Unfortunately, at the time, the supply of the bark was limited and costs were high due to the fact that cinchona trees only grew in the Andes Mountains. Furthermore, harvesting and shipping processes were time consuming and expensive, and Spain had a total monopoly on the product. Not happy with these limitations, other European powers began trying to procure their own supply of the bark by sneaking cinchona seeds out of Peru and attempting to grow the trees elsewhere. Peruvian authorities became wise to the growing threat to their highly profitable export and outlawed foreigners from even going into cinchona forests. Despite their best efforts, Spain and Peru lost their monopoly on the bark in 1865 after a British man named Charles Ledger successfully obtained and shipped a pound of cinchona seed to the Dutch, who proceeded to successfully grow massive quantities of the trees on plantations in Java (in modern-day Indonesia).[26] This increased supply of bark to the market was complemented by major improvements to chemistry and industrialization. For instance, two French pharmacists, Joseph Pelletier and Joseph Bienaimé Caventou, successful purified the active antimalarial ingredient of the bark in 1820 and named it quinine in honor of the native Peruvian name of the bark.[27] They published their purification process and refused to patent their discovery, which enabled others to begin manufacturing

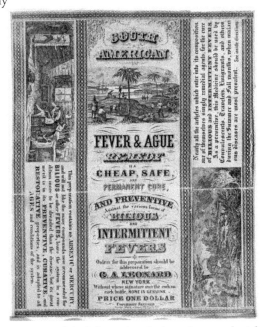

Medicine label for a South American malarial fever remedy. (Library of Congress)

and selling purified quinine extracts and pills in large quantities. Further-more, botanists in the 1860s used selective cultivation and grafting methods to make the trees hardier and increase quinine production in their bark. Clin-ical trials in the 1860s confirmed the efficacy of using purified quinine to treat malaria, and other studies showed that quinine could also be used as a prophylactic to prevent malaria.[28] By the 1870s and 1880s, purified quinine was being distributed to the masses all over the world, and people living in malaria-endemic areas routinely took quinine pills to keep from getting sick. Quinine was often taken in the form of carbonated tonic waters, mixed with sugar and alcohol to offset the bitter taste. Interestingly, common beverages such as soft drinks and gin and tonic were popularized as a result of their use as vehicles to deliver the bitter-tasting quinine to the population (e.g., British living in India).

One of the major by-products of the mass production, distribution, and prophylactic use of quinine in the 1870s and 1880s was an increased interest in Africa. Armed with a near unlimited supply of protective quinine, Euro-pean leaders realized that they could now penetrate the interior of Africa without fear of being wiped out by malaria. They financed a number of expe-ditions in order to map out the land and gain insight into resources and potential roadblocks. The success of explorers like Dr. David Livingstone and Sir Henry Stanley in reaching deep into the heart of Africa further rein-forced the idea that quinine had turned the "White Man's Grave" into a lucra-tive land of opportunity and riches.

This newfound freedom from malaria coincided with several other major political and economic changes to produce one of the largest and devastating land grabs in the history of the world, a mass colonization of Africa that involved eight different European nations taking over roughly 90 percent of the continent in just over 30 years (1881–1914). One major factor that con-tributed to this land grab was the recent outlawing of the slave trade in nearly all of Europe. The slave trade was a very profitable industry for several centu-ries, and its loss left a severe economic void that created a desperate need for new markets and sources of raw materials. Second, several new European powers burst onto the scene around this time. For instance, Germany was finally unified under Prussian control in 1871.[29] Under the initial rule of Otto von Bismarck, Germany preferred to use its power to simply maintain its status quo on the European continent. However, the dismissal of von Bis-marck by Kaiser Wilhelm II in 1890 ushered in a more aggressive foreign policy (called Weltpolitik) that was characterized by an increased focus on acquiring foreign territories. Similarly, after over 50 years of civil wars, the independent states of Italy finally unified into a single kingdom in 1871 (with Rome as its capital).[30] The creation of these two new countries further inten-sified a growing power struggle that existed between European powers like England, France, Spain, Russia, Belgium, and Portugal. When it was clear that malaria had been "conquered" and Africa was up for grabs, everyone wanted to rush in and lay claim to their "piece of the pie." A third major factor that contributed to the rapid colonization of African was the Industrial Revolution. The creation of stronger steel machinery, more reliable ships, and powerful new weapons allowed Europeans to mobilize large numbers of people and overpower native African clans. It also created a huge demand for raw materials to supply the explosion in new products that were being developed all over Europe.

When it became clear that several European powers had interest in moving into Africa permanently, there was a real worry that a world war would erupt between the countries vying for position there. These fears led Portugal and Germany to convene a meeting of 14 countries in Berlin in 1884–1885 to discuss how to fairly subdivide Africa.[31] This conference, known as the Berlin Conference, formerly ushered in the "Scramble for Africa" by laying down ground rules for occupation. It not only established what was meant by "occupation" (e.g., a country could not claim land that they had not step foot in), it also created policies to allow for effective trade between colonies and drew up borders for each country's territory. The conference's delegates also agreed to ban all forms of slavery on the continent. This is ironic considering that the 30 years that followed produced some of the worst examples of human exploitation in history. Following the conclusion of the conference, European colonial powers quickly moved en masse into Africa to claim what was now theirs.

The results of the European invasion and subsequent colonization were absolutely catastrophic for the African continent. Millions of Africans were killed as armies moved in and crushed any type of native resistance. Massive numbers of survivors were forced into deplorable working conditions as they stripped mines, cleared land for plantations, and harvested products like rubber and ivory. Those that were not murdered were often mutilated for not meeting harvesting quotas. In all, scholars believe that about 10–20 million Africans were killed in the Belgian-controlled Congo Free State and another 20–30 million throughout the rest of Africa. The atrocities committed during this time easily rival those perpetrated by the Nazis during World War II or any other mass genocide of the 20th century.

When the colonial period finally ended around 1970, the newly independent African countries faced many more years of violence and civil unrest due to the rather arbitrary country borders that were initially established during the Berlin Conference. Countries were mostly created along longitudinal and latitudinal lines rather than by grouping people according to their common religious affiliations or ethnicities. As a result, people of vastly different backgrounds were forced to coexist in these artificially created countries. Many populations did not handle these differences well, which led to a number of long-lasting and bloody civil wars that left millions dead, maimed, orphaned, and homeless. The stripping of natural resources from the land was equally devastating to the long-term stability of Africa. Billions of dollars' worth of gold, diamonds, oil, and other raw materials were systematically removed from Africa's land and shipped to Europe. Upon gaining their independence, these countries had little left to export, which led to widespread poverty and economic paralysis.

In all, one can make an argument that the development of quinine initiated a destructive chain reaction for Africa that it has yet to recover from. Once malaria was no longer a threat to susceptible European populations, Africa was brutalized and stripped of most of its wealth. Not surprisingly, Africa is currently the most impoverished continent on the planet, leading the world in infant death, lowest life expectancy, and worst quality of life. In a very sad case of irony, Africa still also leads the world in deaths from malaria. In fact, some economists have suggested that the widespread presence of malaria is not only a symptom of African poverty but also a measurable cause of it. It causes a significant loss of income as people are too sick to work, it stunts the education of infected children, and it requires a huge amount of national resources for prevention and treatment. In some parts of Africa, malaria accounts for as much as 50 percent of all hospital admissions and uses up 40 percent of public health expenditures.[32] Some have estimated that malaria by itself results in a 1.3 percent reduction in the gross domestic product (GDP) of some African countries, which compounds every year and prevents those countries from ever experiencing economic growth.

The discovery and production of quinine was also significant for several other reasons unrelated to malaria or Africa. Most importantly, quinine was the first drug to be used in the treatment of a specific infectious disease. It demonstrated that lifesaving drugs could be found in the environment and that they could be isolated and mass produced. It also sparked the chemical industry (e.g., German company Bayer) to begin trying to synthesize chemicals that could kill other infectious agents like bacteria.[33] This research directly led to the discovery of early forms of antibiotics (e.g., Salvarsan and sulfonamides) and to the development of a variety of chemical dyes that were instrumental in the early fields of histology and microbiology. Such discoveries prompted others to search for new drugs, which then prompted others. Quinine was thus the first link in the chain of a long line of chemical discoveries that eventually resulted in the mass production of safe and effective antibiotics and antiviral drugs.

Mosquitoes and the Panama Canal

One of the greatest public works projects in history was the building of a 48-mile-long canal through the middle of the Isthmus of Panama, thereby connecting the Atlantic and Pacific Oceans and saving ships roughly 8,000 miles of travel around the southern tip of South America. Piggybacking off the successful construction of the Suez Canal, which links the Red Sea with the Mediterranean Sea, the French government received permission from Colombia (which controlled Panama at the time) to build a similar waterway in the Americas. Construction of the Panama Canal began on January 1881 with a workforce of several thousand men and a budget of about $120 million.[34] Despite having some of the best minds in France working on the project and having expectations that it would be easier, cheaper, and faster than the building of the Suez Canal, it was doomed from the start. The rocky, mountainous land of Panama made digging very difficult, and the large amount of rain produced deadly mudslides and floods.[35] Furthermore, infectious diseases like dysentery, yellow fever, and malaria were rampant, leading to countless sick and dead workers. One Frenchman living in Panama at the time summed up the general opinion of the project when he said, "If you try to build this canal there will not be trees enough on the isthmus to make crosses for the graves of your laborers."[36] Unfortunately, his prognostication turned out to be accurate as over 20,000 workers lost their lives due to mudslides, accidents, violence, and (most of all) malaria and yellow fever. Thousands more remained chronically sick or injured, which drastically slowed progress of the project. After eight years of frustration and expenses exceeding $250 million, the French finally backed out of the project after completing only about 40 percent of the digging. No progress would be made on the canal for another 15 years.[37]

Following the inauguration of Theodore ("Teddy") Roosevelt in 1901, the United States began expressing interest in finishing what France had started in Panama.[38] In early 1903, the United States proposed a treaty with Colombia to purchase the land and rights to the Panama Canal for $40 million; however, the Colombian Senate refused to accept the terms. The United States responded by giving funds and military support to armed rebels in Panama and encouraging them to seek their independence from Colombia. They were successful in doing so by late 1903 and proceeded to quickly sell control of the canal to the United States for the bargain price of $10 million. By the middle of 1904, the United States had moved into the Panama Canal Zone and began hiring a massive workforce, improving infrastructure, and ultimately resuming construction. However, early leaders of the project worried that the some of the same obstacles that doomed the French attempt would lead to a similar fate for the U.S. project. Of primary importance was addressing the ongoing problem of infectious disease that absolutely decimated the French workforce. For instance, by 1906, over 85 percent of all workers had been hospitalized at some point due to malaria, yellow fever, or dysentery. Of all these diseases, yellow fever was by far the most feared due to its high death rate and the severity of symptoms; however, malaria was much more pervasive and a much bigger issue for the administration.

In an effort to curb the growing threat to the entire project, top officials established an independent sanitation department to deal specifically with health matters of the workers. The leader of this new department, Dr. William Gorgas, was handpicked by Teddy Roosevelt due to his success controlling infectious disease in tropical Cuba.[39] President Roosevelt's personal physician expressed the importance of this decision when he said, "You are facing one of the greatest decisions of your career . . . If you fall back on the old methods you will fail, just as the French failed. If you back Gorgas you will get your canal."[40] Although he was initially limited due to bureaucratic red tape, Dr. Gorgas finally got to work dealing with the malaria problem in February 1905. What followed was one of the greatest public health success stories in history.

A few very important scientific discoveries in the late 19th century were critical to the success of Gorgas's plan for disease control in the Panama Canal region.[41] The first was the discovery that the mosquito was a carrier for yellow fever, a hypothesis first proposed by Carlos Finlay in 1882 and later confirmed in 1900 by a group of scientists led by U.S. Army Major Walter Reed, M.D. This monumental finding was complemented by equally important discoveries with malaria. In 1880, Charles Laveran meticulously examined blood samples of patients who were suffering from malaria and consistently detected the existence of a protozoal parasite that he named *Oscillaria malariae*. It was the first time that a protozoan had been conclusively shown to cause a human disease. Then, in 1897, Dr. Ronald Ross observed the presence of the malaria parasite in the gut of an *Anopheles* mosquito that had fed on the blood of a malaria patient four days previously. He conducted very elegant studies to confirm that mosquitoes were the main vector for malaria and subsequently described the life cycle of the malaria parasite. Ross, an accomplished poet and author, expressed the relief he felt following his discovery when he wrote, "With tears and toiling breath, I find thy cunning seeds, O million-murdering Death."[42]

It is hard not to overstate the enormous impact that these combined discoveries had on the field of tropical medicine. One scientist compared them to Jenner's development of a smallpox vaccine in terms of their importance to the health of all mankind. Malaria and yellow fever were no longer mysteries that were believed to be caused by foul-smelling air emanating from swamps. Their true causes had finally been identified and characterized, which enabled people like Gorgas to finally attack them in an intelligent and scientific way. The possibility of eradicating malaria and yellow fever from tropical environments by systematically controlling the mosquito population now became a reality.

In the years preceding his work in Panama, William Gorgas was sent to Cuba as the chief sanitation officer and charged with controlling the widespread yellow fever and malaria that had plagued the island since the 1700s.

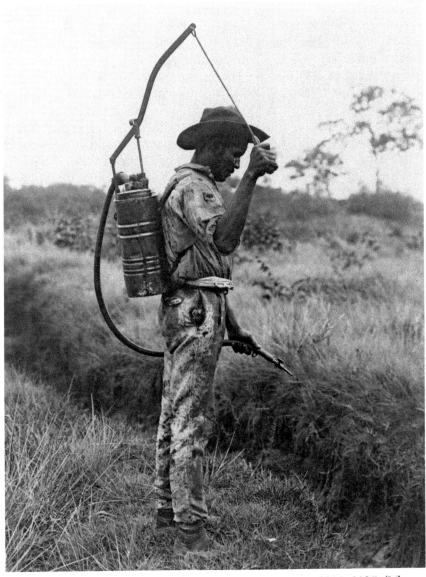

Spraying oil on breeding places of mosquitoes, Panama, ca. 1890–1925. (Library of Congress)

Knowing about the importance of mosquitoes in the transmission of both yellow fever and malaria, Gorgas targeted his efforts on killing the mosquito vectors, preventing their reproduction, and isolating infected people with protective netting. He ordered the drainage of unnecessary standing water and had oil sprayed on the surface of other water sources in order to kill developing mosquito larva. He even went so far as to fine local residents for not covering barrels of water outside of their homes. In the end, his war against mosquitoes was highly effective, allowing his workers to successfully eradicate yellow fever from Cuba and drastically reduce in the incidence of malaria in the process. This was watershed moment in the history of epidemiology because it marked the first time that an infectious agent had been successfully eliminated from any environment by targeting an insect vector. It helped set the stage for the discovery of other disease-carrying insects, and it ushered in a new phase of disease control that focused more on vectors rather than actual causative agents. For instance, the flea was found to be the vector of bubonic plague in 1898, which allowed public health officials to more efficiently slow plague epidemics by targeting rats and the fleas they carry.

After gaining many accolades from his successes in Cuba, Dr. Gorgas was offered and accepted a similar position in the Panama Canal Zone in 1904.[43] Upon arriving there, Gorgas realized that malaria was a much more widespread and frequent problem than yellow fever, which had cyclical outbreaks rather than a continued presence. In some cities along the Canal Zone, as much as one-sixth of the population suffered from malaria each and every week. Gorgas expressed his concern with malaria by saying, "If we can control malaria, I feel very little anxiety about other diseases."[44] Armed with a $1 million budget, a workforce of over 4,000 men, and the full support of the president, Gorgas instituted his multipronged attack against mosquitoes and the conditions that promote their reproduction. For an entire year, his mosquito brigades systemically drained and oiled all standing water, cut high grass and brush, fumigated homes repeated with a natural insecticide made from sulfur and chrysanthemum flowers, handed out prophylactic quinine, screened homes and government buildings, sprayed a larvicide composed of carbolic acid, and killed any adult mosquitoes seen in tents of workers. Although some natives and canal officials were often outraged at the aggressiveness of his tactics, Gorgas was very effective in doing his job.

By 1906, yellow fever had been completely eradicated from the Panama Canal Zone and malaria infections had begun to decline. Although malaria would never fully be eliminated from the area, hospitalizations due to malaria would drop tenfold due to Gorgas's sanitation policies. Workers were healthier than they had ever been before, which allowed them to make great progress on the excavation. On January 7, 1914, the Panama Canal officially opened after a total of 18 years of construction. It remains one of the most important areas of ship traffic in the world, permitting the passage of over 300 million tons of cargo each year. Many question if the canal would have ever been completed if not for Dr. Gorgas and his meticulous control of the mosquito population in the middle of the tropics. He helped defeat two of the deadliest diseases known to man at a time and place that was critical for the future economic growth of two continents. He additionally showed that malaria no longer had to impede human progress. With proper sanitation and quinine, we could drastically reduce the power it holds over us.

Paralysis of 20th-Century Armies

As mentioned previously in this chapter, malaria had a drastic impact in shaping the empires of the ancient world by incapacitating armies, taking the lives of several key world leaders, and making certain regions of Europe and Asia (e.g., Rome, Greece, India) nearly unlivable for foreign aggressors. More modern wars like the American Revolutionary and Civil Wars and Napoleonic wars fared no better and were similarly influenced by malaria outbreaks. A prominent colonel in the British army observed firsthand the effects of malaria in armed conflict in the 19th century and wrote, "The history of malaria in war might almost be taken to be the history of war itself, certainly the history of war in the Christian era."[45] Malaria was something that every military leader feared and had to plan for. For instance, one of the first expenditures made by the newly formed U.S. Continental Congress was to purchase a massive amount of quinine for Washington's army so that they would be healthy enough to fight the British. Such foresight proved to be key in securing victories for the Americans in battles fought in the malarious American South.[46] Malaria may not have killed as many soldiers as had diseases like typhus, typhoid fever, or plague, but it nonetheless affected the outcomes of wars.

One would logically infer that the purification and mass production of protective quinine in the late 19th century would have changed this trend and lessened the impact that malaria had on all subsequent wars of the 20th century. Indeed, infection numbers were down all throughout Europe, and it appeared as if malaria may be defeated for good as the 20th century began. Unfortunately, epidemic diseases like malaria often do not behave in ways that are logical and expected. This fact was sadly confirmed at the commencement of the first great war of the 20th century, World War I.

One of the most malarious and contested regions of Europe at the start of the war was the Balkans.[47] As German forces moved in and began rapidly advancing throughout the region, British and French armies joined forces in support of their Serb allies and established a base in Salonika, Greece, in October of 1915. Unfortunately, a large number of malaria-infected Greek refugees had migrated there about the same time and provided a perfect source of *Plasmodium* for the *Anopheles* mosquitoes living there. What followed was a military campaign marred by three years of unending malaria infections. For instance, an average British contingent of about 160,000 soldiers reported over 162,000 hospital admissions for malaria alone, and about 80 percent of the French forces were also infected. That means that many soldiers developed malaria more than once, and many thousands died as a result. There were several examples of attacks that were canceled because of a lack of healthy soldiers on both sides. Famed British doctor Ronald Ross was even brought into the Balkans in an attempt to control the malaria epidemic there; however, his tried and true methods of using quinine and bed netting failed to stop or even slow the disease. Malaria posed similar problems on several other fronts during World War I, including battles in Africa, Italy, and the Middle East. Unfortunately, many of those who became infected during this time would end up carrying malaria back their home countries at the conclusion of the war. This set the stage for a major reemergence of malaria throughout Europe and Asia in the years leading up to the World War II.

World War II was so significantly impacted by the ongoing presence of malaria in battle zones like the Pacific islands and Africa that it triggered lasting changes to strategies used for preventing and treating the disease. Following the bombing of Pearl Harbor in December 1941, large numbers of Allied troops were sent to the island nations of the Pacific (e.g., Philippines and modern-day Indonesia) in an attempt to free them from Japanese control. Despite attempts to plan for the widespread malaria that soldiers would encounter, it quickly became apparent that officials drastically underestimated the malaria problem and were grossly underprepared to combat it. Some have estimated that the Allies brought less than half of the amount of quinine that they actually needed to keep their soldiers healthy. The Allied commander of the Pacific, General Douglas MacArthur, expressed his frustration with the situation when he famously stated, "This will be a long war if for every division I have facing the enemy I must count on a second division in hospital with malaria and a third division convalescing from this debilitating disease!"[48] What made the situation so dire was that by 1942, Japan had control over 90 percent of the world's supply of cinchona trees (on the islands of the Philippines and Java), and Germany controlled the factories in the Netherlands that were responsible for purifying quinine from the bark.[49] This created a disastrous shortage of quinine that left the entire Pacific force in danger of being wiped out.

The response of the U.S. military to this growing threat was multifaceted. First, the Allies sent teams to Central and South America, purchased large amounts of their cinchona bark, and reached agreements for the creation of new cinchona plantations (especially in Costa Rica).[50] While these efforts yielded over 12 million pounds of bark for the Allies, the time and cost in procuring purified quinine from these sources did little to make up for the major quinine shortage in the Pacific. As a result, the military was forced to rely on alternative methods of control that included draining local water supplies, spraying of larvicides, providing bed netting to soldiers, and promoting education.[51] Soldiers were instructed about the mosquito life cycle and how/when they breed and transmit malaria. They were ordered to bathe and swim at specific times of the day and to avoid any unnecessary standing-water sources. One particularly artistic army captain named Theodor Geisel created a series of educational cartoon pamphlets about malaria that were widely distributed throughout the Pacific. He would later write 46 widely popular children's books under the pseudonym Dr. Seuss.

In 1942, the U.S. War Department called for the creation of a new public health program that would be responsible for controlling malaria around military bases in the southern United States and Caribbean so that soldiers undergoing training would be free of malaria

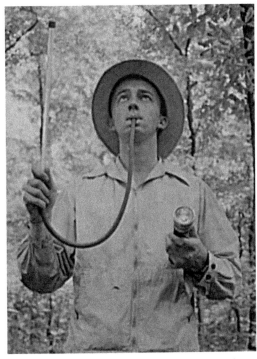

Collecting anopheles mosquitoes in a malaria control area in Alabama, June 1942. (Library of Congress)

and remain healthy enough to be deployed. The Malaria Control in War Areas (MCWA) program was established for this purpose and was so effective in reducing malaria infections that the War Department made it the goal to completely eradicate malaria from the United States after the end of the war.[52] The MCWA program ended in 1946 and was replaced by a more permanent public health institution that was named the Communicable Diseases Center (CDC), based in Atlanta, Georgia. The first mission of the CDC was to finish what the MCWA had started and eliminate malaria domestically. In 1951, the country was declared free from malaria, which prompted the CDC (now called the Centers for Disease Control and Prevention) to shift its focus to surveillance of other infectious diseases and health threats. Since that time, the CDC has grown into one of the premier public health agencies in the world and has personnel stationed throughout the United States and in more than 25 countries.

Despite the best efforts of military leaders to control the spread of malaria among troops in the Pacific and Africa, the shortage of quinine and an inability to control mosquito populations led to the death of 60,000 U.S. troops over the course of World War II. The death toll would have been even worse had it not been for the development of a new and very effective insecticide called DDT near the end of the war. Although it was first created in the 1870s, it was not until 1939 that a Swiss chemist named Paul Müller realized that it had potent activity against both mosquitoes and body lice (which carry deadly typhus). After some initial safety testing, the military ordered widespread spraying of DDT in forests of war zones and directly onto the skin its soldiers.[53] Rates of malaria and typhus infections dropped precipitously as a result. This success led to the continued usage of DDT to control insect populations long after the end of the war. In fact, DDT was the primary weapon used by the WHO when it embarked on a campaign to eradicate malaria from the entire planet in 1955. However, popular opinion of DDT would change drastically in the early 1960s when Rachel Carson published her scathing book *Silent Spring*. It detailed how DDT and other pesticides were destroying the environment, killing large numbers of birds, and posing great risk to human health. Further research by the government and environmental groups confirmed these fears, and DDT was eventually outlawed by the U.S. Environmental Protection Agency in 1972. In addition to the devastation done to the ecosystem, a recent study published in 2014 linked DDT exposure to an increased risk of late-onset Alzheimer's disease.[54] Those with the disease had four times the level of DDT by-products in their tissues than those without the disease. Thus, the desperate need to control malaria during World War II (and later Vietnam) ended up having permanent negative impacts on both the health of people and the environment.

Permanent Changes to Our Genome and Blood

Upon entering the human body and replicating briefly in the liver, *Plasmodium* parasites quickly spread into the blood and infect and kill massive numbers of RBCs. It is the destruction of these red blood cells that causes the majority of pathology associated with malaria and it is within RBCs that *Plasmodium* achieves its highest levels of replication. The quantity and health of one's RBCs is therefore a major determinant of how susceptible a person is to being infected by *Plasmodium* and developing malaria. People with normal amounts of functional RBCs tend to be easily infected by *Plasmodium* due to having healthy target cells for the parasites to replicate in. In contrast, there are some people in the population who harbor natural genetic mutations that change the shape, number, or biochemical composition of their RBCs. While these people can be initially infected by *Plasmodium* parasites, their altered RBCs serve as poor hosts for merozoite replication. As a result, they exhibit some level of resistance to malaria and very often survive large-scale epidemics. Interestingly, a great variety of "malaria resistance" mutations have been identified in people from many different geographical locations, which indicates that malaria has been a powerful force in shaping human evolution throughout the world. In other words, malaria has caused such devastating and widespread epidemics that it has literally shaped the very sequence of the human genome.

Most of the mutations that provide resistance to malaria are found in genes that code for the hemoglobin protein. Hemoglobin is a large, abundant protein that is made up of four different subunits, two alpha chains and two beta chains. It is utilized by our RBCs to carry oxygen to cells throughout our body, which enables them to efficiently extract energy from the nutrients we eat. When *Plasmodium* merozoites infect our RBCs, they break down large amounts of hemoglobin protein and then use its amino acids to make their own proteins. The loss of hemoglobin and subsequent reduction of oxygen levels in the infected cell lead to significant changes in cellular morphology and biochemistry, which trigger death shortly thereafter. Newly made *Plasmodium* merozoites are released from the dying cell and immediately go looking for new RBCs to infect.

The most common hemoglobin mutations that provide malarial resistance are ones that cause changes to the structure of the beta chain. One beta chain variant, called hemoglobin S, binds to oxygen so poorly that it induces changes to the shape of the RBC. Instead of having a normal concave disk shape that allows them to easily move through small blood vessels, these RBCs have a more rigid, sickle shape that causes poor circulation and clumping together. People who inherit the hemoglobin S mutation from both parents (thus harboring two mutant copies) have large numbers of these sickle-shaped RBCs and develop the disease sickle-cell anemia. Sickle-cell anemia is painful and debilitating and very often leads to death, especially for those living in developing countries who lack access to basic medical care. In contrast, people who carry one normal version of the beta chain and only one mutant S version suffer only minor circulatory problems and gain resistance to malaria. In fact, carriers of this sickle trait are 90 percent more resistant to infection with the deadliest form of malaria (caused by *P. falciparum*) than those possessing two normal copies of the beta chain.[55] In areas where *P. falciparum* is endemic, such as most of Africa, the Middle East, and India, as much as 30 percent of the population carries the protective sickle trait. Similarly, certain populations in West Africa harbor another beta chain mutant, called hemoglobin C, that provides similar levels of protection against malaria.[56] This mutation is a bit different from the sickle-cell variant in that a person needs to inherit two copies of hemoglobin C to gain any kind of protection against malaria. A third variant of the beta chain, hemoglobin E, is seen in those living in Southeast Asia. People who express hemoglobin E have enhanced resistance against *P. vivax*, which makes sense considering it has been endemic in that region for thousands of years. In all, it is clear that having an abnormal hemoglobin beta chain can provide an individual with an enormous protective advantage despite causing some circulatory problems for the host.

A second set of hemoglobin mutations that provide malarial resistance do so by causing a decrease in the production of one of the two subunits rather than changing their shape.[57] For instance, when the amount of alpha chain made in a RBC is significantly reduced due to one of these mutations, the hemoglobin protein attempts to assemble itself using only beta chain. Unfortunately, hemoglobin made up of only beta chain is very unstable and is degraded before it can do its job of moving oxygen around. The resulting disease is a severe form of anemia called alpha thalassemia. People can also have mutations that cause a drop in the production of beta chain and corresponding increase in alpha chain levels. As expected, the amount of stable hemoglobin produced is very low, and the circulating RBCs are nearly useless as a result. This disease, which is called beta thalassemia, is extremely dangerous and often results in death if not treated with a bone marrow transplant. In both types of thalassemia, the RBC is so malformed that any further stress placed on it (e.g., infection with *Plasmodium*) triggers the immune system to rapidly destroy it. As a result, parasites don't have enough time to complete their life cycle, and the infection is quickly halted. Similar to the case with the sickle-cell trait, people who inherit a thalassemia mutation from only one parent have the benefits of malaria resistance while only developing minor anemia. Those that inherit thalassemia mutations from both parents often die of the anemia, which makes malaria resistance somewhat of a moot benefit. Thalassemia diseases can be found among populations in nearly every geographical region where malaria has existed for a long period of time. This includes Africa, Middle East, India, Southeast Asia, and most of the Mediterranean. In fact, the thalassemia mutations are some of the most common in our species, which again illustrates how important malaria has been to the evolution of humankind.

Besides changes to hemoglobin, alterations to the outer surface of RBCs can also provide some level of malaria resistance.[58] Most cell types in our body (including RBCs) have thousands of different proteins that are embedded in the outer covering of the cell, called the plasma membrane. These plasma membrane proteins provide a number of functions for our cells, including acting as enzymes, transport channels, adhesion proteins, and receptors. Three such proteins that are relevant to a discussion of malaria are two receptors called Duffy antigen and Gerbich antigen and a transport channel called band 3. All three proteins are found on the surface of RBCs and serve important functions. The Duffy antigen normally helps RBCs communicate with other blood cells, and the band 3 and Gerbich antigen proteins function to transport nutrients and maintain the structural rigidity of RBCs, respectively. Although they perform vastly different functions and have completely different structures, all three can be utilized by *Plasmodium* merozoites during the attachment phase of infection. Once merozoites enter into the bloodstream, they need to specifically find, attach to, and invade RBCs in order to complete the rest of their life cycle. A few of the major ways in which they latch onto the RBC membrane is by binding to the Duffy antigen, Gerbich antigen, or band 3 proteins that are found there. Without this attachment, the parasites fail to enter the RBC and instead float around in the blood until being destroyed by immune cells. Interestingly, scientists have found that some populations have natural mutations in one or more of these genes, which confers those who harbor them with resistance to certain forms of malaria. For instance, a large percentage of people of African descent (as much as 95% in some locations) have mutations in their Duffy antigen genes and are almost completely resistant to *P. vivax* infections. Similarly, people of Melanesian descent (e.g., Papua New Guinea) often carry mutations in the band 3 or Gerbich antigen genes or both, which provides them some resistance to *P. falciparum* infections and severe cases of cerebral malaria.

A third category of RBC genes that are commonly mutated in people who are resistant to malaria are those that code for enzyme proteins. Thousands of chemical reactions take place in our cells, and enzymes are required for each one of them. Without them, our cells would not be able to digest nutrients, grow, divide, protect themselves from toxins, or communicate. They are so important that the loss of a single enzyme can often have lethal effects. For instance, Tay-Sachs disease, phenylketonuria, Gaucher's disease, adrenoleukodystrophy, and alpha-1-antitrypsin deficiency are all caused by the loss of a single enzyme.

Two enzyme deficiencies are particularly dangerous to the life and health of RBCs.[59] People who lack either the glucose-6-phosphate dehydrogenase (G6PD) or pyruvate kinase (PK) enzyme often develop severe hemolytic anemia when they encounter any type of cellular stress. In other words, the loss of these enzymes makes their RBCs more susceptible to destruction if they are exposed to stresses such as low oxygen levels, various chemicals, or infection. For instance, if a person who has inherited either of these deficiencies becomes infected with *Plasmodium* parasites, their infected RBCs are stressed to the point that they undergo changes to their shape and are rapidly killed off by the host spleen. As a result of this rapid killing, merozoites do not have enough time to replicate, and the person never develops malaria. People who inherit one good copy of either enzyme are generally healthy and still exhibit some level of resistance to even the most severe form of malaria (caused by *P. falciparum*). Interestingly, these enzyme deficiencies are two of the most common on Earth, affecting over 400 million people of Mediterranean, Southeast Asian, African, and Indian descent.

Malaria has selected for more permanent mutations in the human genome than any other pathogen in history. While malaria did not cause any of these mutations, it helped increase their presence in the population by killing genetically "normal" people at a higher rate than those with defects in their RBCs. The very structure and function of our RBCs have changed forever in a large percentage of the human population due to the malaria parasite. The story of malaria resistance in humans is a remarkable example of how our species was able to defend itself against devastating epidemics prior to the advent of antibiotics, vaccines, and modern medicine. It shows the amazing plasticity of our genome and demonstrates that humans, like every other living thing on Earth, is capable of evolving in the midst of threats to our survival as a species.

CHAPTER FIVE

Tuberculosis

If the importance of a disease for mankind is measured by the number of fatalities it causes, then tuberculosis must be considered much more important than those most feared infectious diseases, plague, cholera and the like. One in seven of all human beings dies from tuberculosis. If one only considers the productive middle-age groups, tuberculosis carries away one-third, and often more.

— Dr. Robert Koch, 1882, from the speech in which he
had announced the discovery of the causative agent
of tuberculosis (consumption)[1]

Tuberculosis (TB) is arguably the oldest, most feared, and deadliest disease in the history of mankind. It is believed to have made the jump from bovids (e.g., cattle, bison) to humans at least 17,000 years ago and has remained one of the top killers of our species almost continuously ever since.[2] It has been found in Neolithic remains that date back to 9,000 years ago, and it has been found in the bodies of ancient Egyptian mummies.[3] It was mentioned in at least two places in the Old Testament and in the sacred Hindu text Atharvaveda. Although other diseases like plague, smallpox, and influenza have garnered more "fame" in the media due to their production of very destructive cyclical epidemics, TB has been a continuous and ruthless killer that has taken the lives of as many as 2 billion people throughout our history. The only other disease that even comes close to tuberculosis in terms of its seemingly never-ending persistence and ferocity is smallpox, though some have estimated the TB has killed twice as many.

Amazingly, nearly one-third of Earth's population (over 2 billion people) is believed to be currently infected with the causative agent of TB, a small bacterium called Mycobacterium tuberculosis. It continues to kill about 1–2 million people every year and currently ranks as the leading cause of death from infectious disease in the world. Most of the 2 billion people who are infected exhibit few signs of disease due to a rapid and protective immune response that prevents the bacteria from multiplying uncontrollably. This is often referred to as latent TB. However, people who are malnourished or have other diseases (e.g., HIV) that weaken their immune systems will often develop debilitating pneumonia and/or chronic wasting that eventually kills them. The gradual loss of weight and strength is so severe that it appears that the disease literally consumes the person from the inside out. For this reason, active forms of TB were historically referred to as consumption, the White Death, or the White Plague (due to the pale color of skin that accompanies wasting). It is considered to be one of the greatest health threats in the world today, due in large part to the recent appearance of drug-resistant TB strains and prevalence of people co-infected with HIV and TB.

Tuberculosis is acquired through the inhalation of another's infected respiratory secretions. People with active TB release millions of bacteria inside of tiny aerosol droplets (called droplet nuclei) every time they cough, sneeze, spit, or even speak. Amazingly, some of the smaller droplets can remain suspended in the air for several hours after an infected person has left a room or airplane (and remain alive for much longer). That means that a TB patient can cough in a room in the morning and an unsuspecting person can enter that same room in the afternoon and inhale the bacteria. This ability to "hang around" in an enclosed room is especially scary considering the fact that the infectious dose of the TB bacteria is relatively small. Scientists have estimated that as few as 10 actual bacteria cells are needed to initiate an infection in a susceptible person. Thankfully, most people have a strong enough immune system that a quick exposure to a few bacteria usually does little actual harm. However, when individuals are repeatedly exposed to someone with active TB and they have a weakened immune system or lung damage, their risk for contracting the disease goes up immensely. Therefore, TB is very commonly transmitted among family members and in enclosed places like prisons, homeless shelters, and even hospitals.

Upon entering the lung of a person, most bacteria are quickly eaten by immune cells called alveolar macrophages and drawn into membrane-enclosed structures called endosomes or phagosomes. The phagosome acts like a "jail cell" that generally functions to keep bacteria confined and away from the nutrient-rich parts of the cell. The macrophage then fuses other membrane-enclosed structures called lysosomes to the phagosome. Lysosomes contain highly toxic substances such as strong acid, hydrogen peroxide, free radicals, and several different digestive enzymes (e.g., proteases). The result of this fusion event is the direct delivery of deadly toxic products onto the pathogen, which in most cases leads to its quick destruction. The macrophage then usually ships the now-dead pathogen back to its cell surface and releases the parts into the outside fluid.

When *Mycobacterium tuberculosis* bacteria enter the human lung, they are rapidly eaten by alveolar macrophages and exposed to lysosomal toxins. However, unlike most other species, the TB bacteria have an outer surface that is surrounded by a thick layer of a wax-like substance called mycolic acid that prevents most chemicals from passing through. As a result, the bacterial cell surface is protected by this waxy "force field," and the bacteria survive the onslaught. Not only do they survive, the TB bacteria will actually begin to replicate within the phagosome. The infected macrophage senses that it is unable to destroy the bacteria inside of it and sends out chemical distress signals that help attract more macrophages and other immune cells (e.g., T and B cells) to the area. The reinforcements surround the infected macrophage in an attempt to contain the infection. Most of the time this process works and the TB bacteria stay stuck in this mass of immune cells, unable to cause any significant damage to the lung. The mass is usually visible on an X-ray and is referred as a tubercle or granuloma.

About 90 percent of the time, isolated tubercles remain for the remainder of the person's life and cause no visible signs of disease. This is what is called latent TB. However, for people who are immunosuppressed because of other diseases (e.g., HIV), medication, or malnutrition, the TB bacteria break through this immune barricade and begin replicating uncontrollably. This can occur during the initial infection or many years later when a person who has harbored latent TB has experienced a period of immunosuppression. In either case, the inflammation that results from active bacterial replication leads to a persistent pneumonia and cough, night sweats, chest pain, and fatigue. In some cases, the replicating bacteria leave the lung and spill into the lymphatics or blood. They can then disseminate to distant sites such as the kidneys, spleen, and pancreas and establish infections all over the body. This widespread form of TB, often referred to as miliary TB, is almost universally fatal if left untreated and even kills about 20 percent of those who have sought medical attention. Miliary TB causes widespread and persistent inflammation and tissue damage. The patient becomes incapacitated and gradually begins to waste away until dying of pneumonia or organ failure.

Tuberculosis is a slow progressing disease that sometimes takes several years to kill its victims. While this is in large part due to the host's protective immune response described earlier, it is also a result of extremely slow growth kinetics of the TB bacterium itself. Bacteria like Staph and *E. coli* can copy themselves every 18–20 minutes if given proper nutrients and space whereas *M. tuberculosis* takes from 16 to 20 hours to divide just once. While this slowness may seem like a drawback for the pathogen, it is actually beneficial because it gives it time to replicate to high numbers and spread to new hosts before killing its source of nutrients. From the perspective of the infected victim, the slowness of the disease can be cruel, prolonging a life characterized by chronic sickness and despair. Over a period of several years it slowly consumes the physical, emotional, and mental well-being of those infected before finally ending their misery. They are cognizant of their death sentence yet are unable to prevent it.

The Industrial Revolution and the Great White Plague

Despite infecting and killing over a billion people over the course of several thousand years, there is surprisingly little mention of TB in the historical record prior to the 18th century. Unlike almost every other disease in this book, TB was never implicated as being an important factor in any significant historical event or was it ever suggested to have influenced society in any meaningful way. One of the likely reasons for this is that TB has been endemic in the human population for so long that most simply saw it as a normal part of everyday life. It had always been around, slowly and consistently killing people of all different classes and ethnicities for as long as people could remember. There was nothing unusual about people dying of TB, and few historians thought it was necessary to write about it in any great detail. As a result, TB became somewhat of a forgotten plague that flew under the radar for most of history.

The Industrial Revolution that swept across Western Europe and the United States in the 18th century marked an important turning point for TB. Before this time, most of the population lived and worked in rural areas that were relatively isolated from one another. Such natural separation helped limit the spread of TB due to the fact that infection typically requires repeated and prolonged exposure to someone who is already sick. The average person living in the country simply did not travel, work, or cohabitate enough with strangers to ever pick up the disease from them. TB was thus a crowd disease that rarely ever had a crowd. However, this began to change in the 1750s as innovations to iron making, power generation, and mechanization made it much more profitable to make goods in large urban factories than small artisan workshops. As work began to become scarce in rural areas, massive numbers of laborers and their families were forced to uproot their lives and move to one of the many cities that were cropping up near major manufacturing centers. Unfortunately, promises of fair wages were grossly overstated as were prospects for affordable housing in the increasingly overcrowded and filthy slums. People that were previously earning a good salary and living in their own home in the country now had no choice but to share small, single-room apartments with other families in the same situation. In some cases, as many as 20–30 people would sleep together in a single tiny, cramped room. One British pastor, describing his immensely overcrowded parish in 1844, wrote, "It contains 1,400 houses, inhabited by 2,795 families, or about 12,000 persons. The space upon which this large population dwells is less than 400 yards (1,200 feet) square."[4] In other words, it was about 12,000 people living in a space that is equivalent to less than four football fields.

While overcrowding is still dangerous in today's world, it was especially toxic at a time before the advent of modern sanitary practices. Little was done to safely contain or discard the large amounts of human waste and household trash that were generated on a daily basis in these cities. As a result, city streets often turned into horrific cesspools that were filled with rotting garbage, rodents, and foul-smelling excrement. In addition to creating unimaginably awful living conditions, the widespread pollution provided a perfect breeding ground for waterborne diseases like cholera and typhoid. Chronic gastrointestinal illness was complemented by a variety of respiratory diseases that spread well in the cramped and poorly ventilated apartment buildings and factories. TB, in particular, was adept at moving within these buildings due to the fact that the mycobacterial cells are able to remain suspended in the air for long periods of time without dying. As a result, a single person with a persistent cough could spread TB to everyone who happened to be sleeping or working near them on a daily basis. It is a situation that unfortunately became commonplace in industrial cities throughout the 18th and 19th centuries.

Conservative figures estimate that deaths from TB increased two- to threefold during the Industrial Revolution, making it the number-one killer in cities and responsible for about one-quarter of all deaths in Western Europe.[5] The disease was especially deadly to people who were chronically malnourished or sick with other diseases since both tend to weaken a person's immune system and make them more susceptible to infection with TB. In fact, for the first time in its long history, TB had started to be seen as a disease of the poor. Wealthier individuals could afford to live in larger, less crowded homes outside of the city and were thus less likely to come into contact with those suffering from TB. The poor had few options: either share crowded apartments with other families or sleep in even more crowded and prison-like "poor houses" run by the government.[6] Robert Koch once commented about the dire situation facing the poor living in cities when he said, "It is the overcrowded dwellings of the poor that we have to regard as the real breeding places of consumption; it is out of them that the disease always crops up; and it is to the abolition of these conditions that we must first and foremost direct our attention if we wish to attach the evil at its root and wage war against it with effective weapons."[7] Unfortunately, few city governments ever headed Koch's advice to improve the standard of living for the poor who were stuck in these slums. The end result was that TB was transformed from a disease that usually affected small pockets of people in rural towns to one that surpassed plague, smallpox, and cholera as the most serious infectious disease on Earth.

A Romantic Way to Die

A particularly interesting by-product of TB's resurgence during the 18th and 19th centuries was a major shift in how society viewed those suffering from the disease. Prior to the Industrial Revolution, TB was largely seen as some type of supernatural punishment. For instance, in France, some believed that people contracted TB by being attacked by evil fairies at night or being bitten by deceased family members who had returned from the dead as vampires.[8] The most common traits attributed to vampires in popular culture are that of a pale, gaunt figure with reddish eyes and a thirst for blood. People suffering from TB commonly lose a large amount of weight, acquire a whitish pale complexion, have reddish eyes that are sensitive to light, and often cough up a large amount blood. The loss of blood was thought to give them a thirst for new blood, thus triggering them to bite others. Alternatively, some thought TB was caused by personal moral failings such as excessive drinking or prostitution.[9] These almost puritanical beliefs held that an unhealthy soul made a person more susceptible to physical maladies such as TB. Rather than killing the person outright as punishment, TB gave the sinner a chance to purify themselves, repent of their sins, and draw closer to God. As a result, people who contracted TB were often despised, treated with scorn, and subjected to isolation.

The rise of the Romantic Movement in the late 18th century triggered a drastic change in how society viewed TB as a disease and those who contracted it. One of the primary reasons for this shift had to do with the fact that an inordinate number of famous and brilliant poets, artists, composers, and authors succumbed to TB during this time (probably due to the fact that most were poor and lived in cities).[10] A short list of those who died from TB includes John Keats, Elizabeth Barrett Browning, Frederic Chopin (likely), Emily Bronte, Walt Whitman, and Robert Louis Stevenson. As a result, TB started being regarded as a disease that targets only the most gifted and truly artistic individuals. Getting TB was a sign that one was exceptional and chosen. In his book *The Last Crusade: The War on Consumption, 1862–1954*, Mark Caldwell eloquently writes that tuberculosis "was a badge of refinement . . . it led your friends not to mourn your early death so much as to venerate you as one marked out for a fate of special distinction."[11] Some like Lord Byron and the Brazilian poet and playwright Casimiro de Abreu even went as far as almost craving a TB death so that others would view them as being more interesting and artistic.

TB was also thought to put a person more in touch with their emotions, allowing them to forsake worldly materialism and achieve heights of creative genius. Indeed, some of the greatest works of literature and music were written by people who were either suffering from TB themselves or watching loved ones die from it.[12] For instance, Keats wrote many of his poems that had themes of suffering and mortality immediately following the death of his two brothers from TB and during his own battle with the disease. Similarly, Edgar Allan Poe lost both parents and his wife Virginia to TB, and Charlotte Bronte witnessed the death of three sisters (including Emily) and one brother to the disease. Such personal connections to TB led many authors and composers of this period to incorporate sympathetic and almost heroic TB sufferers into their stories, which further romanticized the disease. Some examples include Mimi from *La Bohéme*, Satine from *Moulin Rouge*, and characters from *La Traviata*, *Les Misérables*, *East of Eden*, *Magic Mountain*, and *Wuthering Heights*. The end result of romanticizing TB in such ways was that the general public began to strongly associate TB with a melancholic and almost otherworldly state of being.

Another reason why TB was seen as an "in vogue" disease during the 19th century had to do with the appearance of TB victims themselves. The ideal image of beauty in Europe and much of Asia at the time was that of a thin, fair-skinned figure with rosy cheeks and larger eyes. Lighter skin tones have been associated with wealth and nobility since ancient Roman times as they were a sign of a life of leisure spent indoors out of the scorching sun. Women in the Victorian Era would often apply an array of cosmetics such as powders and creams in order to lighten their skin to an ivory complexion. Corsets were commonly worn to give the appearance of thinness, sometimes being pulled so tight that ribs would be broken. Since the application of brightly colored makeup to the cheeks and lips was associated with loose morals and prostitution, women would pinch their cheeks and bite their lips in order to produce the reddish color. Those suffering with TB were regarded as almost being lucky because the disease produced these visible signs of beauty as part of the natural course of the disease. Chronic wasting creates a trim figure with larger-looking eyes, recurrent nighttime fevers produce flushed cheeks, and the coughing up of large amounts of blood leads to anemia and a pale complexion. Although they lay dying in agony, many viewed them as beautiful, almost angelic figures.

Societal views of TB shifted again near the end of the 19th century when modern science first demonstrated that the disease was caused by infection with a small, rod-shaped bacterium. One acquired TB because they were exposed to a microscopic pathogen and not because they possessed any special personality trait, artistic gift, or intellectual genius. This monumental discovery caused the mystical romanticism of the 19th century to be replaced by science and medicine. Once seen as being sympathetic and beautiful, those dying of consumption were once again viewed with pity and contempt. As a result, they were subjected to much greater levels of isolation that often prevented them from obtaining work, getting married, or interacting with others who were healthy. The shift even caused society to change how it referred to the disease. An increasing number of medical and news reports at

the turn of the 20th century called the disease by the more technical histological term tuberculosis rather than consumption or phthisis. In being characterized scientifically, tuberculosis had come to be viewed by the upper
crust of society as it had always been viewed by the poor in the inner cities—
a dreadful, painful, and drawn-out death sentence.

Convalescent Therapy Is Popularized

People suffering from TB have been prescribed a wide variety of treatments throughout history, including special diets, bloodletting, opium,
mercury-based compounds, and leeches. In the early 1830s, a young British
general practitioner named George Bodington wrote several scathing articles
about these widely accepted treatments for TB and criticized the harm that
they often did to his patients.[13] He also disagreed with the practice of treating
TB patients in cramped, unsanitary, and stuffy city hospitals. Based on his
own clinical observations, he developed an alternative treatment paradigm
that called for cool fresh air, moderate exercise, a healthy diet, and a relaxing
state of mind. He tested his theory by personally caring for six TB patients in
his country home over a period of several years. In 1840, he attempted to
publish an essay that described the success of his limited study and his belief
that special open-air facilities should be built in areas with fair climates and
devoted solely to the treatment of TB patients. Unfortunately, reviewers from
several medical journals, including the prestigious *Lancet*, not only rejected
his article but also directly mocked his ideas and medical credentials.
Although his work was eventually published, the widespread negative back-
lash from his peers led him to switch careers and begin studying psychiatric
disorders.[14]

About 15 years after the publication of Bodington's essay (1854), a German doctor named Hermann Brehmer became so intrigued by this more
natural and holistic treatment strategy that he built the first facility specifically devoted to the treatment of TB, in a small town in modern-day Poland.[15]
This type of facility, known as a sanatorium (or sanitorium), was designed to
be more of a medical health spa than a hospital. Similar to what Bodington
originally proposed in his essay, patients were treated to healthy doses of
cool fresh air, light exercise, a lot of bedrest, positive attitudes, and a diet rich
in nutritious foods. Within a few years, the popularity of these sanatoria
began to skyrocket and thousands of similar facilities were consequently
built in rural areas all over Europe and North America. Some were private
facilities that catered to wealthy patients whereas others were state-run facilities that admitted the poor and minorities. Although it would take nearly two
decades, Bodington eventually gained widespread recognition for his pioneering work in the field, and his essay would go down as one of the more
influential publications in medical history.

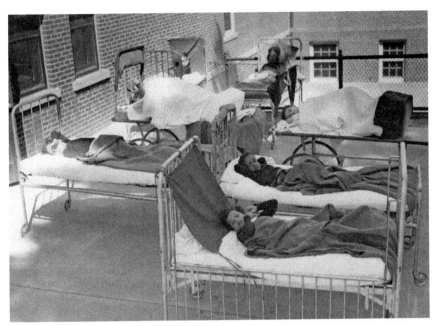

Sanatorium patients on a porch, ca. 1920. (National Archives Record Group 69-PWA)

The actual quality of life of those living in these facilities was paradoxical in that they were places that promoted relaxation, peace of mind, and optimism but also had high levels of death, suffering, and isolation.[16] People entered the sanatoria knowing that there was a good chance that they may one day leave in a casket. In fact, the typical registration process involved a discussion about how their autopsy would be performed and a prepayment of shipping costs if their body needed to be sent home for burial. Upon entering, a significant number of patients failed to regain their health and stayed for as long as 8–10 years without ever leaving. This prolonged isolation from the outside world, combined with an endless monotonous routine that was sometimes compared to that found in a prison, often took its toll on the emotional well-being of the residents. While both the staff and patients were discouraged from discussing death or expressing outward signs of grief when patients died due to its negative effects on morale, death was ever present and pervasive throughout the facility. Faced with their own mortality, people often sought sexual pleasure and other diversions in order to live their possibly limited time to the fullest.

Long-term stays at sanatoria were the most common way to treat TB for nearly 100 years; however, many have questioned whether or not they were actually effective in saving lives. The editor of the *British Journal of Tuberculosis* summarized this debate when, in 1909, he wrote, "Fads and fancies have gathered about so called 'open-air' treatment, and impossible claims have been made by inexperienced enthusiasts as to the almost miraculous efficacy accruing from sanatorium residence. In spite of all exaggerations and failures, there can be no doubt but that the maintenance of a strictly hygienic course of life offers the best means known to modern medical science for dealing effectually with tuberculosis."[17] Several studies conducted during the early 20th century came to much of the same conclusion.[18] They found that patients residing in sanatoria statistically had only a slightly better chance of surviving TB than those residing in city hospitals, and the benefits were largely limited to those who entered sanatoria in the very early stages of the disease. Patients with advanced TB were found to have the same chance of dying no matter where or how they lived. The now-famous Madras experiment conducted in 1956 convincingly confirmed these findings and once and for all demonstrated that healthy diets, rest, and fresh air provided no therapeutic benefit to patients already infected with TB.[19] These studies, together with the discovery of effective antibiotic therapies in the mid-1940s, led to the gradual decline of the entire sanatoria movement. Costly and ineffective sanatoria began closing all over the world in the 1960s, and the trend continued until July 2, 2012, when the last remaining TB sanatorium in the world, in south Florida, officially closed.

Despite not providing many measurable health benefits to infected patients, sanatoria did serve several vital roles during the worst TB pandemic in recorded history. First, it helped reduce the spread of TB in local populations by quarantining those with the disease. Infected patients living in isolated sanatoria had a much lower chance of passing the disease onto friends, family, and coworkers when compared with those who lay dying in their homes or in city hospitals. As a result, countless lives were spared from the horrors of a prolonged TB illness and death. Another interesting by-product of sanatoria is that it drastically improved the quality of life for many who were considered terminally ill. Rather than living their last days in dirty, cramped hospitals, those in sanatoria were allowed to die with dignity in relatively serene and peaceful surroundings. In a way, they functioned as a precursor to the modern-day hospice concept about 100 years before end-of-life palliative care was ever considered as an option.

Medical Microbiology Is Born

For most of its history, TB was thought to be caused by inhalation of filthy, toxic air (miasma) rather than from exposure to some specific infectious agent. It was not until the middle of the 19th century when improvements to microscopy and staining techniques enabled a young German physician named Robert Koch to finally disprove this antiquated theory. With tenacity and ingenuity, Koch brilliantly demonstrated that consumption, the dreaded

White Plague, was caused by infection with a small, slow-growing bacterium and not due to miasma. Complemented by the work of visionaries like Louis Pasteur and John Snow, his findings helped ignite a scientific revolution that is unrivaled in the history of medicine. It forever changed the way that infectious disease research was conducted and ultimately gave rise to the now widely accepted idea that microscopic germs can cause human disease (known as the Germ Theory of Disease).

After graduating from medical school in 1866 and serving in the Franco-Prussian War, Robert Koch eventually settled down and worked as a surgeon in a southern German town. Fueled by a natural curiosity for microorganisms, he constructed a small laboratory in his medical office that was equipped with a homemade incubator and a microscope that he received as a birthday gift from his wife. His microbiology career began modestly with a study of algae; however, following a local outbreak of anthrax, he transitioned to investigating microbes that cause human disease. With almost no funding or formal training, Koch meticulously and accurately described the life cycle of the anthrax bacterium (called *Bacillus anthracis*).[20] He developed new techniques to grow and visualize the bacterium on microscope slides, he elucidated how the bacterial cell produces small protected spores that survive for long periods in soil, and he demonstrated how the bacterium alone could cause anthrax when inoculated into experimental animals. His monumental work, published in 1876, was so well received that one preeminent pathologist of the time wrote, "I regard it as the greatest discovery ever made with bacteria and I believe that this is not the last time that this young Robert Koch will surprise and shame us by the brilliance of his investigations."[21] In addition to laying the groundwork for all future anthrax research, his paper garnered him international recognition, a new governmental position, and permanent research support. It was then that Koch switched his focus to a target that was a bigger killer and more feared than anthrax—tuberculosis.

When Koch and his team decided to search for the causative agent of TB, he had no idea of how incredibly difficult his task would be. As mentioned earlier, *Mycobacterium tuberculosis* is a very slow-growing bacterium that has a waxy outer covering that not only protects it from our immune cells but also provides resistance to almost all known stains. The average bacterium (e.g., *E. coli*, *Staphylococcus aureus*) can replicate fast enough to form a visible mound of cells on the surface of a petri dish (called a colony) in about 18–24 hours; *Mycobacterium tuberculosis* can take over a month to form a colony. Similarly, most human bacterial pathogens can be stained with conventional dyes and visualized with minimal effort or training; *Mycobacterium tuberculosis* has to be stained using multiple dyes in a complex series of steps that is difficult to master even for trained microbiologists. All who had attempted to accomplish this seemingly impossible task before Koch had failed.

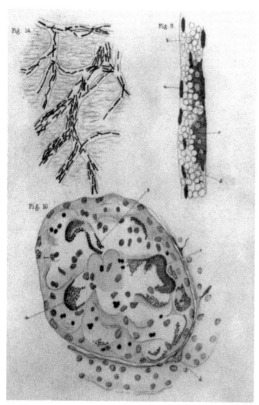

Illustration of bacteria from Robert Koch's *Investigations into the Etiology of Traumatic Infectious Diseases*, 1880. (Library of Congress)

On March 24, 1882, Robert Koch stood at the podium before an audience at the annual meeting of the Berlin Society of Physiology.[22] He started his speech by describing the devastation inflicted on society by TB and then proceeded to describe how he and his team succeeded in isolating, staining, and visualizing the rod-shaped *Mycobacterium tuberculosis* bacterium for the first time in history. After concluding his amazing presentation, he invited members of the audience to come up and look through a microscope to see the results for themselves. The entire audience sat in complete stunned silence. There were no questions and very little applause as Koch quietly walked off the stage. The future Nobel Prize laureate Paul Ehrlich, who was in attendance, later stated, "I hold that evening to be the most important experience of my scientific life."[23] Koch's speech and subsequent publication would go down as one of the most influential in medical history, not only because it identified the greatest of all human killers but also because it provided a road map and various new tools that could be used to identify other human pathogens.

One of the most important innovations that arose from this work was a drastic improvement in how bacteria were grown in the lab.[24] When Koch started his studies on anthrax and tuberculosis, bacteria could only be grown in liquid culture. Typically, one would take a sample from an infected animal or human and use it to inoculate a flask of some nutrient-enriched broth medium. After allowing the bacteria to grow and replicate in this liquid for some fixed period of time (usually 24–48 hours), one could take the resulting dense mixture and either look at the cells under the microscope or use it to infect some other animal. While this method of growth is still extensively used, it has a major flaw in that most samples taken from infected animals or people are mixtures of bacteria, a combination of those that are responsible for the disease and those that normally grow in the individual. As a result, if one were to inoculate a broth culture with this specimen, multiple species of bacteria would grow side by side and result in a mixed final culture. This was a major problem for anyone (like Koch) who wished to demonstrate that one specific bacterial species causes some defined disease.

Koch and his team addressed this issue by spreading clinical specimen onto a solid growth surface and allowing the bacteria to grow as small isolated colonies.[25] In doing so, they would be able to separate each type of bacterial species into distinct mounds of cells, which could then be picked and expanded using broth culture as described above. The team's early attempts involved growing colonies on thin slices of potato or on the surface of coagulated blood serum placed inside of test tubes. When these both failed to yield reproducible results, they shifted to adding gelatin to the growth medium in an attempt to solidify it (kind of like making bacterial Jell-O). Unfortunately, gelatin was found to melt at temperatures needed to grow most bacteria, and many bacteria secrete enzymes that destroy gelatin. As a result, they determined that gelatin was relatively unusable for this purpose. It was at this point that Fanny and Walter Hesse joined Koch's lab and changed the course of medical history.[26] Fanny told Koch about how she used to make jellies and puddings using a different solidifying agent, derived from a type of seaweed. This component, called agar, was then tested in the lab and shown to have a higher melting temperature than gelatin and was impervious to bacterial digestive enzymes. From this point forward, solid nutrient agar became the preferred way of growing isolated colonies of bacteria. With these new plates in hand, Koch was able to separate out the various types of bacteria found in clinical specimen and definitively showed that just one, *Mycobacterium tuberculosis*, was the sole causative agent of TB.

This work also led Koch to describe the set of criteria that he used to convincingly demonstrate that *M. tuberculosis* was the direct cause of human TB. These four guidelines, known collectively as Koch's postulates, later became a kind of standard of proof to be used by scientists who wished to "prove beyond a reasonable doubt" that organism X causes disease Y. Although they do have some limitations (e.g., they cannot be used to identify viral diseases), the postulates proved to be critically important as scientists all over the world raced to identify other disease-causing bacteria. Within about 15 years of Koch's monumental speech, nearly every other human bacterial pathogen had been isolated and identified using Koch's agar plates and postulates.

Another significant development that emerged from Koch's work was an improvement in how dyes were used to stain and visualize bacteria under a microscope. The vast majority of bacterial species are naturally clear and are thus very difficult to see without some form of stain to provide contrast between the bacteria and clear glass microscope slide. The first successful use of a dye to stain bacteria was performed somewhat accidentally by Carl Weigert in 1871.[27] He was examining sections of biopsied skin from patients with smallpox lesions (caused by a virus) when he noticed large aggregations of bacteria in the diseased tissue. They had absorbed and retained the applied dye differently than the surrounding human cells, allowing them to be easily distinguished from the other components of the mixed tissue. Familiar with Weigert's data, Koch and his team got to work methodically testing out different protocols and dyes in order to stain the notoriously resistant TB bacterium. Despite the inherent difficulty, they accomplished their goal in 1882 and forever changed the future of clinical microbiology, histology, and pathology as a result. Koch's triumph in staining one of the most impervious cell types on the planet demonstrated that any cell (bacterial or human) could be stained with enough effort and ingenuity. This inspired other scientists like Paul Ehrlich (Noble laureate mentioned earlier and cousin of Weigert), Hans Christian Gram, Franz Ziehl, Friedrich Neelsen, and Weigert himself to continue perfecting existing staining protocols and to develop new ones like the Gram and H&E stains.

Pasteurization, Chest X-Rays, and Other Tools for Preventing and Diagnosing TB

Attempts to control the spread of tuberculosis in the 19th and 20th centuries led to the implementation and popularization several preventative and diagnostic tools that are still widely used today. One of the earliest such measures was the rapid heating and cooling of milk (pasteurization) in order to prevent the transmission of food-borne TB.[28] Although the vast majority of TB cases are due to inhalation of infected respiratory droplets, it can also be transmitted through the ingestion of infected food products like milk. In fact, three different species of *Mycobacteria* can cause TB food poisoning (*Mycobacterium tuberculosis*, *Mycobacterium paratuberculosis*, and *Mycobacterium bovis*). When Louis Pasteur developed his method of pasteurization in the 1860s, he did so in order to save the failing French wine industry that had succumbed to widespread contamination with bacteria. With TB food poisoning making large numbers of people sick during this time, others began applying Pasteur's heating method to milk in order to make it safer for human consumption. By the turn of the 20th century, most milk producers had begun to pasteurize their product and incidences of food-borne TB plummeted. Furthermore, while TB created the impetus for the initial pasteurization of milk, it also led to the drastic reduction of other diseases spread by milk (e.g., typhoid, foot and mouth disease, anthrax). Thus, the fight to prevent TB ultimately led to broad improvements in food safety.

A second preventative measure implemented during this time was the TB vaccine. The original vaccine was created in the late 19th century using the same approach that was used to produce the smallpox vaccine. A bacterium that causes the bovine form of TB (*Mycobacterium bovis*) was injected into people with the idea that it would provide cross-protection to the human form of the disease in much of the same way that cowpox provided protection against smallpox. Unfortunately, those who conducted these first clinical trials in Italy were unaware that full-strength *M. bovis* is capable of causing human TB nearly as well as *M. tuberculosis*. As a result, many of those who were given the "vaccine" actually ended up developing TB and several died. At this point, two French scientists, Albert Calmette and Camille Guérin, began working together at the Pasteur Institute on a new weakened version of the *M. bovis* vaccine.[29] They took the disease-causing *M. bovis* strain and grew it for a long period of time in medium that was unfavorable for its growth. This caused a gradual accumulation of mutations that rendered the *M. bovis* weakened (attenuated) and unable to thrive in the human body. The new safe, attenuated form of the vaccine, called the bacillus Calmette–Guérin (BCG) vaccine, was first used in humans in 1921 and soon became one of the more widely administered vaccines in the world.

By the early 1930s, studies were being conducted to formally evaluate how well the BCG vaccine actually works over the long term.[30] Interestingly, these trials have produced widely conflicting data that seem to be dependent on where the trial was conducted and what strain of the vaccine was used. In some cases, it was found to provide protection to over 80 percent of its recipients while in others, the efficacy was determined to be less than 10 percent. Similarly, some trials found protection to last for over 50 years whereas others show protection lasting just a few years. Despite such inconsistent findings, the BCG vaccine became increasing more popular following World War II and is now recommended to be given to young children in all at-risk countries. In fact, there are only a handful of countries (including the United States) that still do not routinely give the vaccine to their population. It has no doubt saved countless numbers of lives and prevented the epidemic from spreading more profoundly during the 20th and 21st centuries.

A number of important diagnostic tools developed during this time also helped reduce TB infection rates. For most of history, TB was diagnosed following the onset of symptoms such as pneumonia, coughing up bright-red blood, and progressive weight loss. This is problematic because an infected person can spread the bacteria for months prior to the appearance of severe signs of disease, which means they can transmit the infection to their friends, family, and coworkers long before anyone knows that they are even sick. Being able to identify who is harboring *M. tuberculosis* in a population is critical because it allows for earlier medical interventions and treatments.

One of the earliest such tools developed was the stethoscope.[31] In 1816, a young French physician named Rene Laënnec was called to see a young female patient regarding a potential heart ailment. Realizing it would be inappropriate for him to put his ear directly onto the chest of a young woman (which was the way that physicians commonly listened to sounds inside the body), he rolled up a thick piece of paper into a hollow tube, put it on her chest, and listened to her heartbeat through the other end. He was shocked by how well the sound reverberated through the tube and immediately began thinking about how to refine his new invention. After three years of testing different materials, he eventually decided on a hollow tube of wood of a fixed diameter with an earpiece on one end. With his new tool in hand, Laënnec got to work characterizing the sounds produced by various cardiac and pulmonary conditions at different stages of disease. One disease that he had a particular fascination with was TB because his mother, brother, uncle, and two mentors all died of the disease. His stethoscope allowed him to correlate sounds he was hearing in the lungs of dying patients with pathological changes he observed in the lung tissue following autopsy. It provided a way to hear subtle changes in lung function of TB patients at early stages of disease and allowed for earlier and more proactive intervention. In a sad case of irony, Laënnec himself died of TB just 10 years after inventing the instrument that was later used to diagnose it.

The greatest tool used for diagnosing TB interestingly came about from one the most famous failures in the history of TB research.[32] Following the isolation and characterization of the TB bacterium in 1882, Robert Koch began working on a cure for the disease. He created various protein extracts of several *Mycobacterial* species (*M. tuberculosis*, *M. bovis*, and *M. avium*) and injected them into already-infected animals to see if they could somehow trigger the immune system to begin fighting off the disease. According to modern examination of his lab notebooks, these early experiments failed to demonstrate any type of measurable benefit of the extract injections. Then, in 1890, Koch unexpectedly announced that he had successfully developed a cure for TB, which he called tuberculin. He claimed that once injected into infected patients, some tuberculin component attaches itself to TB granulomas and initiates their destruction by the host immune system. The TB bacteria inside the granulomas are thus killed in the process as a bystander. After much celebration and fanfare, Koch began marketing his miracle cure for widespread distribution in Europe and the United States. Unfortunately, within a few months, it became abundantly clear in the medical literature that tuberculin had little to no therapeutic effect on existing TB lesions in humans and, in some cases, even caused severe inflammatory reactions to take place. When asked to show his original test data or reveal the composition of tuberculin, Koch remained secretive and borderline deceitful. He eventually had to concede that his original tuberculin extract was ineffective as a cure and as were several subsequent modified versions. Robert Koch, a Nobel Prize winner (1905), who had one of the most brilliant careers in the history of medicine, died in 1910 amid great controversy because of tuberculin. Some historians have even questioned whether Koch purposely tried to scam the medical community and profit off his previous, well-deserved fame. Examination of his records strongly suggests that he honestly believed his tuberculin cure could work, and he spent the greater part of 10–15 years trying to prove it. Koch may have been guilty of self-delusion and perpetrating bad science, but he was not a con artist.

Tuberculin could have been remembered in the same light as other famous medical flops like thalidomide, fen-phen, and Vioxx if not for the brilliant work of three physician scientists in first decade of the 20th century. Early in the human trials with tuberculin, Koch had noted that TB-infected patients tended to exhibit very strong local and general inflammatory reactions in response to tuberculin when compared to healthy (uninfected) individuals given the same injection. This was very similar to what was observed by Clemens von Pirquet, who, in 1906, found abnormal inflammatory reactions in people repeatedly given horse serum or the smallpox vaccine. Von Pirquet, along with his Hungarian collaborator Béla Schick, were the first to call this type of response an allergic reaction. Von Pirquet then began working with tuberculin, trying to better characterize why people were having allergic reactions to it and to determine if he could use it as some type of diagnostic indicator of a TB infection.[33] Interestingly, he discovered that injection of a small amount of tuberculin under the skin induced a localized allergic response in only those who have been infected with TB, even if they are not yet exhibiting any symptoms of the disease. This was significant because it allowed physicians to identify people in the population who were harboring TB bacteria in their body long before they became sick and could spread it to others. In the subsequent couple of years, two other scientists, Charles Mantoux and later Felix Mendel, built on von Pirquet's work and refined the composition and delivery of his test.[34] It eventually became widely known as the Mantoux test and was again later improved (by partially purifying the tuberculin extract) into the modern-day PPD test. Since 1907, the Mantoux/PPD test has been used throughout the world to provide early detection for millions of cases of tuberculosis, which has slowed the spread of the epidemic and saved countless lives. Thus, what was once viewed as the greatest blunder in Robert Koch's illustrious career gave rise to a valuable lifesaving diagnostic tool.

Anyone who has been previously exposed to *Mycobacterium* will test positive when given the PPD skin test. This not only includes those who have been naturally infected with the *M. tuberculosis* bacteria but also anyone who has received the attenuated BCG vaccine at some point in their life. Since most countries in the world require the partially effective vaccine, a large number of people in the population will automatically test positive. This represents a major hurdle for local governments that need to be able to track new TB cases during an outbreak, and it is the central reason why countries like the United States and Great Britain do not currently include BCG in their normal immunization schedule. Such problems create a dire need for alternative tests that can distinguish between those who are truly infected from those who just appear to be infected due to their immunization.

In 1895, German physicist and future Nobel Laureate Wilhelm Röntgen produced and detected a unique wavelength of electromagnetic radiation that he termed X-rays. This new powerful form of energy was interesting to physicians because it could easily penetrate human soft tissue (skin, fat, internal organs) and provided photographic images of dense internal structures like bones, teeth, and foreign objects like bomb shrapnel. Early machines were poorly adapted to provide clear images of internal organs like the lungs, heart, or GI tract and so few thought they could ever be employed to detect disease states at those sites. However, modifications to X-ray tubes at the beginning of the 20th century allowed scientists like Francis Williams to peer into the lungs of those harboring latent and active TB infections and detect characteristic pathological abnormalities (e.g., tubercules/granulomas).[35] By the 1920s, public health campaigns initiated by the National Tuberculosis Association and other similar organizations advocated for widespread PPD tests and chest X-rays for all, including those not exhibiting any symptoms. They created mobile X-ray clinics that would tour between cities and offer free chest X-rays for anyone interested. Chest X-rays became so commonplace that they even made their way into some very famous works of literature. For instance, in Thomas Mann's seminal book *The Magic Mountain*, the main character Hans Castorp lives in a sanatorium and vividly describes his moving experience of seeing inside his body for the first time:

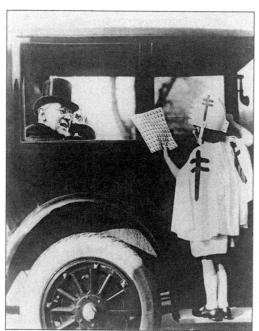

Woodrow Wilson stops on his daily drive to purchase Tuberculosis Seals from Sylvia Suter, a little Health Crusader, 1923. (Library of Congress)

And Hans Castorp saw, precisely what he must have expected, but what it is hardly permitted man to see, and what he had never thought it would be vouchsafed him to see: he looked into his own grave . . . It seemed that in Hans Castorp's case, the test of the eye confirmed that of the ear in a way to add lustre to science. The Hofrat had seen the old as well as the fresh spots, and "strands" ran from the bronchial tubes rather far into the organ itself—"strands" with "nodules."[36]

For the first time in history, we had the ability to both listen (stethoscope) and see (X-ray) inside of diseased lungs. These diagnostic tools, along with the Mantoux/PPD test and preventative measures like pasteurization and the BCG vaccine, helped drastically limit the spread of TB in the population during the 20th century. However, for those who were already infected, this knowledge was of little value. Until the discovery of effective antibiotics in the mid-1950s, there was almost nothing that could be done to stop or even slow the progression of the disease. A TB diagnosis was still as much of a death sentence then as it was centuries before.

Quest for Antibiotics and Their Failure

As mentioned in chapter 4, the discovery and use of quinine as a treatment for malaria proved that microbial diseases could be eliminated from already-infected people. This prompted chemists to begin purposely synthesizing new compounds with the hopes of finding some that may be effective at killing bacteria. In 1909, German chemist Paul Ehrlich and his assistant Sahachiro Hata found that the 606th arsenic-based compound they created and tested, arsphenamine, effectively killed the bacterium that causes syphilis (*Treponema palladium*).[37] After extensive animal testing and numerous human clinical trials, Ehrlich's miracle compound went on the market the following year as Salvarsan, a combination of the words salvation and arsenic. Salvarsan and its slightly better derivative Neosalvarsan quickly became widely popular throughout the world and remained the drug of choice for the treatment of syphilis and African sleeping sickness for nearly four decades. Unfortunately, Salvarsan was relatively toxic to humans and ineffective against most human bacterial diseases, including tuberculosis. It was a great first step in the search for bacterial cures, but it was clearly not the optimal solution.

About 20 years after Ehrlich's monumental work with Salvarsan, a Scottish scientist named Alexander Fleming stumbled upon arguably one of the best lifesaving compounds in medical history. He had spread some *Staphylococcus* (Staph) bacteria on a petri dish and accidentally left the lid off the plate long enough for a mold spore land on it. After letting it sit for several days, he examined it and noticed something strange. There was a single mold colony contaminating his plate, and it seemed to be producing a chemical that was killing the Staph bacteria around it. This compound, which he named penicillin after the mold that produced it (*Penicillium notatum*), was found to be relatively safe for humans and very effective against a large number of human bacterial pathogens. Chemists Howard Florey and Ernst Chain took

Fleming's penicillin and successfully purified, mass produced, and tested it in clinical trials. Penicillin became available to the general public in 1942 and was quickly dubbed a "wonder drug" that could potentially put an end to all bacterial diseases. Hope for this lofty goal quickly faded as penicillin-resistant strains of Staph and other bacteria were discovered within just a few months. Also, to the great disappointment to all of those affected by tuberculosis, penicillin and all other antibiotics isolated in the 1930s and 1940s (e.g., sulfa drugs) were completely ineffective against TB. This would provide a major impetus for a worldwide search for other naturally occurring antibiotics that could possibly be used to defeat the stubborn TB bacterium. An antibiotic revolution had begun and the Holy Grail was a chemical capable of killing the seemingly unkillable *M. tuberculosis*.

Interestingly, the source of this elusive chemical was a small patch of farmland near Rutgers University in rural New Jersey.[38] Professor Selman Waksman and his team had long been interested in soil molds and the chemicals they produce to fight off competing soil bacteria. The observation that *M. tuberculosis* bacteria die very quickly when placed into soil particularly piqued his interest. With the help of a grant from the American National Association against Tuberculosis, the Waksman lab began looking in various soils for antibiotic-producing molds. He had successfully isolated a number of new mold species and even found a few that made antibiotics in his first 10 years on the project. The term antibiotic was actually coined by Waksman during this work. Unfortunately, the first two antibiotics that he discovered (actinomycin and streptothricin) were extremely toxic to animal test subjects and were thus unusable for humans. Then, in 1943, Waksman recruited a young graduate student named Albert Schatz to join his lab and a breakthrough was made within just three months. In just his 11th sampling, Schatz isolated a new strain of a greyish-colored mold called *Streptomyces griseus* from a compost and manure pile near his building at Rutgers. To his surprise, this strain was found to produce a chemical (named streptomycin) that could not only inhibit the growth of his test organism, *E. coli*, but also *M. tuberculosis*. After extensive animal and clinical testing by collaborators at the Mayo Clinic, streptomycin was deemed to be safe for human usage and a patent was subsequently issued in 1946. The world finally had its first-ever treatment for TB. Ironically, the cure for the single greatest killer in the history of mankind came from a pile of manure on a farm and was discovered by a graduate student in just his third month in lab.

The discovery of streptomycin set off a series of very significant firestorms—some scientific and some legal.[39] When Schatz and Waksman jointly patented streptomycin, both agreed in writing to forgo their patent rights and all profits from their discovery so that it could be distributed more inexpensively to the world. Unbeknownst to Schatz at the time, Waksman and Rutgers had made secret agreements with chemical companies (e.g., Merck) to give them 20 percent of all royalties from the sale of streptomycin. Upon realizing he had been misled, Schatz filed a lawsuit against his former mentor and employer for scientific credit and royalties. He won the lawsuit, but the ugliness of the court proceedings and a scandalous attack on his character caused Schatz to become somewhat of a scientific pariah. Selman Waksman, in his Nobel Prize speech in 1952, failed to even mention Schatz by name and for years afterward, refused to give him his due credit. In a 1949 letter to Schatz, Waksman wrote, "you must, therefore, be fully aware of the fact that your own share in the solution of the streptomycin problem was only a small one. You were one of many cogs in a great wheel in the study of antibiotics in this laboratory. There were a large number of graduate students and assistants who helped me in this work; they were my tools, my hands, if you please."[40] Time did eventually heal this rift. Schatz went onto have a very successful scientific career, and Rutgers eventually recognized him with a Medal of Honor in 1994 for his contribution to this history-making discovery. The Schatz-Waksman lawsuit was significant because it was the first to raise questions about intellectual property rights of students who make major discoveries under the supervision of senior mentors.[41] Several similar lawsuits have arisen since, and this issue still very much lingers in labs throughout the world.

The discovery of streptomycin was also important from the scientific perspective because it demonstrated that antibiotics capable of stopping tuberculosis could and do exist. This prompted a feverish search by chemists and soil microbiologists to find other chemicals with similar activity against TB.[42] The second one discovered was an aspirin derivative called 4-aminosalicylic acid (or PAS) that was not as potent as streptomycin and a bit more expensive to make. In 1951, a chemical called isoniazid (INH) was found to be safe, cheap, and 10 times more effective against *M. tuberculosis* than streptomycin. Similar results were seen with the antibiotic rifampicin, which was discovered in 1957. It seemed for a short time that TB had finally met its match with these new antibiotics and would become a disease of the past. Unfortunately, *M. tuberculosis* had another trick up its sleeve that would strike fear into clinicians all over the world.

Interestingly, patients taking these various antibiotic "cures" were still dying of tuberculosis, albeit at much lower rates. The reason for this was that the TB bacteria were acquiring random mutations in their own genes that provided them with resistance to each of the antibiotics. For instance, a survey done in the mid-1950s estimated that as many as 5 percent of all TB strains tested were resistant to one of the three primary TB drugs.[43] As a result, doctors began instructing patients to take multiple, sometimes three or four, antibiotics simultaneously with the idea that they would have an additive effect against the bacteria.[44] Also, the odds of any one strain of *M. tuberculosis* being resistant to multiple antibiotics were very low at the time, so prescribing multiple antibiotics took some of the guesswork out of having to choose the best one. This "shock and awe" method of TB treatment seemed to work for a while, with record low numbers of deaths and new infections being reported. Some government agencies such as the Centers for Disease Control and Prevention even began to cut funding for TB research throughout much of the 1970s. Then, in the mid-1980s, physicians began seeing an increasing number of patients infected with *M. tuberculosis* strains that were resistant to several antibiotics. Even more worrisome was the isolation of some multidrug-resistant (MDR) TB strains that were resistant to all available medications. Such findings prompted the World Health Organization to declare TB a "global emergency" in 1993. Reports published in 2014 confirmed these concerns when it showed that MDR TB was found in over 35 percent of newly infected patients and 76 percent of TB patients who were treated previously with antibiotics.[45] About 14 percent of those patients tested had extensively MDR TB strains (called XDR TB), which means they had almost no treatment options available and little hope for recovery.

What has prompted this distressing rise in antibiotic-resistant *M. tuberculosis*? One factor has been the rapid spread of the human immunodeficiency virus (HIV) over the last 30 years.[46] HIV weakens a person's immune system by targeting and killing the very cells (T cells) that normally protect us from infectious disease. With a suppressed immune system, HIV patients are much more susceptible to being infected and harmed by a variety of other viral, fungal, or bacterial pathogens, including TB. When someone has the misfortune of being infected with both TB and HIV, their immune system is weakened to the point that the TB bacteria are able to replicate uncontrollably throughout their body. As antibiotics are given to this co-infected person, the drugs kill off most of the bacteria but are unable to finish the job because of the person's poor immune response. Bacteria that survive the antibiotic onslaught will live long enough to acquire resistance mutations, which they can pass onto their bacterial offspring. Before long, the HIV-infected person will be filled with antibiotic-resistant TB and will have a much greater chance of transmitting it to others.

A second major factor contributing to this problem is the misuse of antibiotics by those undergoing treatment. With most bacterial infections, patients are required to take antibiotics pills at home for only about 5–10 days. In contrast, those with TB need to take antibiotics every day for several months in order to kill the slow-growing and protected bacterial cells. In extreme cases, patients may be on antibiotics continuously for as long as a full year. The extended treatment regimen is problematic because it is very expensive and difficult to follow faithfully, especially for those who are impoverished and living in unstable environments (e.g., the homeless). Patients may miss days or forget to refill their prescriptions, which allow some bacteria to survive and to acquire resistance mutations. To combat this problem, many hospitals and public health administrators have begun requiring patients to come into a local clinic every day to and take the pill in the presence of medical staff. This specialized treatment program, called directly observed therapy or DOTS, has been shown to successfully reduce the incidence of MDR and XDR TB in some poor and rural communities. For instance, a DOTS program in Lima, Peru, in the early 2000s was found to have a cure rate of over 80 percent.[47]

Despite the advent of modern sanitation, vaccines, various diagnosis tools, and several antibiotics, tuberculosis is still currently the second leading cause of death from infectious disease in the world. Scientific advancements have slowed the epidemic for brief periods of time but none have never really come close to stopping it. In fact, several studies suggest that TB cases are again on the rise and the epidemic may only continue to get worse. The story of TB is clearly not finished and may never be. It was with our species soon after its creation and may be with us until the end.

CHAPTER SIX

Typhus

Soldiers have rarely won wars. They more often mop up after the barrage of epidemics. And typhus, with its brothers and sisters—plague, cholera, typhoid, and dysentery—has decided more campaigns than Caesar, Hannibal, Napoleon, and the inspectors general of history. The epidemics get the blame for defeat, the generals get the credit for victory. It ought to be the other way around.
    —Hans Zinsser, 1935, from the book *Rats, Lice, and History*[1]

Epidemic typhus has had significant impacts on nearly every major war fought on the European and Asian continents for over four-and-a-half centuries. During the course of almost every war, large numbers of soldiers are forced to mobilize to specific locations and live in close contact with one another in overcrowded and often unsanitary tents and barracks for months or even years. In doing so, they will wear the same dirty, unwashed uniform for days on end, share bedding and blankets, and huddle closely in the face of enemy onslaughts and harsh winters. Similarly, violent battles often cause major displacements of civilians and the consequent creation of unimaginably cramped refugee and concentration camps. Food supplies in battlefields and camps were always limiting, creating widespread malnourishment and weakened immune systems. Altogether, the congested and unhealthy living conditions that almost universally result from warfare provide a perfect breeding ground for infectious diseases and the parasites that carry them. One such parasite, the human body louse, is particularly adept at flourishing within the confines of an active war zone. Body lice are able to jump easily from host to host through any direct physical contact or sharing of clothing/bedding. Through its ability to transmit the bacterium that causes epidemic typhus, the simple louse has drastically affected the outcome of several very important battles in history and humbled some of the most brilliant military minds (e.g., Napoleon Bonaparte).

Epidemic typhus is caused by infection with the bacterium *Rickettsia prowazekii*. It is different from other human typhus diseases like murine and scrub typhus in that it has an abnormally high fatality rate and is transmitted by lice rather than by ticks, fleas, or mites. When a louse carrying *R. prowazekii* bites a human, it typically defecates on the skin as it takes its blood meal. Chemicals in the louse saliva cause an inflammatory itching response, which prompts the person to scratch the area. That scratching creates small, microscopic abrasions in the skin and ultimately provides an opening by which the bacteria are able to enter the body. Once inside, *R. prowazekii* bacteria promptly reach the bloodstream and attach to the cells that line the blood vessels (called vascular endothelial cells).

Unlike most bacterial pathogens, which usually do their damage while living outside of our cells, *R. prowazekii* forces its way into the interior of the endothelial cells and begins to replicate there. Overwhelmed with bacteria, infected cells become sickly and eventually burst. Newly made *R. prowazekii* released from these exploding cells can then bind to neighboring endothelial cells and infect them as well. Before long, the death of so many endothelial cells leads to widespread inflammation and the perforation of blood vessels. Patients will experience a rash (due to the internal hemorrhaging), a prolonged high fever that can approach 105°F, and a severe drop in blood pressure. The reduction in blood flow causes internal organ damage and produces localized tissue death in the extremities. The fever, which is one of the highest induced by any infectious agent, often leads to confusion and a state of delirium. If left untreated, the end result of epidemic typhus is death in over 40 percent of the patients.

Early Descriptions of Epidemic Typhus

No one knows exactly when epidemic typhus began causing disease in the human population. One of the earliest descriptions of a typhus-like disease was the epidemic that struck Greeks in 430–426 BCE during the Peloponnesian Wars between Athens and Sparta.[2] The disease, called the Athenian plague, was described by the Greek historian Thucydides and later by the Roman philosopher Titus Lucretius Carus as one that produced a disseminated pustular rash, a high fever that "internally burned so that the patient could not bear to have on him clothing or linen even of the very lightest description,"[3] and bloody vomit and diarrhea. Since this latter symptom, gastrointestinal hemorrhaging, is very uncharacteristic of modern epidemic typhus, many epidemiologists have suggested other possible causes of the disease. Some believe the Athenian plague was instead due to typhoid fever, an unrelated waterborne disease that produces a high fever and gastrointestinal distress. This disease, which was famously spread by Irish immigrant "Typhoid Mary" Mallon, is caused by infection with *Salmonella* bacteria and is spread rapidly in areas with contaminated water sources (like most ancient battlefields). However, Thucydides's observation that small animals were also dying of the same disease suggests that it may not have been typhoid fever after all. Others have since suggested viral hemorrhagic fever or bubonic plague as possible causes of the Athenian plague.

Although vague references to similar typhus-like diseases continued all throughout the Dark Ages, it was not until the late 15th century that we see the first clear and definitive description of the disease. This first recorded epidemic occurred in southern Spain during a time when the Spanish monarchy was attempting to forcibly expel, convert, or kill all of the country's remaining Muslim Moors (a process called The Reconquista). Several hundred years of fighting between Christian crusaders and the Moors had drastically diminished Moorish control in Spain and forced them to seek refuge in the southern Spanish province of Granada.[4] They remained there, occupying 14 fortified cities, in an uneasy truce with the Christian leaders to the north. However, in 1481, when the Moorish king Muley Abul Hassan of Granada surprise-attacked the nearby Christian town of Zahara and then subsequently refused to pay King Ferdinand II of Aragon his yearly tribute of gold, Ferdinand vowed to rid Spain of all Moors once and for all. He is famously quoted as saying he would go into Granada (which means pomegranate in Spanish) and "pick out the seeds of this pomegranate one by one."[5]

By 1489, a Christian army of about 25,000 soldiers had surrounded the Moors in a single city in Granada and began attacking it with nonstop cannon fire. When a quick Christian victory seemed imminent, an epidemic of typhus erupted in the Spanish army and killed over 17,000 of their troops within just a few months.[6] Such devastation had an enormously negative impact on their ability to mount an overpowering offensive against the last Moorish stronghold. As a result, the weakened Christian fighting force took another three years to gain administrative control of the city, and pockets of Muslim resistance would remain for another 100 years. The victorious soldiers eventually returned to their native countries and brought epidemic typhus with them. This caused widespread dissemination of the disease throughout Europe, which laid the groundwork for all future Eurasian epidemics. Similar to start of the Black Death epidemic at Caffa in 1343 (see chapter 2), a war between Christians and Muslims had given a somewhat rare disease a perfect opportunity to enter new populations and become a permanent fixture. As a result, nearly every war fought on the continent for the next 500 years would be altered in some way by epidemic typhus.

Typhus and the Protestant Reformation

Following the deaths of his grandfathers King Ferdinand II of Spain in 1516 and Holy Roman Emperor Maximilian I in 1519, a teenager named Charles V became both the king of Spain and unquestioned political leader of the Catholic Church. These titles gave him control over an enormous amount of land in Europe and the Americas and provided him with access to a large number of Christian fighters who were ready go to battle whenever he required them to do so. Within just a few years of taking the throne, Charles V was embroiled in an extensive series of military campaigns against three of his key adversaries—the French, Ottoman Turks, and followers of the newly formed Protestant religion. These wars, which were plagued by the ongoing presence of epidemic typhus, ultimately defined the reign of Charles V and forever altered the history of Eurasia and several of the world's major religions.

When Charles V was declared the Holy Roman Emperor in 1519, he immediately gained a number of powerful enemies who felt that they were unfairly passed over for the job. One such rival was the reigning King of France, Francis I. By 1521, Francis I had formed an alliance with the Republic of Venice and attacked the army of Charles V in northern Spain. The fighting soon spilled over into France, the Low Countries (e.g., Belgium and Netherlands), and Italy and continued for another four years.[7] Just as the French forces were moving into northern Italy and heading toward Rome (1525), they were ambushed by the army of Charles V in a small town called Pavia. Within just four hours, the French army was split and utterly destroyed. Most of the French nobles present were killed, and Francis I himself was taken prisoner by Charles V. After being forced to sign the humiliating Treaty of Madrid and surrendering all rights to lands in Italy and elsewhere, Francis I was freed and allowed to return to France in 1526.

Within weeks of being released from his Spanish captors, Francis I had regrouped his army and formed alliances with the new pope (Clement VII), Henry VIII of England, many of the independent Italian republics, and Suleiman the Magnificent of the Ottoman Empire. When Charles V learned that Pope Clement VII had betrayed him and joined forces with his most hated rival (and the Muslim Ottoman Turks), he sent an army into Rome to formally capture the city.[8] Unfortunately, his men disobeyed direct orders to not sack the city and completely pillaged it in March 1527. They made off with most of the valuable treasures of the Vatican and forced the pope to flee for his life. The news of this blatant disrespect for the sanctity of the Western "Holy Land" led the French alliance to reinvade Italy and once again attack Charles V. With a force of over 30,000 troops, the French had surrounded an overmatched Spanish army of 11,000 in Naples and controlled the ports that supplied the region. Also, bubonic plague had struck Naples and killed or sickened most of the waiting Spanish combatants. The Prince of Orange, who was the leading Spanish commander in Naples at the time, snuck out of the city and sent word to Charles V that he was planning on surrendering their position in Italy.

When all looked lost for the Spanish, "General Typhus" stepped in and changed the course of the war.[9] Within just about a month, over 20,000 of the French soldiers succumbed to the disease. The remaining sickened troops fled, which gave the Spanish army renewed life and an easy victory over the French. Epidemic typhus had accomplished what Spanish guns and swords could not. It was seen a miraculous gift from God, an agent of salvation for Spain and for Charles V. As a result, Charles V maintained unquestioned and absolute control over the Holy Roman Empire, most of Italy, and Pope Clement VII. The pope was eventually freed from his imprisonment at the Castel Sant'Angelo and allowed to return to his role as the head of the Catholic Church. However, he served his remaining time as pope under constant fear that Charles could have him killed at any time.

One of the other people most affected by the typhus epidemic and resulting Spanish victory in 1527 was King Henry VIII of England. He was an important supporter of Charles V in the early part of the Italian Wars (1521–1526) and even helped him fight Francis I on several occasions. However, in 1526, he betrayed Charles and joined forces with the pope and Francis following his release from Spanish imprisonment. This betrayal was interesting because at the time, Henry was married to Charles's aunt, Catherine of Aragon.[10] The situation became even more uncomfortable in July 1530 when Henry formally asked Pope Clement VII for an annulment of his marriage to Catherine. He claimed that this request was based on a passage from Leviticus, which states that marrying the wife of your deceased brother is "unclean." (Catherine was formerly married to Henry's brother Arthur.) In reality, Catherine had failed to bear him a male heir despite five pregnancies, and he wanted to marry his mistress Anne Boleyn.

The pope was now put into a difficult position. Does he side with his political ally Henry and risk angering Catherine's nephew Charles, or does he deny the request in order to preserve his own life? After a lengthy series of proceedings, the pope made the safe decision and denied Henry's request. This posed a major problem for Henry, who, in late 1532, learned that Anne was pregnant, and his heir would be illegitimate without a proper marriage. Faced with mounting pressure and feeling personally insulted by the pope's refusal, Henry responded by breaking away the Roman Catholic Church and starting a new church under the direct control of the English king himself.[11] Doing so gave him the freedom to legally divorce Catherine under English law and marry Anne. This new religion, the Church of England (Anglican Church), maintained most of the Catholic doctrines and liturgies initially but became progressively more Protestant under the reign of Henry's eventual heir Edward VI. Had typhus not helped Charles save his throne in 1527, it is likely that the pope would have granted the annulment to his ally Henry, and the English Reformation may have never happened.

The rise of Protestantism in other European countries was also significantly affected by epidemic typhus during the 16th century. In an effort to control the spread of the new religion, Charles V and his successors enacted laws to limit heretical Protestant teachings, held local tribunals called inquisitions to identify and eliminate religious heretics, and raised sizable armies to defend Catholicism. For instance, Charles V, in his now-famous denunciation of Martin Luther at the Diet of Worms assembly in 1521, decreed that he "forbid anyone from this time forward to dare, either by words or by deeds, to receive, defend, sustain, or favour the said Martin Luther. On the contrary, we want him to be apprehended and punished as a notorious heretic."[12] Protestant leaders in Germany, Scandinavia, and Eastern Europe responded by forming their own political and military allegiances against what they considered to be tyrannical control by Charles. Formal associations like the League of Torgau and Schmalkaldic League enabled disparate Protestant groups to combine forces and mount a more unified resistance to advancing powerful Catholic armies.

In many of the early battles between the two, it looked as if Catholics would be successful in systematically weeding out the growing Protestant threat. For instance, Catholic forces led by Charles completely decimated the Protestant army in Mühlberg, Germany, in 1547 and triggered the dissolution of Schmalkaldic League.[13] That defeat nearly destroyed the Protestant Reformation and left only two cities in Germany that openly opposed the authority of the Holy Roman Empire. Five years later, when a powerful Catholic army was again preparing to attack an overmatched Protestant force in Metz, France, it looked as if the Protestant movement may be dealt a final crushing blow.[14] However, a few months into the battle, Charles had to call off the siege because as many as 30,000 of his men had died of typhus. Reports of the retreat describe rows of dead bodies and sickened Catholic soldiers lining the streets leading out of the city. This enabled Protestantism to persist in the region and continue spreading throughout Europe at a time when the movement was militarily and politically very weak. The significance of this cannot be overstated when one considers that the two groups would continue to fight off and on for the next 65 years until finally engaging in one of the longest, bloodiest wars in the history of Europe, the Thirty Years' War (1618–1648). It is during this war (discussed below) that typhus finally spread to epidemic levels and became endemic throughout the European continent. Thus the perpetual and almost pathological insistence on going to war over religious beliefs is what allowed typhus to flourish and create an epidemic nightmare.

Taken together, it is clear that one cannot properly discuss the Protestant Reformation without mentioning the role that epidemic typhus played in shaping key battles during the early years of the movement. Influential leaders like Charles V, Francis I, Henry VIII, and various German princes looked almost powerless against epidemic typhus. They planned and schemed tirelessly only to have the disease seemingly decide the victor of key battles randomly. In the end, both sides benefited from and were harmed by typhus at different times. It was an equal opportunity killer that was neither Catholic nor Protestant.

The Thirty Years' War

The Holy Roman Empire in the early 17th century consisted of hundreds of semiautonomous political states that exercised some measure of religious freedom. Since the signing of the Peace of Augsburg in 1555, leaders of the German provinces were permitted to adopt Lutheranism as the *de facto* religion of their land, and those Lutherans living in Catholic-controlled regions were allowed to freely practice their religion without fear of reprisal from the empire.[15] This began to change in 1617, when Ferdinand II, a devout Catholic and staunch anti-Protestant, was chosen as the king of the heavily Protestant region of Bohemia (in modern-day Hungary and the Czech Republic). As a leader of the Counter-Reformation movement and the Catholic League, Ferdinand sought to create more religious uniformity in Bohemia, and in doing so, he hoped to root out Protestantism from the region. He initiated a series of restrictive policies against Protestants early in his reign, which created a great deal of resentment and fear among the Bohemians.[16] When Ferdinand sent representatives to Prague (Bohemia) in May 1618 to discuss these policies, members of the Protestant assembly threw several of the representatives out of a third-story window. (Amazingly, they all survived the fall.) This formal revolt against Ferdinand, known as the Second Defenestration of Prague, marked the official start of the Thirty Years' War.

Several events over the next year caused a relatively minor local skirmish to escalate into a vicious, transcontinental war.[17] One of the most significant was that Ferdinand II was chosen as the King of Hungary in 1618 and then Holy Roman Emperor in 1619 following the death of his cousin Matthias. This gave him firm command of an enormous amount of land, subjects, and resources with which to impose his will on the rebellious Protestants. Meanwhile, Protestant nobles in Bohemia had formed an alliance and decided to sever all ties with Ferdinand and the Holy Roman Empire. In August 1619, they made Protestantism the state religion, ousted Ferdinand as the King of Bohemia, and elected Frederick V as the new king. Ferdinand, understandably incensed by these events, obtained military support from the Catholic League and launched a series of attacks against the Bohemians. With a force that outnumbered the Bohemians three to one, Ferdinand's army crushed the rebellion in November of 1620. However, in doing so, he sparked fear into Protestants all throughout Europe that the Catholic army would begin invading other Protestant lands. As a result, a large alliance of Protestant states, called the Protestant Union, soon became directly involved in fighting. Over the next 25 years, countries like Sweden, England, France, Denmark, and Saxony declared war on the Holy Roman Empire, Spain, Austria, and Hungary. Although the fighting was largely centered in the German states, nearly the whole of Europe became embroiled in what can be considered the first true world war.

The Thirty Years' War caused devastation to the land and population of central Europe. Some have estimated that nearly 10 million people lost their lives as a direct result of the war, with only about 400,000 of those resulting from combat.[18] Mass movements of soldiers from all over Europe and the widespread destruction of homes combined to produce a perfect environment for typhus and bubonic plague to flourish in the armies and among civilians. In fact, this war was the first time in which typhus moved from the battlefields and barracks to towns and homes. Typhus truly reached epidemic proportions during this war and moved in the general population all throughout Europe. In his book *Rats, Lice, and History*, Zinsser elegantly writes, "The Thirty Years' War was the most gigantic natural experiment in epidemiology to which mankind has ever been subjected."[19] Typhus was able to move like it had never before, which gave it an opportunity to establish itself as an endemic disease in jails, schools, and other crowded environments all over Europe. In doing so, it served as the source for several even more deadly typhus epidemics over the next three centuries.

A Thorn in Napoleon's Side

French emperor Napoleon Bonaparte, perhaps more than any other leader in modern history, had his reign and reputation destroyed by epidemic typhus. After a series of military conquests in revolutionary France, Italy, and Egypt, Napoleon returned to France in 1799 and seized political control of the country by overthrowing the ruling French Directory. As first consul, Napoleon led France in a series of military victories over Austria and restored order domestically by instituting reforms to the French government, legal system, and economy. In 1802, Napoleon helped formalize a change to the constitution that made him the leader of France for life, and he was crowned as emperor two years later. He continued to terrorize most of Europe and Russia for the next eight years through a series of very costly wars. At the height of the Napoleon's empire in 1810, France controlled most of continental Europe (except the Balkans) through direct occupation or through alliances with puppet governments that were subservient to Napoleon. It looked as if Napoleon was poised to take control of all of Eurasia when he decided to march through Poland and invade Russia in 1812.

France and Russia had an uneasy partnership since signing the Treaties of Tilsit in July of 1807.[20] In these agreements, Russia committed to only trade within the Continental System (those countries in Europe friendly to France), and France in turn allowed Russia to retain nearly all of its land. The two also agreed to support one another militarily as France continued to fight with Britain and Russia with Ottoman Turkey. However, within a few years, tensions began growing between the two as France became increasingly involved with Russia's neighbor, Poland, and Russian merchants continued to trade with France's enemy, England. Also, Napoleon had his sights on British-controlled India. The powerful British navy prevented him from invading India by sea thus forcing him to march his forces overland through Russia. Once it was clear that an invasion of Russia was needed to force it "back into line," Napoleon assembled a massive army of approximately 690,000 men that included about 270,000 French soldiers and men from the various territories that were controlled by Napoleon (Italy, Poland, Austria, and modern-day Germany).[21] On June 24, 1812, Napoleon moved this Grand Armée to the shores Niemen River and officially declared his intention to cross the border into Russian-controlled territory.[22] They took several days to cross the river and began marching through Poland with no resistance from the Russian army.

As the enormous Grande Armée pushed deeper into Poland, it soon began facing a number of costly logistical problems.[23] First, the roads in rural Poland were not built for the transport of heavy equipment or large numbers of troops, which greatly hindered the supply wagons that provided the Grand Armée with food, clean water, and fresh clothing. This obstacle was further exacerbated by Napoleon's insistence on pushing the cavalry and ground troops on toward Moscow as fast as possible. As a result, within just a few weeks, the army was almost completely separated from a reliable source of supplies, and those supplies were already running dangerously low. Finding little relief in the drought-ravaged Polish countryside, troops were ordered to go into local villages in search of help. Napoleon's chief surgeon Dominique-Jean Larrey warned those foraging to have minimal contact with local peasants for fear that they may contract dangerous diseases from them. Unfortunately, most of the men conscripted into the Grand Armée from other countries had little experience in obtaining provisions in this way and many lacked the necessary discipline to do so responsibly. As a result, many of the soldiers who raided Polish towns and stole whatever goods they could find ended up having brief, but consequential, interactions with the local residents. What resulted from these encounters was infinitely worse than Dominique-Jean Larrey could have ever imagined.

One of the diseases that were endemic in Poland during this time was typhus. Men returning from these excursions unknowingly brought back typhus-infected lice on their clothes and introduced them to the rest of the army.[24] The filthy and cramped living conditions in the barracks, combined with the soldiers' inability to properly wash or change their clothes, allowed the invading lice to spread uncontrollably among the troops. Infested men were bitten continuously throughout the day and night, which drastically limited their ability to sleep at a time when they were exhausted, sick, and starving. By the end of their first month in Poland, an estimated 80,000 men (and thousands of horses) had died or become incapacitated largely because of typhus and dysentery. Rather than slowing the advance and allowing Larrey to set up proper field hospitals, Napoleon ordered the army to keep moving deeper into Russia. As early fall approached, thousands of men continued to die, and many others became incapacitated by illness or left by desertion. In fact, some have estimated that Napoleon had lost nearly half his fighting force by the time they faced the Russians at the fierce Battle of Borodino, a battle that caused the loss of an additional 30,000 troops.[25]

Following the somewhat hollow victory at Bordino, the depleted Grand Armée, which now had just under 100,000 troops, marched just 75 miles and arrived in Moscow on September 14.[26] What they found there had to be an absolutely disheartening sight for all those sick and weary soldiers: an abandoned city that had been burned and stripped of its food, water, and other lifesaving resources. They had marched and fought almost continuously for three straight months over several hundred miles of rough terrain. They battled endless hunger, thirst, exhaustion, louse infestation, and disease. They watched several hundred thousand of their friends suffer in agony as they lay dying from typhus and dysentery. There they were, standing victorious at the gates of one of the greatest cities in the world, the crown jewel of the Russian Empire, and they had to feel defeated. Nearly 80 percent of their force had been depleted in just three months in order to conquer a now useless city. They were still hungry and still sick.

The Grand Armée remained encamped in Moscow for another month, eagerly waiting for the arrival of fresh supplies and troops and waiting in vain for Alexander to formally surrender. Unfortunately for Napoleon, the 15,000 new soldiers that joined his ranks in September and October was roughly equaled by the number who died of typhus during that time.[27] Also, Alexander used this time to strengthen his own army and position his troops in order to thwart a potential French retreat. Leo Tolstoy eloquently described the difficulties faced by the French army while in Moscow when he wrote in his classic *War and Peace*, "The army, like a herd of cattle run wild and trampling underfoot the fodder which might have saved it from starvation, was disintegrating and perishing with every day it remained in Moscow."[28] By mid-October, Napoleon realized that he would lose his entire army if he remained in Moscow any longer and ordered a full retreat. Leaving behind over 10,000 typhus-infected troops, Napoleon officially abandoned Moscow on October 19, 1812, and headed southwest toward Paris with the remnants of his once Grand Armée.[29]

The retreat that followed was even more devastating than the march into Moscow because the troops had two additional foes to contend with—the bitter cold and a reinvigorated Russian army. Men continued to die by the thousands as they trudged back through the desolate and diseased Russian countryside. The Russian army continually harassed the rear flank of the retreating army, and local townspeople refused to provide aid. There were reports of helpless, dying men, so hungry that they often resorted to chewing on leather or the flesh of their fallen comrades. By the time they reached the German border later that winter, only about 30,000–40,000 of the fighting force remained. Of those that made it all the way back to Paris months later, only about 1,000 were healthy enough to ever fight again.[30]

A comprehensive analysis of Napoleon's catastrophic 1812 invasion of Russia reveals that it failed as a result of the interplay of many different factors and not just because of typhus. Poor leadership decisions, arrogance, drought, disease, a brutally cold winter, and a tenacious Russian army all worked together to doom Napoleon and his dream of expanding his empire into Asia. However, one cannot deny that losing an estimated 200,000 men to typhus had to have had a profound impact on the power and morale of the army, especially considering that typhus killed over five times more men than did Russian bullets or exposure to the cold. Typhus decimated the Grand Armée long before it faced any significant action on the battlefield or marched through the unforgiving Russian winter. It had accomplished in six months what no military leader had done in the previous 20 years: it humbled the military genius of Napoleon and forever destroyed his aura of invincibility. In the years that immediately followed the disastrous 1812 campaign, Napoleon gradually lost his control over Europe until he was finally defeated at Waterloo in 1815.

The Irish Potato Famine and Immigration

The Great Famine of Ireland (a.k.a. the Irish Potato Famine) began in 1845 and lasted more than seven years, claiming a million lives and forcing another 1.5–2 million to emigrate from the country.[31] In the years preceding the famine, daily control of the farmable land had passed from the hands of the landowners to a group of landlord middlemen who subdivided the land into extremely small plots and then rented them to tenant farmers. The farmers, in turn, were responsible for planting a crop that would yield a harvest sufficient enough to both pay the rent and feed their family. Unfortunately, the relative small size of the plots and poor nutrient content of the overgrazed Irish soil severely limited the type of crop that they could use. By the early 1840s, most of these tenant farmers had begun to rely on a single species of potato (the Irish Lumper) as their sole source of food and income because potatoes were very nutritious and could grow well in relatively poor-quality soil. Such dependence on a single, genetically uniform crop would prove to be devastating when, in 1844, a new plant disease arrived from the Americas and began destroying large numbers of potatoes throughout Europe. The causative agent of this potato blight, a water mold referred to as *Phytophthora infestans*, infects potatoes and causes them to turn black and become inedible. By 1847, *P. infestans* had completely overtaken the potato industry of Ireland, causing an amazing drop of more than 80 percent in the annual potato yield.

The near total loss of their primary crop had immediate and severe impacts on the Irish people. With almost no income coming in, large numbers of struggling tenant farmers and their families were evicted by unsympathetic landlords. Some estimate that nearly 500,000 people were kicked off their land during the early years of the famine, with many forced to watch their homes be leveled to the ground.[32] The resulting widespread homelessness led many families to begin sharing small residences in order to pool their limited resources and avoid starvation. Unfortunately, cramping increasing numbers of poor and malnourished people into small spaces provided an ideal situation for infectious diseases like typhus, dysentery, and cholera to flourish. Of the roughly 1 million Irish who perished during the famine, it is believed that typhus caused several hundred thousand of those deaths, and other diseases and starvation collectively caused most of the rest.[33] In fact, census data from 1851 suggest that about 20 times more Irish died from disease than starvation during the worst years of the famine.

The starving and sick masses now faced a life and death decision: stay and try to rebuild their lives in the midst of unprecedented suffering or leave in search of new opportunities elsewhere in Europe or the Americas. Unfortunately, the million or so Irish who chose to immigrate to North America found that the diseases ravaging the Irish population would follow them on their journey across the ocean aboard unsanitary and overcrowded ships.

Ships leaving western Irish ports typically had one of three destinations—Europe (e.g., Great Britain), the United States, or Canada. Fares for ships leaving for the United States and most of Europe were intentionally made higher than those heading to Canada in order to purposely funnel the poor immigrants into British-controlled Canada. Unfortunately, low fares typically led shipowners to provide the bare minimum amount of food, water, and space for the travelers despite the existence of several laws designed to protect passengers (e.g., Passenger Acts of 1842).[34] Some ships were packed with nearly twice the number of passengers that they were designed for and most provided no food and only two pints of unclean water per day per passenger. Such horrific conditions enabled typhus ("ship fever") and dysentery to spread at an alarming rate during the 40-day journey. Ship manifests indicate that about 30 percent of all people who set sail for the Americas during the years of the famine succumbed to disease while at sea. Those who perished during the voyage were often callously tossed overboard to hungry sharks that commonly followed the ships. One passenger traveling to Quebec in May 1847 described the hopelessness felt by passengers aboard these "coffin ships" when he wrote,

> We thought we couldn't be worse off than we war; but now to our sorrow we know the differ; for sure supposin we were dyin of starvation, or if the sickness overtuk us. We had a chance of a doctor, and if he could do no good for our bodies, sure the priest could for our souls; and then we'd be buried wid our own people; in the ould churchyard, with the green sod over us; instead of dying like rotten sheep thrown into a pit, and the minit the breath is out of our bodies, flung into the sea to be eaten up by them horrid sharks.[35]

Sentiments and stories like this were unfortunately very common among those fleeing the famine during the peak years of the blight.

Arrival in the Americas did not bring the immediate salvation from the horrors of famine or typhus that many hoped for. Port cities in Canada and the United States were unprepared to handle the constant influx of large numbers of ships filled with immigrants sick with typhus. By mid-1847, hospitals in cities like Grosse Isle (Quebec), Toronto, Montreal, and New York were so inundated with typhus victims that they were forced to construct makeshift tents or sheds in order to quarantine them.[36] Most of these "fever sheds" were as crowded, filthy, and ill equipped as the passenger holds of the coffin ships that they had just escaped from. As a result, typhus continued to spread among the immigrants in epidemic proportions, claiming the lives of thousands of quarantined Irish in just a matter of months (1847–1848).

The situation in many port cities became so dire that local authorities began requiring passengers to stay on the infested ships for at least 15 days prior to disembarking in order to ensure that any ongoing typhus cases had a chance to "run their course." For the healthy passengers aboard these ships, that meant another 15 days of being surrounded by filth and sickness. As one may expect, the result of such a policy was that large numbers of passengers who were healthy upon arriving in the Americas ended up contracting typhus and dying while waiting to exit the ships. One particularly stark example of this nightmare was seen in the major Canadian immigration depot at Grosse Isle in Quebec.[37] At one point in the summer of 1847, over 40 ships filled with sick passengers were lined up for over two miles in the middle of the St. Lawrence River. Some of the ships' passengers, in a desperate attempt to clear the boats of typhus, began throwing the dead overboard into the river, and others placed the sick into small boats and released them toward the shore. Local residents described seeing dead bodies floating aimlessly down the heavily traveled St. Lawrence like lifeless logs and sick people clawing in the mud and rocks as they frantically tried to make it to shore. It was a horrific scene that continued until Grosse Isle medical officers decided to lift the ineffective and unsustainable quarantine.

While typhus obviously did not cause the devastation in Ireland, it did compound the misery of those already facing unimaginable suffering there, and it continued to torment those who attempted to escape and start over. It was an opportunistic killer, waiting for a perfect event like the Great Famine to be unleashed on a helpless population.

World War I

The Russo-Japanese War fought in 1905 was the first large-scale war in which more soldiers died of combat wounds than of disease.[38] This amazing accomplishment of medical science led some to believe that we now had enough knowledge and technology to be able to defend ourselves against wartime scourges like typhus and dysentery. Many hoped that this was a sign that typhus had finished wreaking havoc on helpless armies and thwarting the plans of brilliant military strategists. Unfortunately, one of largest and deadliest wars in history was on the horizon. World War I would soon prove to the world that typhus was every bit as dangerous as it always had been. In fact, the war and the political destabilization that resulted from it provided the perfect backdrop for the two worst typhus epidemics in human history.

World War I erupted in Eastern Europe on July 28, 1914, following the assassination of the heir to the Austro-Hungarian throne by a Serbian nationalist. Austria-Hungary, responding to this perceived act of war, proceeded to launch a massive ground invasion into Serbia. Countries who were political allies of Serbia (e.g., Russia) responded by quickly coming to their defense militarily, which triggered allies of Austria-Hungary (e.g., Germany) to also join the war. Before long, nearly 70 million combatants from over 20 countries became embroiled in a brutal, four-year-long trench war on two different fronts: one located in Eastern Europe near Russia and the Balkans and the other in the west near Italy, France, and Belgium. At both locations, soldiers fought for days or even weeks at a time in unsanitary and damp trenches, where cold and crowding led to the rapid spread of body lice and the diseases they carry (typhus and other trench fevers).

Although typhus is not credited with formally influencing the outcome of any major battle during World War I, it did play a significant role in determining when some of those battles would take place. This was especially true on the Eastern front in Serbia, an area hit hard by a major typhus epidemic during the fall of 1914.[39] Following the invasion and subsequent retreat by the Austro-Hungarian army in November of that year, a typhus epidemic broke out among the 60,000 Austro-Hungarian prisoners of war and their Serb captors. It spread quickly to the rest of the Serbian army and to many of the surrounding cities to the south. As temperatures began to drop, the typhus epidemic only grew worse, incapacitating over 6,000 people a day and killing about one-quarter of the entire Serbian army. Some estimates have total fatalities at over 200,000, making it one of the worst typhus epidemics in history.

With such drastic reductions in the number of healthy soldiers available to fight, the Serbs would have been helpless had the Austro-Hungarian and German armies decided to invade again in the winter of 1914–1915. However, the leaders of the Central Powers saw the devastation that typhus had inflicted upon the Serbian forces and decided not to risk their own armies by invading at the height of the epidemic. Instead, they waited over six months before finally crossing the Danube in October 1915. Two days after entering Serbia, the Austro-Hungarian and Germany armies took control of Belgrade and forced the Serbs to flee to the south. The Bulgarian army proceeded to attack southern Serbia one week later, capturing it with relatively little trouble. While this may seem like a total victory for the Central Powers, the delays they faced in Serbia while waiting for the typhus epidemic to subside would later prove to have significant impacts on the outcome of the war.

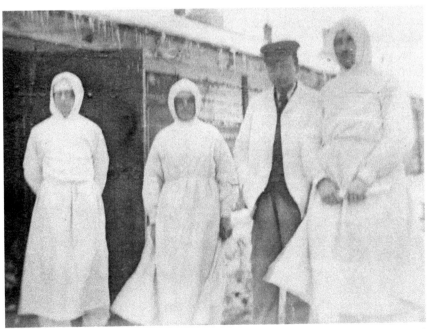

American Red Cross workers disinfecting barracks filled with refugees and "typhus bugs." (Library of Congress)

The prolonged fighting on the Eastern front ended in early March 1918 when Russia formally surrendered to the Central Powers with the signing of the Treaty of Brest-Litovsk. Following its victory, Germany began the arduous process of relocating massive numbers of troops to Western Europe in order to strengthen their planned offensive for later that spring. Unfortunately for them, most soldiers stationed on the Eastern front had become infested with body lice and exposed to typhus while fighting in cramped and unsanitary trenches there. As a result, hundreds of thousands of German troops from over 50 divisions had to be meticulously deloused prior to being transported to France over a thousand miles away. The slowed western migration of German troops provided the Allies with time to bolster their lines with millions of freshly arriving troops from the United States, Britain, and France. Those troops would prove to be the difference that enabled the Allies to survive the onslaught of four German offensive attacks on the Western line and ultimately defeat the Central Powers in November 1918.

Historians and scientists have long debated the role that typhus played in determining the outcome of the events described above. Some have speculated that if the Central Powers had been able to invade and defeat the Serbs prior to the typhus epidemic in 1914, they may have been able to maneuver themselves into a position where they could have attacked Russia from both the north and south.[40] This may have led to an earlier Russian capitulation, which would have given the Central Powers the ability to focus its entire fighting force along the Western front prior to the United States entering the war. Instead, typhus helped prolong the existence of the Eastern front and forced the Central Powers into fighting a very costly two-front war for a longer period of time. Although it did not affect the outcome of even a single battle in World War I, the ever-present fear of typhus paralyzed military leaders and caused them to abandon plans that may have changed the final outcome of the entire war.

An interesting paradox that emerged following the war was that typhus was almost nonexistent on the Western front despite terrible living conditions and very similar levels of louse infestation among the troops on the two fronts. Although the exact reason for this remains a mystery, most epidemiologists believe that soldiers in the west may have been partially protected from contracting typhus due to being previously infected with another louse-borne bacterium named *Bartonella quintana*.[41] Originally mischaracterized as a type of *Rickettsia*, this species causes a nonfatal relapsing fever (known as trench fever) that leaves its sufferers with skin lesions and debilitating leg pain following any type of exercise. While millions of troops on both fronts were suspected of having trench fever at some point, those fighting in the warmer French climate in the west were particularly susceptible to it. For instance, an estimated one-quarter of the entire British army contracted it between the years of 1915 and 1918. Upon recovering from trench fever, it is thought that these soldiers developed an immune response that partially protected them from subsequent reinfections with *B. quintana*. Interestingly, it is thought that this immune response may have also inadvertently cross-protected soldiers from becoming infected with other similar bacteria, including the deadly typhus bacterium *R. prowazekii*. Thus, *B. quintana* (trench fever) seemed to have worked like a natural "vaccine" for the *R. prowazekii*. The mechanism by which it did this still remains to be elucidated.

The Russian Revolution

Following the conclusion of World War I, typhus spread rapidly through-out Eastern Europe as millions of louse-infested troop returned home. One area particularly hard hit in the postwar era was Russia, which experienced enormous losses during the war, two violent political revolutions in 1917, an even more deadly civil war in 1918, and the great Influenza pandemic of 1918 (see chapter 9). Collectively, these events produced levels of poverty, suffering, and chaos that may be unmatched in modern history, and in doing so, they provided ideal conditions for the single worst typhus epidemic to ever hit mankind.

Over 6.5 million Russian soldiers were killed or wounded in World War I. Such staggering losses exacerbated a growing discontent with the reigning monarch Tsar Nicholas II and his perceived indifference to the rising levels of poverty and hunger throughout the country. By 1917, soldiers began defecting in ever-increasing numbers, and workers (men and women) started organizing large protests in the capital city of Petrograd (St. Petersburg) to demand higher pay and better working conditions.[42] When those demonstrations morphed into more violent riots in February of that year, Nicholas mobilized over 100,000 troops and ordered them to quell the rebellion by any means necessary. Not wanting to fire on the large mobs, dispatched troops largely refused to intervene, went into hiding, or even joined in with the protestors. By the time Nicholas returned to Petrograd in March 1917, most of his administrative buildings had been destroyed by the rioters, and his government was in shambles. Following advice from his top officials, Nicholas abdicated his throne on March 15 with the hope of saving his life and the lives of his family. He was promptly placed under house arrest by the new provisional government and remained there until he was executed 16 months later.

The disintegration of the monarchy created a power vacuum in Russia during a time of enormous economic and social turmoil.[43] When the dust settled, two groups emerged from the February Revolution sharing political control over the country. The Provisional Government, formed the day after Nicholas's abdication, was composed of moderate aristocrats who originally sought to restore order and set up democratic elections for later that year. Opposing the Provisional Government was a large council of factory workers and former soldiers that became known as the Petrograd Soviet. Although it initially worked like a political lobby group trying to exert pressure on the Provisional Government to implement social reforms to improve the lives of the working poor, the Petrograd Soviet gradually sought more control over decision making after having major disagreements with the Provisional Government over the war and other domestic issues.

As summer of 1917 began, the Soviet began to strongly align itself with the rising leftist Bolshevik party headed by Vladimir Lenin and Leon Trotsky.[44] The Bolsheviks, like many other popular leftist groups in Russia at the time, believed that the power of the government should be in the hands of the workers and peasants rather than the wealthy bourgeoisie. Seeing little improvement in their standard of living since the dissolution of the monarchy and wanting an end to the war with Germany, these leftist groups, led by the Bolsheviks, overthrew the Provisional Government in October 1917. This second revolution put the Bolsheviks in control of all governmental agencies and allowed them to spread their ideology throughout the entirety of Russia. However, it did not give them support of the majority of the population. For instance, those on the right, the upper and middle classes, monarchists, Cossacks, and some leftist groups were not happy with how the Bolsheviks restructured the government and aligned themselves against the Bolsheviks, forming what many referred to as the White Army (as opposed to the Bolshevik Red Army). What ensued over the next five years remains one of the bloodiest civil wars in Eurasian history.

The Russian Civil War claimed the lives of an estimated 8 million people and left the country in ruins. Both sides tortured, terrorized, and massacred millions of civilians in order to crush what they considered to be a rebellion by traitors to the Russian state. Such brutality was not only condoned but actively encouraged by leaders such as Lenin. For instance, in a 1918 telegram he sent to Bolsheviks in the town of Panza, he wrote,

> Comrades! The kulak uprising in your five districts must be crushed without pity . . . You must make example of these people. (1) Hang (I mean hang publicly, so that people see it) at least 100 kulaks, rich bastards, and known bloodsuckers. (2) Publish their names. (3) Seize all their grain. (4) Single out the hostages per my instructions in yesterday's telegram. Do all this so that for miles around people see it all, understand it, tremble, and tell themselves that we are killing the bloodthirsty kulaks and that we will continue to do so . . . Yours, Lenin. P.S. Find tougher people.[45]

In addition to the killings, millions of homes were burned and thousands of acres of fertile farmland destroyed. Collectively, this resulted in widespread food shortages and homelessness for tens of millions of people, including 7 million children who were left as street orphans. As a result, most of the Russian population was forced to live in such deplorable conditions that infectious diseases like influenza, dysentery, and typhus were almost a certainty.

It is estimated that 25 million Russians, one-quarter of the population, contracted typhus between 1918 to 1922, and as many as 3 million died from it.[46] While the enormity and suffering caused by this epidemic is unimaginable, most historians do not think that it had significant impact on the final outcome of the civil war. The likely reason for this is that typhus showed no favorites. It ravaged both the Reds and the Whites, those in cities and those living in the country, and people in every level of society. It was everywhere, spreading rapidly aboard overcrowded trains as millions of desperate people fled dangerous cities. Although leaders on both sides were concerned that typhus could single-handedly cause them to lose the war, in the end it did not. Lenin once famously stated, "All attention to this problem, comrades. Either lice will conquer socialism, or socialism will conquer lice."[47] Typhus did not defeat socialism but it did cause immeasurable suffering during the birth of it as a movement. Socialism likewise failed to defeat typhus. However, some have suggested that the Russian people's belief that it could may have led them more readily accept the victorious Bolshevik (communist) government in 1922. The Russian people had experienced over eight years of continuous war, hunger, chaos, and disease. They were desperate for it to end, to be free of violence and free of typhus. It is possible that the social order provided by communist government may have convinced them they it represented the best hope for an end to their suffering.

World War II

Several preventative measures developed after World War I helped limit the spread of typhus in the large armies engaged in World War II. First, the discovery of the body louse as the vector for typhus and the subsequent identification of the bacterium *Rickettsia prowazeki* as the causative agent of typhus in 1916 provided epidemiologists with the tools needed to effectively control the disease.[48] Early measures involved the removal and boiling of louse-infested clothing and bedding, extensive bathing, and prevention of overcrowding and other conditions that promote louse infestation. These measures were shown to be effective in controlling small-scale typhus outbreaks (e.g., in Serbia and North Africa in late 1910s); however, the expensive and time-consuming nature of the methods proved to be impractical for large populations. Many of those who were deloused quickly became reinfested as they returned to their normal impoverished surroundings and interacted with others that still had lice. This changed drastically when, in 1939, the insecticide DDT was shown to not only effectively kill the body louse but also to prevent reinfestation for several weeks after application. The subsequent invention of a power duster by the U.S. military in the early 1940s allowed for the efficient delousing of troops and refugees that flooded out of war-torn areas.

The distribution of an effective typhus vaccine also helped to limit typhus infections during World War II. The vaccine was developed in the mid-1930s by a Polish scientist named Rudolf Stefan Weigl.[49] After successfully testing his vaccine in places like China and Ethiopia prior to start of World War II, Weigl began mass producing it by infecting millions of live lice with *R. prowazekii* in a lab and then harvesting the bacteria from the same lice after they had a chance to replicate. In an amazingly dangerous protocol, infected lice were then crushed to release its bacteria, and those bacteria were destroyed with toxic phenol prior to being injected into humans. The vaccine became an immediate success, being praised by all who witnessed its almost miraculous efficacy. A Belgian missionary working in China in the 1930s once noted that

> typhus was one of the greatest human enemies killing at that time more victims then all other epidemics combined. Of 130 Fathers active in China, 70% died of typhus in the years of 1908 to 1931. When news reached us that a Polish Professor has developed a vaccine, we were first very skeptical, since many "cures" were proposed or sold to us before, but all of these failed. Anyway, we decided to try the Polish vaccine and the results turned out to be dramatic. During the past 7 years, since we started using the Weigl's vaccine, not a single of our missionaries or of the vaccinated Chinese patients died of typhus. Your Polish vaccine saved lives not only of missionaries but also of many thousands of Chinese.[50]

Unfortunately, the amazing potential of Weigl's vaccine would not be fully realized initially due to the invasion and subsequent occupation of Poland by the Nazis in 1939. Not wanting to take over his operation or risk being exposed to typhus themselves, the Nazis allowed Weigl to continue his work under their supervision as long as he supplied their troops with the lifesaving vaccine.[51] He was permitted to bring in his own workers to assist with the massive operation, which gave him the opportunity to recruit many of the local intellectuals who would have otherwise been killed by the Nazis. Many of the most brilliant mathematicians, artists, and scientists in all of Poland worked for Weigl as lice feeders. Boxes of hungry (uninfected) lice were strapped to their legs and allowed to bite until their guts were filled with the donor blood. Convincing the local SS that he needed a large number of healthy individuals to produce enough vaccine to supply the Nazis, Weigl procured extra rations for his workers and a special designation so that they would not deported to the death camps. Furthermore, a number of eyewitness accounts indicate that Weigl smuggled tens of thousands of doses of his typhus vaccine out of the lab and administered them to Jews living in the Warsaw ghetto. Knowing that he would be arrested or even killed if he were caught doing this, Weigl risked his life on a daily basis and saved the lives of an untold number of Jews. For this reason, Dr. Weigl was designated by Yad Vashem as "Righteous Among the Nations."

While Dr. Weigl was secretly saving the lives of Jews with his typhus vaccine, one of his former students, a Jew named Dr. Ludwig Fleck, began producing a slightly different typhus vaccine while living as a prisoner in the confines of a Jewish ghetto.[52] His vaccine was initially produced by purifying typhus antigens from the urine of those who had been exposed to the bacterium. This amazingly effective vaccine was noticed by the local SS, who proceeded to send Fleck to the Buchenwald concentration camp so he could mass produce his vaccine for Nazi personnel. When Fleck arrived at Buchenwald, he quickly realized that those already working on typhus there had little understanding of microbiology or immunology. In fact, the workers had been unknowingly using the wrong bacterium for their typhus vaccine, which made it completely ineffective. In one of the best known cases of microbiological sabotage in modern history, Fleck purposely allowed tons of this bad vaccine to be produced and administered to the unsuspecting Nazi elite. Meanwhile, Fleck produced much smaller amounts of an effective typhus vaccine, which he mostly gave to the prisoners of the camp and to anyone who was sending his vaccine off for testing. Amazingly, this went on for nearly 16 months and Fleck was never caught. However, Fleck continued to struggle with his decision throughout the war and for many years afterward because of his oath as a physician to do no harm to his "patients." In the end, he felt that the Nazis receiving his bogus vaccine were his captors rather than his patients, and none of them were actually being harmed by the fake vaccine.

Despite having Weigl's vaccine and powerful insecticides to control the spread of typhus, certain populations remained susceptible to devastating outbreaks during the entirety of World War II. In particular, the overcrowded and unsanitary conditions experienced by the Jews in ghettos, transport trains, and concentration/death camps provided a perfect breeding ground for lice and typhus.[53] For instance, the large Warsaw ghetto, before being liquidated by the Nazi military in 1943, held an estimated 400,000 severely malnourished Jews in area of just 1.2 square miles. Typhus outbreaks were so widespread there that some estimate as many as 100,000 Jews died of typhus within a three-year period. When confronted with this public health emergency, local Nazi doctors and administrators refused to intervene and responded by shooting any Jew attempting to escape the Warsaw ghetto in search of food or other provisions. They were largely content with allowing typhus to exterminate the Jews in the confines of the ghetto as long as it posed little risk to themselves or the surrounding population.

Similar to the ghettos, cases of typhus were also extremely common in concentration camps despite efforts by Nazi administrators to control its spread. Prisoners were stripped, shaved, and disinfected upon arriving at the camp, and regular inspections were performed in order to minimize the threat of typhus to the SS officials working there. Unfortunately for the prisoners, such meager measures would prove to be insufficient to counteract the horrendous conditions in the camps. Many hundreds of thousands of imprisoned Jews succumbed to typhus, including Anne Frank and her sister Margot, who died in the Bergen-Belsen concentration camp in 1945.[54] Several camp survivors who knew the Frank sisters recall seeing them both exhibit clear signs of typhus early in February, about two weeks before they are believed to have passed away from the disease.

While the Nazi leadership seemingly turned a blind eye when typhus was ravaging their enemies, they were intensely concerned about typhus and its potential effects on the German population and military. In addition to forcing soldiers to undergo rigorous screenings and other preventative measures (e.g., vaccinations and DDT spraying), Nazis routinely used the media to remind its own population to practice proper hygiene and seek medical attention if experiencing typhus-like symptoms. Furthermore, they imposed strict quarantines on towns experiencing suspected typhus outbreaks. Whenever local health officials were alerted to cases of typhus, they would send blood samples for testing and confirmation before imposing travel sanctions in those neighborhoods.

One particularly astute Polish doctor named Eugene Lazowski was aware of these policies and decided to use the Nazi fear of typhus against them.[55] Together with his friend and fellow physician, Stanisław Matulewicz, Dr. Lazowski began injecting heat-killed typhus bacteria into residents of 12 different local ghettos around the Polish cities of Rozwadów and Zbydniów. These residents began exhibiting mild typhus-like symptoms soon after being injected, which led Nazi officials to have their blood tested for the bacterium. When those tests came back positive (since they were injected with typhus proteins), the Nazi officials, fearing a full-blown typhus outbreak, imposed a strict quarantine on the whole area surrounding these towns. As a result, none of the residents (including the Jews inside) were deported to concentration camps, and none were murdered. It is estimated that this fake typhus epidemic saved the lives of at least 8,000 Jews who would have no doubt been killed during the "Final Solution."

Another interesting aspect of typhus during World War II is how the disease and its vector closely coincided with Nazi ideology pertaining to the Jews. A review of both early and later Nazi writings reveals that they believed

Jews to be subhuman parasites that spread "disease" to all nations. Such beliefs were clearly defined in a 1944 Nazi pamphlet entitled *Jew as World Parasite*:

> The German people has recognized that the Jew has crept in like a parasite not only into our people, but into all the peoples of the earth, and that it is attempting to corrupt the original racial characteristics of the peoples in order to destroy them both racially and as states, and thereby rule over them . . . The Jew is the parasite of humanity. He can be a parasite for an individual person, a social parasite for whole peoples, and the world parasite of humanity.[56]

Early attempts at controlling the Jewish problem revolved around taking away their rights and possessions and then removing them from German society through relocation and deportation. When Nazi leadership realized that such measures were not working in the way they had hoped, they came up with a more permanent solution to their "parasite" problem. In 1941, Hitler and the architect of the Holocaust, Heinrich Himmler, devised a plan to exterminate the "parasites" in Germany and the whole of Eurasia. New types of camps were built called death camps whose sole focus was to industrialize the mass killing of Jews and other undesirable parasites (e.g., gypsies, homosexuals, and handicapped). Heinrich Himmler gave a speech to an assembly of SS officers in 1943 in which he said, "Getting rid of lice is not a question of ideology. It is a matter of cleanliness. In just the same way, anti-Semitism, for us, has not been a question of ideology, but a matter of cleanliness, which now will soon have been dealt with. We shall soon be deloused. We have only 20,000 lice left, and then the matter is finished in the whole of Germany."[57]

Nazis thus equated Jews with lice and disease, which was supported by the fact that Jews in ghettos and camps were contracting typhus at a high rate. As a result, Nazis were able to effective use various forms of propaganda to convince the general population of this association. One such poster shows a stereotypical Jewish-shaped skull surrounded by a crawling louse with the caption "Jews-typhus-lice." The goal of such propaganda was to equate Jews with typhus so that populace would fear the Jews in the same way that they had feared typhus for so many generations. This would lessen the emotional effect of seeing Jews discriminated against or harmed. Preying on such natural fear proved to be an effective strategy when considering the atrocious things that ordinary citizens did to their Jewish neighbors with relatively little provocation in many cases.

CHAPTER SEVEN

Yellow Fever

A man cannot work hard here without risking his life and it is quite impossible for me to remain here for more than six months . . . my health is so wretched that I would consider myself lucky if I could last for that time! The mortality continues and makes fearful ravages . . . You will see that the army which you calculated at twenty-six thousand men is reduced at this moment to twelve thousand.

—French General Victor Emmanuel Charles LeClerc (Napoleon's brother-in-law), written in 1802 from Haiti[1]

Despite causing significantly fewer deaths than the rest of the diseases discussed in this book, yellow fever is one of the most feared diseases in history due to the particularly horrific symptoms it produces in its victims. Most individuals who contract it experience severe flu-like symptoms (fever, muscle ache, nausea) for a few days and then ultimately recover with minimal long-term complications. However, in roughly 15–20 percent of the cases, those afflicted take a sudden and drastic downturn following an apparent recovery. They most often experience severe liver failure, which produces jaundice (yellowing of the skin), abdominal pain and swelling, and high fever. Like other hemorrhagic fevers such as Ebola and Marburg, it usually then progresses into widespread internal hemorrhaging and bleeding out of the eyes, nose, and mouth. Excessive bleeding into the stomach can cause the individual to vomit up large amounts of black, partially digested blood. The shocking sight of this latter symptom gives yellow fever one of its most infamous nicknames, "vomito negro." The extensive blood loss also causes a major drop in blood pressure, which subsequently leads to severe fatigue, multiple organ failure, delirium, and finally death. It is a terrifying and excruciating way to die that no doubt strikes fear into all those who witness it.

Yellow fever is caused by a small virus that is transmitted to humans through the bite of a female mosquito belonging to the genus *Aedes*. This virus, appropriately named yellow fever virus (YFV), is a member of a group of viruses (called flaviviruses) that also includes the Zika, Dengue, and West Nile viruses. Flaviviruses share a propensity to be transmitted between vertebrate hosts by some arthropod vector (mosquito or tick), and most cause severe internal hemorrhaging and/or encephalitis. In the case of YFV, the mosquito species that is most commonly involved in spreading the virus during large-scale epidemics is *Aedes aegypti*.

Upon entering a mosquito, YFV replicates in the epithelial cells of the gut and then eventually spreads to its blood and salivary glands. When the infected mosquito bites a human, the virus is transmitted from the mosquito saliva into the host tissue near the bite wound. The virus is rapidly eaten by local immune cells called dendritic cells and is then transported to the nearest lymph nodes. Rather than being destroyed by immune cells in the lymph nodes, YFV actually has the ability to replicate in these cells and kill them. Doing so allows large quantities of the virus to spill into the blood and disseminate to the liver, spleen, heart, kidneys, and several other organs. After reaching those sites, YFV infects local tissues and begins the process of replication all over again. The host immune system detects that this is occurring and sends immune cell reinforcements to the infected areas. Trying to stop or at least slow the progression of the virus, arriving immune cells release massive quantities of toxic inflammatory chemicals called cytokines into the infected tissues. Although such a response is normally very protective against viral infections, the sheer quantity of inflammatory mediators released creates a toxic environment for host cells and accidentally starts to kill them. Dying host cells release more inflammatory chemicals, which causes a further amplification of the damaging immune response. The end result is that both YFV and host immune response kill a great deal of host cells in a variety of tissues. Such damage leads to fever, liver destruction, shock, and the rest of the symptoms mentioned previously.

Yellow fever has killed several million people since first being described in the 1640s. Although mosquito-control measures and an effective vaccine currently limit the epidemic potential of YFV, it continues to infect about 200,000 people a year and kill 30,000 of them. Most cases of yellow fever occur in tropical regions of central Africa and South America due to their plentiful rainfall and abundant sources of warm water that serve as breeding grounds for the *Aedes aegypti* mosquito vector. Unfortunately for those living in these endemic areas, *Aedes aegypti* is adept at surviving in both urban and rural environments.

Yellow fever can spread very rapidly in densely populated cities as long as mosquitoes have enough open water sources in which to lay their eggs. Periods of excessive rain or disruptions in city services or infrastructure can be enough to trigger an explosion in the mosquito population and cause an outbreak of yellow fever. This exact situation occurred in Angola's capital city of Luanda in 2016.[2] Despite not having any cases of yellow fever for over 30 years, Angola experienced a reemergence of the disease because of disruptions in the city's garbage collection. The excessive trash buildup served as a reservoir for rainwater and provided the perfect environment for *Aedes aegypti* larvae to develop. Within just a few months, hundreds of people died and thousands of others became sick throughout the city. It was a stark reminder that yellow fever is still an extremely dangerous disease that will continue to plague humankind as long as we ignore lessons learned from the past.

The Arrival of the Great American Plague

The origin of yellow fever has been one of the most hotly debated topics in epidemiology over the last 50 years. One reason for this is that there is no mention of a disease that resembles modern-day yellow fever in any ancient record from Europe, Asia, or the Middle East. Famed physicians Hippocrates and Galen fail to mention yellow fever in the Corpus or any other comprehensive medical texts of ancient Greece. Similarly, there are no clinical descriptions of yellow fever in historical writings from the Turks, Chinese, or Romans. As a result, there is little information to draw from when trying to create a model to explain how yellow fever arose and spread to two continents on separate sides of the world. Another issue regarding yellow fever's origins has to do with the fact that it is equally endemic on those two continents. Many have cited the glaring lack of yellow fever in the writings of Portuguese explorers and slave traders who colonized much of the west coast of Africa and use it as evidence that it probably did not originate there. Additionally, proponents of an American origin of yellow fever also point to its widespread distribution in the jungles of the Amazon basin by the 18th century as evidence that it was likely there for many centuries before.

While such explanations sound perfectly logical, a genetic analysis of over 130 different YFV strains done in the early 2000s strongly suggest that yellow fever did in fact originate in Africa and later spread to the Americas.[3] These studies compared the genome sequences of YFV strains from all over Africa and South America in an effort to ascertain which gave rise to the other. Interestingly, the strains from East Africa appeared to be "older" and genetically distinct from those isolated from West Africa or South America. Taken together, the data suggest that yellow fever likely evolved from some other flavivirus in East Africa, spread to West Africa, and then moved to the Americas during the transatlantic slave trade about 500 years ago.

Some have speculated that yellow fever made its first appearance in the Americas in March 1495 when Christopher Columbus attacked and enslaved the native Taino population on the Caribbean island of Hispaniola.[4] Vague accounts of the Battle of Vega Real indicate that many of the Taino natives and some of the Spanish colonizers died of the same disease during and after the battle. However, other than the mention of a fever, few of these descriptions lead one to a firm conclusion that it was yellow fever and not measles, smallpox, influenza, or one of many other European diseases.

Yellow fever likely made the journey to the Americas aboard one of the many slave ships that crossed the Atlantic Ocean during the early 16th century. These ships likely carried stowaway *Aedes aegypti* mosquitoes infected with YFV that had unlimited access to hundreds of malnourished slaves packed tightly into poorly ventilated cargo holds. Upon arriving at the various tropical Caribbean islands, mosquitoes escaped the ships and found a climate that was very similar to that of western Africa. Before long, *Aedes aegypti* established itself in the Caribbean and began to regularly feed on the large, dense populations of Amerindians and European colonizers in those locations. This gave YFV its first opportunity to firmly establish itself in the human population and begin the process of producing large-scale epidemics.

The first truly definitive description of yellow fever was in 1647 during an outbreak of the disease on the island of Barbados.[5] A Jesuit priest named Father Dutertre, who was an eyewitness of the new "plague," described a disease that produced extreme head and muscle aches, fever, and "continual vomiting." This latter symptom, the black vomit, distinguished the 1647 Barbados outbreak from all previous mentions of New World fevers introduced by the Europeans (e.g., the unknown fever in Guadeloupe in 1643). His account is supported by several others who were either witnesses or had received reports from colonists. For instance, the governor of Massachusetts at the time, John Winthrop, wrote in his journal in 1647 about a "great mortality," a "pestilent fever" that killed over 6,000 Barbadians prior to moving on to other nearby islands like St. Christopher (St. Kitts) and Guadeloupe.[6]

Yellow fever traveled rapidly through the rest of the Caribbean islands and finally made it onto the North American mainland in 1648 (Yucatan). Cuba suffered an especially devastating yellow fever outbreak in 1649. According to the historian Pezuela, Cuba "was pitilessly attacked by an unknown and horrible epidemic, imported from the American continent, one third of its population being devoured by a sort of a putrid fever."[7] Yellow fever was now in the Americas to stay. It would continue to jump from the Caribbean islands to various port cities in the Americas for over 200 years, wreaking havoc everywhere it went. It was so commonly spread via cargo vessels during this time that ships had to develop a special yellow flag that they would fly if someone on board had come down with yellow fever while at sea. That flag, and the disease in general, soon gained the nickname "Yellow Jack."

Despite the fact that yellow fever originated in Africa and killed millions there over the course of its history, the disease, historically, has been thought of as an "American plague." This is due in large part to the fact that it has been endemic in sub-Saharan Africa since the 17th century. Continual exposure to YFV has provided enough immunity in the African population to limit large-scale epidemics. In contrast, most of the Europeans who colonized the Americas had little exposure to YFV. They were a virgin population that was highly susceptible to being wiped out by the virus. As a result, yellow fever was able to play an enormous role in shaping the history of European colonial rule in the Americas, and it drastically impacted the growth and development of the young United States.

Philadelphia Epidemic of 1793

Philadelphia was one of the most important cities in the United States in the late 18th century. It had served as the site of the Constitutional Convention in 1787 and became the temporary capital of the new nation in December 1790. During this time, it was home to many founding fathers, including Washington, Adams, Jefferson, Franklin, and Hamilton, and it housed the first U.S. Congress, Supreme Court, and Mint. As a center of commerce, Philadelphia had one of the most active ports in the country, trading goods with cities all over the United States, Europe, and the West Indies. It was unusually tolerant of different religious traditions and accepting of former (freed) slaves and so it became a popular destination city for refugees. As a result, by 1790, Philadelphia (with its suburbs) had become the most populous city in the nation, a thriving, culturally rich mecca that served as a shining example of what the new United States could become. It was unthinkable that this political and economic nerve center of the new nation could be brought to its knees by the arrival of a simple mosquito, but in 1793, that is exactly what happened.

Ships carrying roughly 2,000 colonial refugees and slaves arrived in Philadelphia from the Caribbean island of St. Domingue (Haiti) in June 1793.[8] A violent slave rebellion had erupted there in 1791 and subsequently plunged the entire colony into civil war. Slaves fought for independence while several of the colonial powers there (e.g., Great Britain, France, Spain) fought with one another. It created a dangerous environment that led many of the white European colonists to flee and seek refuge in cities like Philadelphia, Charleston, and New Orleans. Philadelphians were generally welcoming of the refugees, even raising $16,000 for their support. However, their hospitality began to wane as news emerged that a yellow fever epidemic had hit the city, and the source was likely the ships that carried the refugees from St. Domingue.

As the disease began to spread throughout the city in early August, a group of prominent physicians led by Benjamin Rush met to discuss how to best contain, or at least slow, the epidemic.[9] They published a series of suggested measures in the local newspaper and recommended that anyone with the means should leave the city at once. By early September, the epidemic showed no signs of slowing and panic soon set in. Thousands of people fled the city, including George Washington and most of the federal government. Thomas Jefferson, in a letter written to James Madison on September 1, 1793, accurately describes the panic in the city when he stated,

> A malignant fever has been generated in the filth of Water Street which gives great alarm. About 70. people had died of it two days ago, & as many more were ill of it. It has now got into most parts of the city & is considerably infectious. At first 3. out of 4. died. Now about 1. out of 3. It comes on with a pain in the head, sick stomach, then a little chill, fever, black vomiting & stools, & death from the 2d. to the 8th. day. Everybody, who can, is flying from the city, and the panic of the country people is likely to add famine to disease. Tho becoming less mortal, it is still spreading, and the heat of the weather is very unpropitious. I have withdrawn my daughter from the city, but am obliged to go to it every day myself.[10]

Nearly 20,000 Philadelphia residents left the city that summer (40% of the population) and over 4,000 died from yellow fever (around 10% of the population). The epidemic finally subsided in early November due to the cool fall temperatures reducing the size of the mosquito population. Residents gradually returned to the city and the federal government resumed its normal functions. However, the psyche of the city, and the nation as a whole, had been wounded by the yellow fever epidemic of 1793. It glaringly exposed the new nation's inability to effectively respond to crisis. Leaders fled, health officials argued, and citizens turned on one another as the capital of the United States was essentially abandoned in a matter of just a couple of months.

One of the more interesting long-term impacts of the 1793 yellow fever epidemic was how it affected race relations in Philadelphia. The city had become a destination for African Americans in the years that followed the Revolutionary War. Many had earned their freedom by fighting for the Continental Army, some had been freed by slave owners who were moved by the ideals of the revolution, and still others had escaped slavery and fled north. By the time the 1793 epidemic hit, over 2,000 free African Americans were living in Philadelphia.[11] Many had organized into civic organizations that provided social and employment services to the growing African American community. One of the most influential of such groups was the Free African Society, which was founded in 1787 and led by ministers Richard Allen and Absalom Jones. They met regularly as a group to decide how to best educate their children, obtain jobs for the unemployed, care for widows and orphans, and empower members of their community to become truly independent. They were the central voice of the African American community in Philadelphia for many decades.

At the time of the epidemic, there was a popular belief that people of African descent were "genetically" resistant to yellow fever infection.[12] This idea came about from observations during a 1742 yellow fever outbreak in Charleston, South Carolina, in which African slaves living in affected areas seemed to rarely contract the disease themselves. This was likely due to the fact that many of those slaves were born and raised in Africa where yellow fever was endemic. As a result, they were likely exposed to YFV at an early age and gained some level of immunity to it. The situation was quite a bit different in Philadelphia 50 years later. Most of the African Americans living in the United States then were born in the United States. Such individuals had little to no exposure to YFV and were therefore no more protected against the disease than anyone else. This disconnect between what the medical community believed, that all African Americans had intrinsic resistance to yellow fever, and the reality, which was that they did not, would prove to be significant for the African American community living in Philadelphia in 1793.

When yellow fever broke out in the city, Benjamin Rush and other physicians publicly reached out to leaders of the Free African Society seeking help with taking care of the thousands of sick.[13] Absalom Jones and Richard Allen discussed the matter with others in the group and ultimately decided that "it was our duty to do all the good we could to our suffering fellow mortals. We set out to see where we could be useful."[14] Encouraged by the false belief that they were protected, hundreds of African Americans began working throughout the city as emergency nurses and body transporters. While most of the city's residents were either fleeing or isolating themselves from anyone they believe to be infected (including their own family members), the African American community stayed and diligently served the sick. Benjamin Rush once observed that "in every room you enter you see no person but a solitary black man or woman near the sick."[15] Even as increasing numbers of African Americans became sick and died themselves, they stayed and kept caring for the afflicted. They stayed despite working in unimaginably dreadful conditions and receiving relatively little compensation in return.[16] By the time the epidemic was over, nearly 250 African Americans had died of yellow fever. This represented about 10 percent of their population in Philadelphia, which was about the same death rate for whites living there.

One may think that the heroic sacrifices made by the African American community during the 1793 yellow fever epidemic would have earned them acceptance by the white establishment in Philadelphia. Unfortunately, it ended up having the opposite effect. An extremely popular and widely distributed pamphlet published in November 1793 suggested that African

American caretakers financially took advantage of the victims of the epidemic. The author, a prominent publisher named Mathew Carey who fled the city early in the epidemic, claimed, "The great demand for nurses, afforded an opportunity for imposition, which was eagerly seized by some of those who acted in that capacity, both coloured and white. They extorted two, three, four, and even five dollars a night for such attendance, as would have been well paid for, by a single dollar. Some of them were even detected in plundering the houses of the sick."[17] Accusations of extortion and theft led to great public resentment against the Free African Society and those it employed during the epidemic. Despite little actual evidence that African Americans profited dishonestly from their service, Carey's *A Short Account of the Malignant Fever* caused irreparable damage to the reputation of the entire community. His pamphlet successfully destroyed any good will that had developed between the races during those five months and caused African Americans to be even more reviled in Philadelphia after the epidemic than before it.

In response, Jones and Allen published their own account of the epidemic in an attempt to refute Carey's slanderous claims.[18] In it, they provided a scathing criticism of Carey for inaccurately reporting events that he was not there to witness and even suggested that he profited more from the misery of the epidemic than all the extortionists put together. They go on to convincingly refute claims of price gouging by their nurses and state that they "buried several hundreds of poor persons and strangers, for which service we have never received nor never asked any compensation."[19] Unfortunately, their logical and well-defended rebuttal largely fell on deaf ears due in part to the fact that Carey had already published four editions of his pamphlet before theirs was written. The damage had been done. Many in Philadelphia had now come to despise the same African Americans who were caring for them just months earlier.

The 1793 yellow fever epidemic also triggered a great debate as to what caused it. One of the prevailing theories among medical professionals like Benjamin Rush was that the epidemic was caused by widespread filth that had contaminated both the air and water of the city. The stench produced by pooling sewage and garbage, combined with the hot, stagnant air in Philadelphia that summer, was thought to have produced a toxic combination of miasma that gave rise to the disease. Architect Benjamin Latrobe echoed these sentiments when he stated, "we have a proof that there does exist in the mode by which the city is supplied by water a very abundant source of disease, independent of the noxious exhalations of the narrow and filthy alleys and lanes."[20] In contrast to the unsanitary state of the city, some prominent religious leaders in Philadelphia pointed to moral filth as the primary cause of the epidemic. Groups like the Quakers believed Pennsylvania's refusal to formally abolish slavery or prohibit "immoral" theatrical performances contaminated the spiritual health of the city and led to God's judgment in the form of yellow fever. The recent arrival of colonial refugees, who often owned slaves themselves or supported the extreme violence of the French Revolution, only further exacerbated this moral decay in their eyes. The fact that yellow fever seemed to strike port cities at a much higher rate than others only strengthened the idea that refugees, because of their "poor constitution," were the ones who carried yellow fever to Philadelphia in 1793.

The collective response from these theories was a major push to clean up Philadelphia following the epidemic. A committee led by the mayor Matthew Clarkson first called for major improvements in public sanitation, which included bringing in clean water from outside of the city, improving the sewer system, and disinfecting the homes of the poor. While such measures had no impact on yellow fever outbreaks since it is spread by mosquitoes and not poor sanitation, they did indirectly help with other diseases such as typhoid and cholera.

When yellow fever returned to Philadelphia in 1797, 1798, and 1799, city officials began looking at ways to monitor the large number of immigrants who were pouring into the city and believed to be carrying the disease with them. Normal ship quarantines were clearly not working to prevent the introduction of yellow fever and so the Philadelphia Board of Health decided

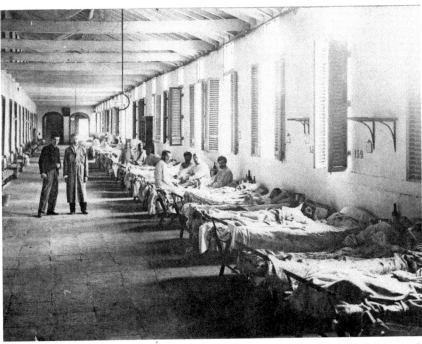

Patients in yellow fever hospital in Havana, Cuba, ca. 1899. (Library of Congress)

to address the problem by constructing a permanent, 10-acre quarantine hospital on the banks of the Delaware River.[21] This facility, called the Lazaretto, had a hospital run by qualified medical personnel and residence halls for large numbers of people. It was designed to receive all immigrants who were entering into Philadelphia, inspect them and their cargo for disease, and then release them into the city only after deeming them to be "clean." It was the virtual gatekeeper of the city, screening millions of immigrants from all over the world for many different types of infectious disease. Opening in 1799, the Lazaretto was the first of its kind in the United States. It revolutionized how the country received and processed immigrants and created the model that was eventually used by other, more famous quarantine hospitals like Ellis Island (NY) and Angel Island (CA). It is impossible to estimate how many epidemics were averted and lives saved as a result of Lazaretto and the other similar quarantine hospitals. Although Lazaretto was built in direct response to multiple yellow fever epidemics, it likely saved the lives of millions who would have died had other diseases like typhus, cholera, smallpox, and plague reached Philadelphia and other large U.S. cities.

The Haitian Revolution and Louisiana Purchase

The French colonial empire in the Americas began when explorers founded several cities along the St. Lawrence River at the start of the 17th century. Fur traders arrived soon thereafter and established business partnerships with many of the native tribes already living in the new French colony. Such relationships enabled the French to maintain some level of administrative control over its sparsely populated Canadian territory while also providing them with the means by which to expand their operations westward toward the Great Lakes and Mississippi River. By the 1680s, the French had set up trading posts and forts all along the Mississippi River and formally established a new colonial territory in the South known as Louisiana. With Canada, Newfoundland, and Acadia in the north, the new Southern colony gave France a total of three million square miles of land in North America. At its height in the early 18th century, this expansive territory, known as New France, stretched over half of modern-day Canada in the north, as far west as the Rocky Mountains, and all the way south to the Gulf of Mexico.

Following the lead of Spain and Great Britain, France also laid claim to several small islands in the West Indies during this time.[22] Upon arriving on islands like Martinique, Guadeloupe, St. Kitts, St. Lucia, and Hispaniola/Saint-Domingue (Haiti), French settlers enslaved or killed most of the indigenous populations (e.g., Caribs) and then imported large numbers of African slaves to work on newly built plantations. Despite their small size when compared to New France, these island colonies were extremely profitable for

France. For instance, nearly 40 percent of all the sugar and 75 percent of all the coffee sold on the entire continent of Europe was produced on French-owned plantations in the West Indies. Together with its lucrative fur industry in North America, these West Indian plantations helped make France one of the richest nations in the world in the 17th and 18th centuries.

Most of the French colonial empire in the Americas was lost to Great Britain and Spain as a result of several wars fought in the mid-18th century. Tensions began rising between French and British colonists as large numbers of new British settlers flooded into the Americas at about the same time that the French were building forts very close to British-controlled territories. Fearing eventual military action by the French or their Native American allies, a local British militia led by George Washington preemptively ambushed a small French camp near Pittsburgh, Pennsylvania, in May of 1754, sparking the French and Indian War.[23] This action led to a strong military response by local French troops, which resulted in a quick surrender by Washington. British and French authorities in Europe, realizing that they may be on the brink of a full-scale war in the Americas, reached out to one another soon thereafter to discuss potential peaceful solutions to these border skirmishes. Unable to come to an agreement, both parties dispatched large numbers of troops from Europe to fight over what they believed to be their rightful claims in North America. This war lasted about nine years and ended when France surrendered in the signing of the Treaty of Paris. In doing so, France gave up its territorial rights to all of New France, including Canada and Louisiana, and most of its West Indian island colonies. Great Britain took control of most of the land east of the Mississippi River whereas Spain, Great Britain's military ally, took control of lands in the west. France eventually regained a small amount territory in the West Indies through its involvement in the American Revolution.

The most important colonial territory held by France during the tumultuous 18th century was Saint-Domingue (Haiti) on the western side of Hispaniola. It was arguably the richest European colony in the world at the time, supplying enormous amounts of sugar and coffee to the Americas, Europe, and Asia. During its peak in the 1780s, it contained roughly 800 independent plantations that were worked by over 465,000 slaves.[24] Amazingly, Saint-Domingue and two other French island colonies (Martinique and Guadeloupe) held as many slaves as the entire original 13 states of the United States put together (roughly 700,000). Thousands of new West African slaves arrived in Saint-Domingue every year, and thousands more were born on the island. By the time the French Revolution began in 1789, Saint-Domingue had become a virtual melting pot of both African- and Caribbean-born slaves, white colonists, runaway slaves living free in the mountains, and about 25,000 free persons of color called *gens de couleur libres*. This latter group consisted mostly of the mixed-race descendants of French slave owners and their female slaves. They were often educated, and some had inherited great wealth from their French fathers.

The French Revolution caused a major stir among the inhabitants of Saint-Domingue.[25] For white plantation owners, the Revolution provided an opportunity to escape the administrative grip of the French government and become more autonomous when trading their goods with other countries. They saw it as a welcomed chance to increase their profit margin while exerting greater control over their slaves and product. In contrast, slaves and freed people of color on the island read the revolutionary Declaration of the Rights of Man and of the Citizen and its assertion that "men are born and remain free and equal in rights" as hope for their own freedom and equal rights.[26] They were supported by many in the newly formed French General Assembly, who had seen the horrors of slavery and believed it should be abolished throughout the empire. Several of the wealthy freed men of color (e.g., Julien Raimond and Vincent Ogé) also traveled from Saint-Domingue to Paris to appear before the General Assembly and speak on behalf of all the discriminated people on their island. Upon returning to Saint-Domingue, they found colonial governors and plantation owners unwilling to give up their free source of labor or grant increased rights to anyone that may threaten their power over the island. This disconnect between the wealthy, white minority on Saint-Domingue and the people of color that outnumbered them 10 to 1 set the stage for one of the most significant events in the history of the Americas, the Haitian Revolution.

The Haitian Revolution began in August of 1791 when slaves in the Northern Province of the island mounted an armed revolt against white plantation owners in the region. They burned hundreds of plantations, killed thousands of white colonists, and confiscated millions of dollars of property.[27] Within a few months, over 100,000 slaves had joined in the revolt and together they gained control over a third of the colony. At the same time the slaves were revolting in the north, free people of color began moving against white plantation owners in the west. In an attempt to appease the revolutionaries and hopefully quell the rebellion, the French General (Legislative) Assembly granted full political rights to the free people of color in 1792. Despite this olive branch, the violence escalated in 1793 when plantation owners formed an alliance with Great Britain and slaves joined the invading Spanish to force the French off of the island. This gave the British military virtual control of most of Saint-Domingue. Fearing that a multipronged war may lead to a total loss of the island, local French administrators responded by unilaterally declaring an end to slavery on Saint-Domingue. As a result, many of the newly freed slaves, led by the brilliant military general (and former slave) Toussaint L'Ouverture, switched alliances back to the French. For the next five years, France, Great Britain, Spain, freed slaves, and white colonists engaged in a prolonged and bloody war that resulted in several hundred thousand deaths.

Historical records indicate that a great many of the deaths on the British side came at the hands of a yellow fever outbreak that was occurring in the West Indies during the 1790s. In fact, some have estimated that nearly 70 percent of the British force, or roughly 100,000 soldiers, became sickened by yellow fever between 1793 and 1798.[28] Weakened by chronic illness and ongoing fighting with L'Ouverture's army, the British finally agreed to leave Saint-Domingue in 1798. L'Ouverture followed this victory by invading and conquering the Spanish-controlled eastern side of Hispaniola in 1800. Although L'Ouverture essentially had political control of the entire island at this point, he had yet to achieve full sovereignty and total independence from France. Unfortunately for L'Ouverture, a new ruler by the name of Napoleon Bonaparte had just ascended to power in France and had aspirations for the reemergence of a colonial empire in the Americas.

In early 1802, Napoleon sent about 60,000 troops to Saint-Domingue with the purpose of regaining administrative control of the island and its very profitable sugar plantations.[29] Beyond simply taking over the land, Napoleon had planned on crushing the revolt and restoring slavery on Saint-Domingue (which he had already done on several other West Indian islands). Upon arriving on Saint-Domingue, the sizable French force, led by Napoleon's brother-in-law Charles Leclerc, quickly took over most of the port cities on the island and had the *de facto* leader L'Ouverture secretly arrested and deported to Europe (where he would die of tuberculosis in prison). The loss of L'Ouverture caused many of the other resistance leaders to desert their posts and join forces with the French. The slave revolt, which had been going on for over 11 years at this point, looked to be on the verge of total collapse. Those who had lived and fought as free men for so long were now facing the very real possibility of becoming enslaved once again. When all looked lost for the inhabitants of Saint-Domingue, a change in weather occurred that essentially saved their movement and altered the course of history.

The start of spring in 1802 brought major increases in rainfall and an explosion in the *Aedes* mosquito population.[30] By May of that year, a full-blown yellow fever epidemic had struck the island. As it had previously done with the British occupiers, yellow fever decimated the French due to the fact they had almost no previous exposure to the disease. As many as 50,000 French soldiers died of yellow fever over the next one-and-a-half years, which wiped out nearly 80 percent of their fighting force. Among the many victims of the 1802–1803 epidemic were Leclerc and five of his generals.[31] Leaderless, sick, and facing fierce resistance from an increasingly powerful native army, most the remaining French troops began withdrawing from the island in fall of 1803. The last French forces were defeated by L'Ouverture's successor Jean-Jacques Dessalines soon thereafter, and the new, sovereign nation of Haiti formally declared its independence on January 1, 1804. Without yellow fever as their ally, it is highly possible that the Haitian people would have been defeated by the overpowering French army and been returned to slavery. Instead, they completed the only successful slave revolt in history that resulted in the creation of a new sovereign state.

The successful slave revolt on Saint-Domingue had other very important long-term consequences in the Americas. Historians largely believe that Napoleon sent troops to the West Indies in order to set up an eventual invasion of the North American mainland.[32] In 1801, France had secretly acquired all of the Louisiana territory from the Spanish that had been lost as a result of the French and Indian War. Napoleon did this with the intention of eventually sending his military to regain control of New Orleans and the lucrative Mississippi Valley, which had become increasingly infiltrated with traders from the new United States. In a correspondence to one of his defense ministers, Napoleon made it clear that the invasion of Saint-Domingue was just a front for his true goal of a restored North American empire. In this letter, he wrote, "My intention, Citizen Minister, is that we take possession of Louisiana with the shortest possible delay, that this expedition be organized in the greatest secrecy, and that it have the appearance of being directed on St. Domingo."[33] Thomas Jefferson and others in the U.S. government saw Napoleon's move into the West Indies and Louisiana as a threat to their own sovereignty. Based on his actions in Europe, it is quite reasonable to believe that Napoleon would have eventually tried to expand his empire beyond the borders of Louisiana. Unfortunately for him, the unprecedented yellow fever epidemic on Saint-Domingue destroyed any possibility of a North American invasion. Napoleon needed the profitable sugar plantations on the island in order to fund the next steps in his plan. Without that money, an invasion of North America could not proceed. Realizing that there was no way to outmaneuver, out-strategize, or overpower yellow fever, Napoleon decided to cut his losses in the Americas. At the height of the epidemic in 1803, Napoleon agreed to sell the entirety of the Louisiana territory to the United States for the ridiculously low price of just $15 million. In doing so, the United States roughly doubled its size and France was out of the Americas for good. Soon thereafter, Thomas Jefferson sent Meriwether Lewis and William Clark on an expedition to explore this new western territory.

Plague of the American South

With the opening up of the Louisiana territory in the early 19th century, growing Southern cities saw significant increases in trade with the West Indies and other ports along the Gulf of Mexico and Mississippi River. While such maritime trade was critical to growth of the Southern economy, it had the unwelcomed drawback of repeatedly exposing the population to yellow fever. As mentioned previously, the disease had become endemic throughout the West Indies by the 18th century due to its tropical climate and ongoing role in the Atlantic slave trade. Ships arriving from the West Indies very often carried people infected with yellow fever or cargo infiltrated with stowaway mosquitoes. As a result, epidemics arose in the South on almost a yearly basis in areas all along the Mississippi River, Gulf coast, and southern Atlantic seaboard. Unlike the sporadic epidemics experienced in northern cities like Philadelphia and New York, the continuously warm, moist climate of the American South provided a perfect breeding ground for yellow fever to become almost endemic in many of cities there. One of the hardest hit cities, New Orleans, experienced 12 epidemics in the years leading up to the American Civil War. Its 1853 epidemic is believed to

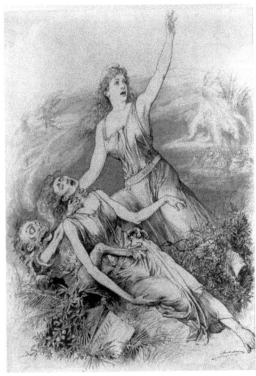

Illustration of a woman representing the state of Florida laying on the ground in the clutches of a monster labeled "Yellow Jack." (Library of Congress)

have infected nearly 40 percent of the city's population and claimed the lives of about 7,800 people.[34] Twenty-five years later, another major epidemic swept through New Orleans and gradually moved up the Mississippi River aboard steamboats. The 1878 Lower Mississippi Valley epidemic sickened over 120,000 people in over 200 different cities and killed as many as 20,000.[35] Similar, less destructive, epidemics also arose in Charleston, Norfolk, Memphis, Savannah, Galveston, and many other Southern cities in the middle of the 19th century. Although death rates of these epidemics pale in comparison to those of typhus, smallpox, and other diseases discussed in this book, they caused widespread panic and had profound effects on all aspects of life in the South.

One of the more interesting by-products of the ongoing yellow fever presence in the American South is how it affected attitudes toward those living there. The epidemics spiked in the South in the years immediately preceding the Civil War when the country was embroiled in fierce debates about slavery. The fact that Northern states, which had abolished slavery decades earlier, saw concurrent declines in yellow fever outbreaks during this same time period led many abolitionists to conclude that yellow fever was acting as an agent of divine punishment against the South and its inhabitants for the evil of slavery. To them, the widespread presence of yellow fever served as proof that slavery was wrong and the Southern way of life was inferior to their own. Such sinfulness was amplified by the perceived debauchery and depravity found in many Southern cities at the time. Bars, brothels, gambling houses, and the annual celebration of Mardi Gras were commonly blamed for yellow fever. A prayer written in 1853 by a Southern bishop named Leonidas Polk nicely illustrates this sentiment when he stated that "Our sins justly provoked thy wrath and indignation against us . . . and mercifully grant . . . that this fatherly correction, may teach us . . . hereafter to be mindful of thy righteous judgement."[36] Cities like New Orleans were increasingly portrayed in the Northern media as sinful cesspools filled with disease, chaos, and filth. Sensationalized articles and graphic engravings illustrating people in the throes of yellow fever also began appearing in newspapers throughout the country. The result of such reporting was that many of those in the North came to view the victims of these Southern epidemics with a mixture of righteous indignation and disgust.

To white Southerners, these yellow fever epidemics served to reinforce their predetermined belief that African slaves were better suited for work outdoors than whites because they seemed to die less frequently from the disease. As was the case in the 1793 Philadelphia epidemic, many at the time incorrectly believed that people of African descent had some sort of innate genetic resistance to yellow fever. Despite evidence from that epidemic that showed the contrary, many continued to assert that Africans were designed, through thousands years of evolution and exposure, to tolerate yellow fever better than other races.[37] The observation that Africans often had innate resistance to malaria led to the assumption that the same must also be true for yellow fever since both diseases arose in Africa. Such ideas allowed Southerners to justify the continued use of African slaves in areas experiencing frequent yellow fever outbreaks (which was most of the South). According to proslavery advocates, work outdoors was just too dangerous for whites and so they had no choice but to keep using slaves. Slavery was thus presented as being a necessary institution because of yellow fever. In actuality, slavery and yellow fever had quite the converse relationship. Yellow fever only existed in the Americas because of the slave trade. Without the continued illegal importation of slaves into the West Indies and America, the South would have likely experienced significantly fewer yellow fever epidemics.

The 1853 and 1878 epidemics also had a tremendously destructive impact on the economies of Southern cities that were trying to establish themselves as centers of commerce.[38] The death and incapacitation of so many people in a largely agricultural region led to the loss of millions of dollars worth of produce and cash crops that either went unharvested or unsold or became rotten. This created significant food shortages that further stressed already depleted municipal and state budgets. Tourism also saw precipitous declines during this time period due to the South's growing negative reputation among Northerners and due to the use of quarantines that restricted travel into affected cities. Quarantines, though somewhat effective in slowing the spread of yellow fever, were devastating to trade and commerce in the South. Many cities forced local businesses to shut down for extended periods until epidemics subsided, and merchants often experienced great difficulty in selling their goods to unaffected areas. As a result, quarantines were often bitterly opposed by local businesses and those politicians loyal to them. This created unnecessary factional tension among city leaders when they needed to be unified against what many referred to at the time as "the worst urban disaster in American history." No one knows the true economic cost of the many yellow fever epidemics that hit the South in the 19th century. However, one report published in 1879 estimated the cost of the 1878 epidemic alone to be over $200 million (about $4 billion in today's dollars). This unbelievable cost is even more staggering when considering the fact that the Southern economy was crippled by the Civil War just 13 years earlier and was already struggling to rebuild and industrialize.

Probably the most significant long-term consequence of these epidemics was a reassessment of who is responsible for the health of the population. Up until this point, all decisions regarding sanitation, quarantines, and public health were made at the local level by city officials. State and federal governments had almost no power to make or enforce policies related to public health or did they have much regulatory oversight as to how cities responded to epidemics. This led to great inconsistencies between cities and even in cities depending on who held political office that year. A poor response to an outbreak by one city often allowed yellow fever to spread to towns nearby, which created further opportunities for the disease to disseminate throughout the country. For instance, in the 1878 epidemic, yellow fever first arrived in the United States when a ship from Cuba docked in New Orleans carrying an infected crew member.[39] The disease quickly spread to others in the city and a full-blown epidemic emerged by middle of the summer. Although a quarantine was enacted by city officials, thousands fled to the surrounding Mississippi Valley without any real screening beforehand. Unfortunately, several infected individuals boarded a towboat for Vicksburg, Mississippi, and delivered the disease there. From there, it moved onto Memphis (on another boat) and eventually to 200 other cities throughout the South via railroads and river traffic. Some cities resorted to setting up armed barricades to prevent anyone who had fled the epidemic from coming into their town whereas others destroyed railroad lines or stopped ships from docking in their ports. In the end, such local measures proved to be grossly ineffective at stopping a disease that could literally spread with the wind. To make matters worse, it was extremely common for municipal leaders to flee from cities in the grips of the epidemic. This made enforcement of any sanitation or quarantine measures nearly impossible.

The inability of cities to effectively prevent or manage yellow fever (and cholera) in the middle of the 19th century led to the creation of a number of regional, state, and federal boards of health. These committees were charged with collecting and disseminating data regarding local outbreaks and then deciding on proper quarantine measures independent of local business interests. They also sought to stop cities from hiding the presence of yellow fever (so not to hurt its own business interests) and compel local health agencies to work with one another. The most significant such board, the National Board of Health, was created in 1879 as a result of broad public outcry following the devastation of 1878.[40] One congressman, speaking about the need for a federal board that oversees public health, said, "The experience of the past has taught us that no seaport town having any commerce will ever adopt and adhere to any quarantine regulation which will interfere to any great extent with their commercial interests."[41] The Surgeon General of Marine Hospital Service at the time, John Woodworth, added, "Yellow fever should be dealt with as an enemy which imperils life and cripples commerce and industry. To no other great nation of the earth is yellow fever so calamitous as to the United States of America."[42]

After some deliberation about fine details, the U.S. Congress passed a bill on March 3, 1879, that created a national board of civilian and military experts that would oversee and advise local health boards, investigate public health issues, disseminate funds to areas experiencing public health crises, and standardize quarantine procedures. It was hoped that this board would identify all of the mistakes that occurred during the widespread 1878 epidemic and fix them to prevent future outbreaks. Although it was funded for only four years and never fully achieved all of its goals, the National Board of Health did help initiate a nationwide improvement in public sanitation, which helped reduce outbreaks of cholera and typhoid.[43] It also created a model that would be used later by more permanent agencies like the U.S. Public Health Service.

The creation of the National Board was a significant turning point because it represented the first step in fighting epidemic disease as a nation rather than as disparate cities and states in the years immediately following the Civil War. In a way, yellow fever helped unify the country against a common enemy, making people realize that the health of individuals is truly dependent on the health of the whole.

Identifying the Carrier

The single most significant barrier to controlling yellow fever in the 19th century was not knowing how it was being transmitted. Most physicians and health officials at the time believed it was spread by poor sanitation and the resulting buildup of toxic miasma. Since mosquito-borne diseases like yellow fever, malaria, and dengue fever are relatively unaffected by environmental filth, attempts by health boards to prevent or limit the spread of YFV through improved sanitation had little to no effect on its prevalence in the population. As a result, it continued to plague much of the southern United States, Latin America, Caribbean, and West Africa for many years after the great 1878 epidemic. However, as microbiological methods began to improve near the end of the century and the United States became embroiled in a war that was being hindered by yellow fever, scientists and politicians made a renewed push to elucidate how the disease was being transmitted.

The epicenter of yellow fever research during this time was the Caribbean island of Cuba, which was only 90 miles away from the United States and was one of its major suppliers of sugar, tobacco, coffee, and various other cash crops. The relationship between the United States and Cuba in the 19th century was complex. On the one hand, the two were mutually dependent for their economic prosperity.[44] A staggering 90 percent of all Cuban exports were shipped to the United States during the 1890s, and roughly 38 percent of all Cuban imports came from the United States. About $50 million worth of U.S. capital had been invested into Cuba for the purchase and modernization of failing mines and sugar plantations there and American workers were flooding into Cuba at an unprecedented rate. While this seems to have been an ideal business partnership for everyone involved, it was complicated by the fact that Cuba was still under the political control of the Spanish Empire during the 19th century. Spain had the power to change trading laws, impose tariffs, and control the way business was conducted in Cuba. As a result, those in the United States were forced to constantly walk a tightrope between keeping Spanish politicians happy and maintaining strong business relationships with Cubans who were being subjugated by them.

The delicate relationship between the United States, Cuba, and Spain became severely strained in 1895 when Cuban rebels took up arms against the Spanish government in an effort to gain their independence.[45] Fearing that a successful Cuban revolt may pave the way for other, less friendly European powers to move into Cuba, the U.S. government initially refused to aid the rebels and even used its navy to block the illegal shipment of supplies and weapons onto the island. However, as the revolt intensified and descriptions of Spanish atrocities in Cuba reached the American people through almost nonstop reporting in the media, public sentiment began to shift in favor of the revolutionaries. Many in the United States, including those whose business interests were being negatively impacted by the ongoing violence, began pushing for the U.S. government to intervene militarily if the conflict were not resolved quickly. By early 1898, the situation had become increasingly dangerous for all those living in Cuba. Although rebels had successfully taken total control of the island and established their own autonomous government by this time, Spanish loyalists remaining there continued to incite riots and destroy property. The U.S. Consul-General living in Havana saw the escalating violence and sent word to Washington that the lives of American citizens were in grave danger. This prompted the U.S. government to send a battleship, the USS *Maine*, to Havana in January of 1898 in order to protect its interests on the unstable island. Just three weeks after arriving in Cuba, the USS *Maine* was rocked by an explosion as it sat in the Havana harbor and sank, killing 268 men. Despite not knowing the cause of the explosion or who was responsible for it, those in the United States saw this as an attack on its military and demanded retribution.

The loudest voices clamoring for war against Spain for its perceived role in sinking the *Maine* came from two prominent New York publishers. Joseph Pulitzer, who owned the *New York World* newspaper, and William Randolph Hearst, who owned the *New York Journal*, began publishing oversensationalized and oftentimes fabricated stories about Spanish cruelty and oppression of the Cuban people several years before the *Maine* incident.[46] Such propaganda and yellow journalism succeeded in enraging the American public and increased demand for increasingly outlandish stories. The sinking of the *Maine* provided the perfect opportunity for Pulitzer and Hearst to increase their readership. They created false illustrations and wrote fictional accounts about how the treacherous Spanish planted mines and shot torpedoes at the *Maine*. They published slogans like "Remember the Maine. To Hell with Spain!" and even offered a $50,000 reward for the capture of the Spanish perpetrators. Their fake stories were so convincing that some who actually survived the explosion and watched the ship sink into the Havana harbor believed the Spanish were responsible. Despite absolutely no evidence to suggest that to be the case (either then or now), public and political pressure forced U.S. president McKinley to issue an ultimatum to Spain on April 20, 1898, requiring their immediate withdrawal from Cuba. They refused, which prompted the United States to begin a full naval blockade of Cuba and issue a formal declaration of war against Spain.

The Spanish-American War lasted only three months and resulted in less than 400 U.S. combat deaths.[47] The combination of a powerful naval assault and over 270,000 ground troops enabled the U.S. military to take control of a number of Spanish territories, including Cuba, Puerto Rico, Guam, and the Philippines. Referred to by some as a "splendid little war," it was a near flawless display of American military might that helped it gain much with relatively little sacrifice. However, as the war began to wind down in late July, outbreaks of yellow fever, malaria, and typhoid started to take its toll on the main U.S. force in Cuba. Tens of thousands became sick and incapacitated with disease and nearly 2,000 died in just those few months. Lieutenant Colonel Theodore Roosevelt, in a letter written to the U.S. secretary of war, expressed his fear that "if we are kept here it will in all human possibility mean an appalling disaster, for the surgeons here estimate that over half the army, if kept here during the sickly season, will die."[48] Military leadership headed these warnings and started a massive withdrawal of troops from Cuba in early August 1898. However, it was necessary to keep 50,000 U.S. troops on the island in order to maintain order and stability while the government transitioned to Cuban leadership. With so many troops stationed indefinitely on an island that was prone to yellow fever epidemics, the U.S. government decided to take proactive measures to prevent a potential disaster. They assembled a team of four microbiology experts that was led by U.S. Army medical researcher Walter Reed and sent them to Cuba to investigate the cause and transmission of yellow fever.

Prior to being dispatched to Cuba, Reed and his colleague James Carroll had been working to confirm a recent study by an Italian scientist (Giuseppe Sanarelli) that claimed to have found the cause of yellow fever—a bacterium named *Bacillus icteroides*—that was reportedly transmitted through respiratory secretions. Through rigorous testing, they had accumulated strong evidence to suggest that Sanarelli's bacillus bacterium was not the cause of yellow fever and was instead a form of hog cholera that had randomly infected some of his test patients. Despite attempts by Sanarelli to discredit their report, Reed and Carroll soon gained experimental support from another physician named Aristides Agramonte, who had also failed to see a connection between *Bacillus icteroides* and yellow fever.[49]

After disproving Sanarelli's finding, the Yellow Fever Board, which consisted of Reed, Carroll, Agramonte, and a young physician named Jesse Lazear, traveled to Cuba to meet with a local doctor and epidemiologist named Carlos Finlay who had been studying yellow fever on the island since 1879.[50] Finlay had worked closely with a team of U.S. scientists following the great 1878 Mississippi Valley epidemic and gained critical insight into the pathogenesis of the disease. He examined tissue samples from infected individuals under the microscope and found that the yellow fever agent seemed to be targeting cells that make up the blood vessels (called the vascular endothelium) rather than the red blood cells themselves. From this, he inferred that "in order to inoculate yellow fever it would be necessary to pick out the inoculable material from in the blood vessels of a yellow fever patient and to carry it likewise into the interior of a blood vessel of the person who was to be inoculated. All of which conditions the mosquito satisfies most admirably through its bite."[51] Finlay made this statement during a presentation at a scientific meeting on August 14, 1881, 19 years before Walter Reed's Yellow

Fever Board arrived in Cuba. In that same presentation, Finlay also described an experiment in which he took *Aedes Aegypti* mosquitoes (known then as Culex) and allowed them to feed on individuals suffering from yellow fever. Those mosquitoes were then placed on the skin of five people who recently arrived on Cuba and had never been exposed to yellow fever before. All five individuals who were bitten by these infected mosquitoes developed some form of yellow fever. Although such findings strongly supported Finlay's mosquito theory of transmission, much of the scientific community in Cuba and the United States believed he was wrong. In fact, even after he successfully repeated the same inoculation experiment with 99 additional individuals over the next two decades, people (including Reed) remained unconvinced by Finlay's methodologies and data.[52]

When Reed's team arrived in Cuba in 1900, they were anxious to meet with Finlay to discuss his experiments. Finlay was extremely accommodating, giving the Yellow Fever Board total access to his notebooks, showing them how he conducted his experiments and even providing them with a sample of his infected mosquitoes. With these materials in hand, Reed placed Jesse Lazear in charge of verifying Finlay's results while he was away in Washington, D.C.

The experiments conducted by Lazear over the next several months helped provide strong support for the mosquito theory. Using Finlay's established methodology for growing and inoculating mosquitoes, Lazear designed experiments to test whether or not mosquitoes could transmit yellow fever and, if so, whether that transmission is dependent upon the severity of disease in the source patient or the length of time that the mosquito is allowed to incubate prior to biting the next person. James Carroll, who was not a supporter of the mosquito theory, agreed to be one of the initial test subjects for Lazear's experiment.[53] After being bitten by a mosquito that had fed on someone with a severe form of yellow fever 12 days prior, Carroll developed the symptoms of yellow fever and nearly died of it. A number of other test subjects were either bitten by mosquitoes that had fed on people with more mild forms of the disease or were bitten by mosquitoes who fed less than 12 days before. None of those individuals were found to develop yellow fever. Thus, it appeared that the yellow fever agent had to incubate inside of a mosquito for at least 12 days in order to effectively cause disease when entering a second person. This was one of the key findings missing from Finlay's earlier experiments and one of the reasons why he often got confusing and contradictory results. Knowing that he had not acquired yellow fever from any other source, Carroll later celebrated the fact that he "was the first person to whom the mosquito was proved to convey the disease."[54] Unfortunately, the excitement of these results would not last long. Lazear, who had also been bitten by a mosquito during the course of the experiment, tragically died of yellow fever on September 26, 1900.

The death of Lazear marked a major turning point in the work of the Yellow Fever Board. Reed returned to Cuba in October with a renewed commitment to furthering Lazear's research and establishing better experimental protocols.[55] Now a believer in the mosquito theory, Reed decided to set up a well-controlled experiment in a camp on the outskirts of Havana that would test whether yellow fever was transmitted by mosquitoes or by contaminated objects and filth. In this camp, which was named Camp Lazear to honor their fallen colleague, Reed set up two different buildings. One building contained all manner of disgusting materials that had been contaminated with blood and vomit from people who had previously died from yellow fever; however, it was treated to be completely free from mosquitoes. The second building was set up to be clean and free from any potential yellow fever–contaminated objects; however, it was sealed off with netting and inoculated with mosquitoes that had fed on people dying of yellow fever. Volunteers were placed into each building and required to sleep there for 20 nights. During the days, the two groups of test volunteers were kept isolated from one another in tents nearby in order to control what they were exposed to during the course of the experiment.

The findings of this three-week study were convincing and clear.[56] All of the individuals who were kept in the filthy building remained perfectly healthy for the course of the entire experiment whereas six of the eight people exposed to infected mosquitoes in the clean building developed yellow fever. Subsequent experiments also demonstrated that direct injection of blood from yellow fever patients into healthy volunteers failed to transmit the disease if the blood was removed after three days postinfection. This suggested that the yellow fever agent does not spread directly between humans in nature. Taken together, such stark results finally disproved the longstanding theory that yellow fever was acquired through exposure to contaminated objects or miasma. In doing so, it also provided an explanation as to why efforts to improve sanitation in Cuba and the American South had little effect on yellow fever transmission rates. Additionally, these studies provided validation for Finlay and his 20 years of dedicated research and conclusively demonstrated the critical role of the *Aedes* mosquito in the transmission of the disease.

The short- and long-term implications of these findings were immense. First, knowing how yellow fever was being transmitted finally gave public health officials a target to stop future epidemics. For instance, the Chief Sanitary Officer in Cuba, William Gorgas, immediately got to work to eliminate the mosquito vector from the island. As mentioned in chapter 4 (malaria), Gorgas employed various methods of mosquito control, which included oiling the surface of lakes, emptying water reservoirs, fumigating homes, and providing nets for residents to sleep under. Such interventions proved to be extremely successful and yellow fever was eradicated from Cuba within about a year. Similar mosquito-control measures were subsequently applied to eliminate yellow fever in the Panama Canal Zone and reduce its prevalence in Latin America and the United States. Yellow fever was eliminated from much of the world within just five years following the publication of Reed's results.

Reed's experiments also garnered a great deal of attention for their innovative design. He was one of the first scientists to provide research volunteers with a written informed consent document that outlined the potential risks of study participation.[57] Unlike previous experiments that usually kept human test subjects uninformed about what was being done to them, Reed provided full disclosure about the dangers of his yellow fever experiments. He refused to force or trick vulnerable people into participating, and he compensated volunteers very generously for their service. Such ethics was in stark contrast to most studies of his day, which typically utilized children, prisoners, and the poor as dispensable, unwitting test subjects. For instance, in the Tuskegee syphilis experiments, poor and illiterate African American sharecroppers were purposely given syphilis and allowed to remain sick for nearly 40 years (1932–1972) in order to study the progression of the disease. At no point were the men informed that they had syphilis, and none were given penicillin even after it had been proven to be an effective treatment for the disease. The compensation for these awful long-term experiments was free medical care (ironically), some meals, and burial insurance. Such outrageous exploitation of minorities and the poor highlighted the need for massive changes in how medical experimentation was performed in the United States. Thankfully, the fallout over the Tuskegee study finally pushed the U.S. government to establish a National Commission for the Protection of Human Subjects and to develop federal regulations that required informed consent for all tests done on humans. It is sad that the medical community failed to follow the example of Walter Reed, who had voluntarily established ethical protocols a full 80 years before informed consent became required by law.

The identification of the mosquito as the vector for yellow fever allowed Reed and Carroll to shift their focus to the search for the etiological agent responsible for the disease. Most scientists at the time believed yellow fever was caused by a bacterium or parasite since no virus had ever been associated with a human disease. To test this theory, they obtained patient samples that they knew contained the yellow fever agent and passed them through a porcelain filter that could trap bacteria and larger particles. They then took the liquid that passed through the filter and injected it into healthy volunteers. To their surprise, all the individuals who received the injections ended up developing yellow fever. This suggested to them that whatever was causing yellow fever had to be small enough to fit through the pores of the filter. The only infectious agent known at that time that had this property was a virus. Subsequent experiments by Reed and Carroll in 1901 confirmed the viral etiology of yellow fever, which marked the first time in history that a human disease was found to be caused by a virus.[58] This was a monumental discovery because it demonstrated a proof of principle; namely, that viruses could infect humans. As a result of Reed's pioneering work, scientists began looking into the possibility that other human diseases were also caused by viruses. What followed over the next decade was an explosion in viral research. Diseases like measles, influenza, rabies, and smallpox that had long remained mysteries to the medical community were found to have a viral cause. For some of these, this information proved to be absolutely essential as scientists attempted to develop effective vaccines and accurate diagnostic tests.

The Search for a Vaccine

In the years that followed the discovery of the yellow fever vector and virus, public health officials largely focused on controlling the mosquito population as a way of preventing epidemics. It was so successful in the early years that a Yellow Fever Commission made up of international experts convened in 1915 to discuss the possibility of eradicating the disease from the planet. Funded by the Rockefeller Foundation and chaired by Gorgas, this group systematically entered endemic regions in South America and Africa and employed the same mosquito control methodologies that worked so well in Cuba, Panama, and the United States. While this worked well in some areas, other locations continued to experience intermittent outbreaks of yellow fever even after rigorous attempts to eliminate *Aedes* mosquitoes there. Such difficulties baffled scientists for a long time until it was finally discovered, in the 1930s, that YFV could also infect monkeys and spread between them via different species of mosquitoes. Control efforts that focused on disrupting the life cycle of *Aedes* species in urban environments thus had little effect on mosquitoes and monkeys harboring the virus deep in jungles. As a result, the risk of yellow fever epidemics remained since it was impossible to prevent the virus from randomly jumping between monkeys and humans when both live in close proximity. Since there was no way to fully eliminate YFV from the environment, scientists began working on the next best alternative—developing a safe and effective vaccine that could be administered to people living in endemic areas.

Standard methodologies for creating viral vaccines in the 1920s typically involved destroying purified virus with heat or chemicals or weakening it by growing it in tissue of some non-host organism. Injecting destroyed virus into a person has the benefit of being completely safe since there is no possibility of the pathogen coming back to life and causing disease. However, this type of vaccine, called a killed vaccine, often induces a relatively poor immune response because the immune system of the recipient is presented with a limited amount of fragmented viral parts rather than a more natural intact, replicating virus. In contrast, weakened forms of live viruses, known as attenuated vaccines, have the benefit of inducing better long-term immunity but do so at a greater risk to the recipient. Attenuated vaccines have the potential to cause an actual infection if the virus undergoes some type of mutation that allows it to regain its strength or the person receiving the vaccine has a weak immune system.

Early attempts at creating YFV vaccine involved treating virally infected liver tissue with formalin in order to inactivate ("kill") the virus. Unfortunately, administration of this type of vaccine failed to elicit any type of protective immune response, leading scientists to focus on the creation of an attenuated vaccine. Attenuation of YFV was initially fraught with difficulties since it could not be successfully grown outside of a human host (or mosquito vector). As mentioned above, a breakthrough came when it was discovered that the virus could be propagated in both wild and lab-raised monkeys like rhesus macaques. This allowed scientists, for the very first time, to take YFV research out of the dangerous medical clinic and move it into a better controlled lab environment. Replication of YFV in rhesus monkeys was very successful; however, the virus particles that resulted were not sufficiently weakened to be of use for any type of vaccine. This prompted scientists to begin looking for alternative types of non-host tissues in which to grow the virus.

In 1930, a young scientist, Max Theiler, discovered that YFV could replicate in the central nervous system tissue of mice.[59] After allowing it to do so for many viral generations, Theiler found that the YFV that emerged from the mouse brain tissue was extremely weakened in its ability to cause liver disease in monkeys and humans. In other words, growing YFV in the mouse tissue seemed to have selected for mutant forms of the virus that lost their ability to destroy liver or vascular endothelial cells. Furthermore, injection of this attenuated YFV into new hosts provided them with long-term protection against future challenges with full-strength YFV. Although it appeared that Theiler might be successful in creating a safe and effective YFV vaccine in the early 1930s, a new complication arose during the animal testing phase of his experiment. The constant growth of the virus in mouse brains had also inadvertently selected for new variants of YFV that showed a preference for growth in nervous tissue.[60] As a result, when rhesus monkeys were injected with the attenuated vaccine, many of them developed severe neurological dysfunction as the virus spread to the brain and replicated there. This was of course a devastating setback to the entire project. A vaccine that prevents one form of the disease but causes another is not what Theiler was hoping to create.

It was at this stage in vaccine development that two separate research groups emerged on opposite sides of the Atlantic Ocean. One was led by

Wilbur Sawyer and Theiler at the Rockefeller Institute in New York and the other was headed by Andrew Watson Sellards and Jean Laigret, who were working at the Pasteur Institute in Paris. Theiler's group continued to work on the vaccine that was created in mouse brains and discovered that they could significantly reduce its tendency to spread to the recipient's nervous system by co-injecting it with small amounts of protective antibodies obtained from people who naturally recovered from YFV.[61] While this worked in terms of giving recipients immunity to YFV, it was not ideal since it involved having to inject blood derivatives from one person into another person every time the vaccine was given. Doing so was expensive and potentially dangerous if the antibody serum donor happened to be infected with something else. Unfortunately, this danger was realized in 1942, when as many as 50,000 U.S. Army recruits who were given the vaccine with human serum developed jaundice. Analysis of the vaccination protocol and reagents revealed that the vaccine itself was not responsible for this widespread outbreak of liver disease.[62] Instead, they found that the human serum co-injected with the vaccine (to make it safer) was accidentally contaminated with another pathogenic virus, hepatitis B virus (HBV). This huge mistake caused the Rockefeller group to reassess the inclusion of human serum in their vaccination protocol.

Meanwhile, the French group was experiencing its own difficulties. Despite also deriving their vaccine from infected mouse brains, they chose to not use human serum with it. Instead, they just accepted the increased risk of neuropathogenic side effects and attempted to further attenuate it through drying, mixing it with egg yolks or oil, or inoculating it via scarification rather than injection. The latter method, scratching it into the skin, proved to reduce the neurotropism of the French vaccine to some extent but never fully eliminated the risk.

The early work with the two vaccines demonstrated that neither was sufficiently safe and inexpensive to serve as a long-term YFV vaccine. Something needed to be done to eliminate the vaccine's neurotropism and dependence on human serum. The answer came a short time later as a result of the diligent and tireless work of Max Theiler. After determining that YFV could also be propagated in tissue from chicken embryos, Theiler began growing the mouse brain–derived vaccine strain in embryonic tissue that lacked a central nervous system. The rationale was that he hoped the vaccine strain would acquire mutations while replicating in the absence of nervous tissue and as a result lose its neurotropism. Theiler continually infected chicken embryo tissue, tested the YFV emerging from it for neurotropism, and then injected it into fresh chicken embryo tissue if it failed his test. After repeating this process over 100 times, Theiler finally made the breakthrough he had been waiting for. One particular strain, named 17D, emerged from the chicken embryo tissue with an inability to infect the central nervous system when injected into a live animal.[63] The 17D strain was also found to still be attenuated in terms of its ability to cause damage to the liver and endothelial cells, and it sparked a great immune response when given to recipient animals and humans. In short, Theiler had succeeded in creating a truly safe and effective vaccine strain that could be administered inexpensively without need for human serum. Other scientists tested his 17D strain with similar results and soon all YFV vaccines administered worldwide were derived in some way from 17D.

The innovative and revolutionary approach used by Theiler to create the YFV vaccine would later earn him the Nobel Prize in Physiology and Medicine in 1951, the only time that a Nobel Prize has been given for the development of a vaccine.[64] He set the benchmark for vaccine design in cases where crude attenuation techniques were found to be insufficient and ineffective. His approach was later modeled by researchers who developed some of the most important viral vaccines in history, including those for polio, measles, HBV, and influenza. Additionally, his 17D vaccine helped arm public health officials with a powerful weapon against future yellow fever epidemics. Together with mosquito control measures, the development of YFV vaccine in 1937 marked the unofficial end to yellow fever's reign of terror. It no longer held the power to paralyze cities or send thousands of people fleeing for their lives. The disease was finally understood and could be controlled in multiple ways. Despite still killing tens of thousands of people a year, yellow fever no longer holds the same potential for global mayhem as it once did.

CHAPTER EIGHT

Cholera

No barriers are sufficient to obstruct its progress. It crosses mountains, deserts, and oceans. Opposing winds do not check it. All classes of persons, male and female, young and old, the robust and the feeble, are exposed to its assault; and even those whom it has once visited are not always subsequently exempt; yet as a general rule it selects its victims preferably from among those already pressed down by the various miseries of life and leaves the rich and prosperous to their sunshine and their fears.

—Written by Dr. George Wood after observing
the horrors of the 1832 cholera epidemic[1]

One of the most common and graphic depictions of cholera in the 19th century shows the Angel of Death arriving to a city from across an ocean and then slaughtering masses of frightened victims with a wide sweep of his sickle. Reminiscent of paintings created during the 14th-century Black Death, these images perfectly captured the fear and sense of helplessness that was so pervasive in cities following the news that cholera had once again reached their shores. Unfortunately, these feelings were a common occurrence during the 19th and 20th centuries, when seven cholera pandemics collectively claimed the lives of over 50 million people worldwide. Although it is currently preventable and treatable, cholera continues to infect as many as four million people every year and kill over 100,000.

Upon consuming food or water contaminated with cholera bacteria, victims experience sudden and persistent watery diarrhea that can lead to a dangerous loss of fluid and electrolytes in just a few hours. In severe cases (about 2–5% of the time), patients may lose over one liter of fluid per hour. The diarrhea can be so extensive that many clinics place patients on special "cholera

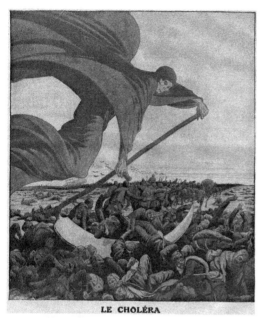

LE CHOLÉRA

Illustration of cholera as the Angel of Death in *Le Petit Journal*, ca. 1912. (*Le Petit Journal*, December 1, 1912)

beds" that have a hole in them and a bucket underneath to catch the almost continuous flow of fluid. The dehydration that ensues can cause severe muscle cramps, irregular heartbeat, lethargy, and a dangerous reduction in blood volume and pressure. Additionally, cholera victims will typically have dark, sunken eyes and a characteristically blue tint to their shriveled skin. If not given intravenous fluid and electrolyte replacement therapy at this point, victims will progress into shock, which leads to coma and death about 30–50 percent of the time. Amazingly, all of the clinical stages of the disease just described can occur in a single day. A person can complain of mild abdominal discomfort in the morning and be dead by evening. In fact, cholera is one of the fastest killers in the microbial world, rivaling such diseases as Ebola and necrotizing fasciitis.

Cholera is caused by infection with a small, comma-shaped bacterium named *Vibrio cholerae*. The bacteria naturally live and replicate in warm bodies of water in areas with poor sanitation. They can grow independently in the water or in small crustaceans called zooplankton. Since a number of aquatic animals (e.g., oysters) feed on zooplankton, *V. cholerae* can also accumulate to high concentrations in some foods that are consumed by humans. In normal situations, the amount of *V. cholerae* in a given water source is naturally kept low by viruses called phages that target and kill the bacteria. (Recall that viruses can infect all forms of life, including bacteria.) However, when there is an excessive amount of rainfall, the phage viruses that normally kill *V. cholerae* become diluted and are unable to destroy the bacteria as effectively. As a result, the amount of bacteria in that water source increases significantly, making it much more likely that a person drinking, washing, or swimming in the water will become infected. Since *V. cholerae* is not well protected in terms of its outer structure, a person needs to ingest about 100 million cells in order to ensure that enough survive through the harsh stomach acid. Those that make it into the intestines will attach to the tissue and begin replicating.

Interestingly, the sheer presence of cholera bacteria in the intestine does very little harm to the host since the bacteria are not overly invasive nor do they spark any type of inflammation. What makes *V. cholerae* such an effective human pathogen is its ability to produce a powerful toxin that disrupts the normal functioning of host intestinal cells. This toxin, appropriately named cholera toxin (CT), attaches to the surface of host cells and gains entry into them. Once inside, the toxin triggers a chain reaction of enzyme activation events that culminates in the opening of protein channels found in the outer membrane of the cell. In particular, the toxin forces a channel called CFTR to open and release large amounts of chloride (Cl^-) ion into the main part of the intestine. Unfortunately, when chloride is transported out of the cell, sodium (Na^+) ions and water will tend to follow it. The end result is a massive accumulation of water and ions (electrolytes) in the intestine that has nowhere to go but out of the body. As the cholera bacteria continue to make CT, more CFTR channels are opened up, and more fluid is lost. If the infected person begins to experience these symptoms in an area without proper sanitation, the billions of bacteria released in their diarrhea can contaminate a new water source, and the whole cycle begins over again.

Unlike most of the other pathogens discussed in this book, cholera causes what are often called common-source epidemics because the pathogen is acquired from some shared environmental source like a lake or a well rather than being transmitted directly between hosts. In common-source epidemics, large numbers of individuals exposed to the same contaminated source can become infected simultaneously and unexpectedly. For instance, if a well becomes contaminated with *V. cholerae* the day before 1,000 people drink from it, every person may come down with symptoms at the same time. Unlike host-to-host epidemics, which often have a slower lag period as the infectious agent progressively spreads through the population, common-source epidemics can seemingly arise out of nowhere and claim the lives of thousands before health officials even have time to react. Since transmission is not directly between people, quarantines are usually minimally effective as are attempts at improving personal hygiene. The only way to truly stop a common-source epidemic is to identify the contaminated source and then either remove the contaminant or prevent people from accessing it. Common-source epidemics can be prevented altogether by maintaining a clean water supply and requiring that standard food safety measures are followed.

The central problem that arises when trying to control cholera and other waterborne illnesses like typhoid and dysentery is that individuals infected from a common source can travel to distant sites and then contaminate local sources there. Now instead of having a single area of contamination to contend with, there are possibly thousands of foci distributed over hundreds of miles. For instance, a person picking up cholera from a river in one city can deposit the bacteria in 10 other cities as they travel home with uncontrollable diarrhea. As you will see throughout the chapter, this pattern of dispersal has been critical for the success of cholera as an epidemic disease for the past 200 years.

Origins and Overview of the Seven Pandemics

The first use of the word cholera comes from the writings of Hippocrates who, in the fifth century BCE, used the Greek word for bile (cholē) to describe a number of different sporadic diarrheal diseases.[2] Based on his somewhat vague clinical description of these diseases, it is likely that Hippocrates never actually witnessed epidemic cholera. Similarly, there are no clear descriptions of cholera in the writings of Galen or any other ancient European medical historian, which suggests that the disease either did not arise in Europe or it did not cause any significant epidemic there during those times.

Although no one knows exactly where, when, or how *V. cholerae* entered into the human population, most epidemiologists believe that it arose somewhere on the Indian subcontinent at least a couple of thousand years ago. One of the more convincing pieces of evidence that supports this theory comes from writings on ancient stone monoliths found in some Hindu temples. For instance, there is a monolith at a shrine in western India dating back to the fourth century BCE that contains the inscription, "The lips blue, the face haggard, the eyes hollow, the stomach sunk in, the limbs contracted and shrumpled as if by fire, those are the signs of the great illness which, invoked by a malediction of the priests, comes down to slay the braves."[3] While one may argue that this could have been referencing any number of diseases, symptoms like blue skin, sunken eyes, and perpetually contracted muscles are much more indicative of cholera than other diarrheal diseases like typhoid fever or dysentery. Similarly, people had been worshiping a Hindu goddess devoted to cholera (Oladevi) at a shrine near Calcutta for hundreds of years before any mention of the disease in the medical literature.[4] This, combined with the fact that the first six cholera pandemics all began near the Ganges River delta in India/Bangladesh, strongly suggest that *V. cholerae* was endemic to the warm waters there for some time.

The first definitive written account of cholera came in the middle of the 16th century when Portuguese historian Gaspar Correia wrote about separate outbreaks of the disease in Calcutta in 1503 and 1543. In his 1556 book *Lendas da Índia* (Legends of India), Correia provided a vivid description of the many horrifying physical manifestations of cholera and characterized the deadly disease as one that "struck with pain in the belly, so that a man did not last out eight hours' time."[5] Many other European explorers who visited India over the next 250 years described an additional 62 outbreaks of cholera during that time. Medical historians have examined these accounts and determined that 10 of them could be classified as epidemics based on how extensively the disease spread in India. Despite clearly recognizing that endemic cholera in India was a ticking time bomb, none of the European colonists who controlled India from the 16th to the 18th centuries made much of an effort to control or study the disease. As a result, cholera remained firmly entrenched in warm waters of the Ganges waiting for someone or something to move it beyond the confines of India.

The first true cholera pandemic began in 1817 following the Hindu Kumbh Mela festival that takes place in the Ganges every few years.[6] During this festival, millions of Hindus from all over the world make a pilgrimage there in order to bathe in its sacred waters. In 1817, a particularly rainy monsoon season hit India as a result of unusual weather anomalies the year before (1816 was known as the year without a summer). This triggered a major increase in bacterial counts in the Ganges just as the festival began. Widespread cholera infections began popping up among the pilgrims in September and then subsequently traveled with them as they made the trek back to their homes. Before long, cholera had spread all throughout the Indian subcontinent, killing tens of thousands of natives and many of the British colonists who lived among them. However, unlike previous smaller outbreaks and epidemics, this one did not stop in India. Instead, it traveled with the British as they shipped cargo and military supplies to colonial possessions in Asia and the Middle East. Appearing for the first time in cities like Bangkok, Manila, and Baghdad, cholera wreaked havoc everywhere it went. Over the next few years, it had spread all the way to the coast of Africa (Zanzibar),

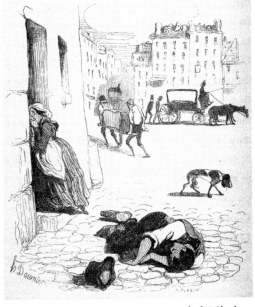

Illustration by Honoré Daumier titled "Cholera in Paris." It appeared in *Némésis médicale illustrée* (1840), Volume 1, p. 69. (National Library of Medicine)

north into Russia, and east into Japan. Such unfettered spread continued until 1824, when an exceptionally cold winter killed off most of the *V. cholerae* bacteria living in Asian water sources. The seven-year pandemic was finally over, but the damage had already been done. The deadly combination of poor sanitation, a religious pilgrimage, and colonialism helped move cholera from a local disease to a worldwide threat. Cholera had truly gone global for the first time in its history, and unfortunately it was just the beginning.

The second cholera pandemic struck just five years later (1829) and lasted roughly 20 years.[7] Like the first, it began along the Ganges delta in India and spread rapidly to cities all over Asia via colonial trade routes. By the early 1830s, cholera had moved from Russia into Eastern Europe and then made its way to Western Europe for the first time. Many of the larger European cities like London and Paris were hit especially hard due to widespread overcrowding and poor sanitation. Some of those infected in Great Britain boarded ships to the Americas and brought cholera to New York City in June 1832. From there it spread to Philadelphia, Boston, New Orleans, and into Mexico. In Asia, cholera also flourished outside of cities at the many Hindu festivals and Muslim Hajj pilgrimages to Mecca and Medina. Some have estimated that as many as 30,000 people died from cholera during the Hajj in 1831, and many more thousands died at the event every year. Infecting so many religious pilgrims also allowed cholera to move into most of the Middle East and even into northern Africa. By the time it finally subsided, the second pandemic of cholera had claimed the lives of hundreds of thousands of people and spread throughout the world at speeds that may only be rivaled by the 1918 influenza pandemic.

The third (1852–1860), fourth (1863–1875), fifth (1881–1896), and sixth (1899–1923) cholera pandemics all started along the Ganges and followed similar patterns of spread as was observed in the second pandemic. However, each was a bit different in terms of which regions were most severely affected. For instance, the third pandemic hit Russia harder than the rest of Asia, killing an estimated 1 million people, whereas the fourth pandemic caused mass casualties in Africa. Interestingly, the fourth pandemic was also the last time that cholera had significant impacts in Western Europe or the Americas due to improvements in sanitation that helped to eliminate cholera from municipal water supplies (see later in the chapter). The sixth epidemic largely stayed in Asia and killed 10 million people in India and another 500,000 in Russia. Such statistics clearly show why cholera was regarded as the single most prevalent and feared microbial killer of the 19th century.

The current cholera pandemic, the seventh, began in 1961 in Indonesia. It marked the first time that a cholera pandemic began outside the confines of the Ganges delta, and it was the first that had a relatively low mortality rate. Major improvements to sanitation, antibiotic usage, oral rehydration therapy,

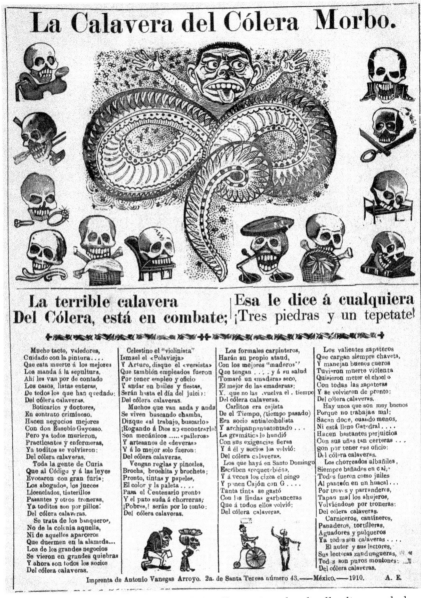

A poster published in Mexico in 1910 illustrating the deadly disease cholera. (Library of Congress)

and the appearance of less virulent strains of the bacteria (e.g., El Tor) collectively helped limit cholera's impact on the population. However, whenever there has been a disruption to sanitation infrastructure following a natural disaster or war, cholera has reappeared and wreaked havoc.

Cause of Social Unrest

The industrialization and urbanization that occurred in the early 19th century led to the creation of several new social classes. The first was a prosperous middle class that was composed mostly of educated professionals (e.g., doctors, lawyers), shopkeepers, factory owners, managers, and small landowners. These individuals gained enormous wealth and political influence as a result of the economic boom that accompanied the Industrial Revolution. In addition to boosting their social status, this newfound wealth also improved their quality of life by enabling them to move to areas outside of the increasingly dangerous and crowded cities. Living in suburban estates helped keep the middle class relatively isolated from most epidemic diseases and allowed them to set up their own better quality schools, hospitals, and places to partake in leisure activities. As a result, they enjoyed longer, happier lives than they had just decades earlier.

In stark contrast to the gains experienced by the middle class during this time, the large number of rural laborers and immigrants who migrated to cities in search of work endured poverty and misery that is unrivaled in modern history. Most worked in jobs that required them to put in very long hours in unsafe environments for almost no pay. Barely making enough money to support themselves, the urban working poor were usually forced to live in overcrowded and unsanitary slums that were rife with violence, hopelessness, and infectious disease. Their immense suffering was often magnified by chronic mistreatment and exploitation by the wealthier classes, who tended to view the poor with a sort of apathetic contempt. The poor, in turn, tended to be distrustful of the powerful aristocracy. Such disparity in the outlook and standard of living between the upper, middle, and working classes created a ticking time bomb that was ready to explode if given the right spark. Unfortunately, the dreaded cholera that spread uncontrollably through cities in the 19th century provided just the right trigger for major clashes to occur between the classes.

When cholera first reached industrialized cities during the second pandemic (1830–1832), the disease quickly entered into the slums and began killing large numbers of the poor living there. For instance, in New York City, most of the 3,500 people who died of cholera in 1832 were poor Irish immigrants and free African Americans living in the Five Points slum.[8] Similarly, over 100,000 people succumbed to cholera in the slums of St. Petersburg and other Russian cities, and several thousand more died in the poorer areas of Paris, Liverpool, and London.[9] As cholera swept through these cities and killed an alarming number of working-class laborers, the upper and middle classes for the most part did relatively little to alleviate their suffering. While some philanthropists did establish soup kitchens and workhouses during the worst of the epidemic, most simply sat back and watched as the poor died in record numbers. A major reason for this is that many had come to associate the physical filth of the slums with that of the people who lived there. The poor were increasingly portrayed in the media as being responsible for the epidemic because of how they "chose" to live.[10] The result of such vilification was that community leaders in many cities purposely withheld humanitarian aid using the rationale that it would only serve to keep alive the very people thought to be causing the spread of the disease. One prominent civic leader in New York City voiced this opinion in an 1832 letter when he wrote, "those that are sickened must be cured or die off, and being chiefly of the very scum of the city, the quicker their dispatch the sooner the malady will cease."[11] According to this almost Malthusian model of infection control, the best way to stop the epidemic was to let cholera kill off the "vector" of the disease, the poor "scum" that resided in the filthy slums.

Not wanting the epidemic to spread beyond the confines of these areas, many cities imposed strict quarantines to prevent the movement of people into and out of the affected neighborhoods. To the poor living (and dying) there, such restrictions were seen as an unwanted intrusion by the government, a cruel policy that significantly amplified their suffering. As the death toll from cholera continued to rise, the growing resentment and distrust between the classes began to boil over and result in several violent conflicts. These local skirmishes, known collectively as the "cholera riots," occurred in cities all over the world and resulted in significant destruction of property and several deaths.

The first set of cholera riots occurred in Russia in 1830–1831.[12] The disease reached Russia for the first time in September 1823, but it died out during the cold winter just a few months later and never really caused a significant number of deaths. However, when it returned six years later, it was a much different story. It arrived in the city of Orenburg from the south and quickly spread throughout the country by 1830. Widespread panic set in as the disease reached larger cities like Moscow and St. Petersburg and began devastating the populations there. In an effort to prevent further spread of cholera in major urban centers, the government led by Tsar Nicholas I set up very strict quarantines and armed checkpoints to prevent unnecessary travel within and between cities. In some places, people were prevented from going to work or leaving their homes even when seeking out medical attention. As the epidemic grew worse, Nicholas and other top government officials fled the capital city (St. Petersburg) and virtually cut off communication with the populace. Local health officials made the situation worse by indiscriminately putting anyone who had health issues or were indigent into the same facilities as those dying of cholera. One person living in St. Petersburg at the time noted that the police were not much better. He wrote, "our police, who have always been noted for their insolence and extortionary practices, have become even more shameful, instead of being helpful in these sad times."[13]

Rumors began to fly that doctors were purposely trying poison the sick and that Polish and German immigrants were conspiring with the Russian government to kill off the poor. Feeling trapped by the quarantines and abandoned and abused by all who were in the position to help them, the poor in St. Petersburg and several other Russian cities began to lash out.

The riots began on June 21, 1831, in St. Petersburg, as protestors assembled in Sennaya Square and started attacking medical carriages that were transporting the sick. In the days that followed, rioters destroyed several local clinics and killed many of the doctors who were working inside of them. One rioter came back from the fighting and proudly stated that a doctor "got a coupl've rocks in the neck; he sure won't forget us for a long time."[14] The Russian government responded by sending two army regiments into Sennaya Square to restore the peace. Shortly after the rioters were halted by the threat of cannon fire, Nicholas himself entered the middle of the city and spoke to the crowd. Accounts vary dramatically as to what he said on that day; however, most suggest that he ordered the crowd to kneel before him and remove their hats in submission. Whatever he said worked, and the riot dissipated on June 23. Although the riots of 1831 failed to drastically change how the Russian government responded to the cholera epidemic, they did alert the leadership that the poor were not going to sit idly by and die without having their voices heard.

Another country that experienced a significant number of violent uprisings during the second cholera epidemic was Great Britain. Unlike the Russian riots, which were triggered by a general discontent with restrictive government quarantines and poor leadership, the violence in Britain was caused by the buildup of anger over how the upper classes had been mistreating the deceased bodies of poor people. The issue first entered into the national spotlight in October 1826 when the *Liverpool Mercury* published an article about the discovery of 33 dead bodies that were awaiting shipment to Scotland.[15] These bodies had been stolen from local graveyards, put into a salt preservative, and sold to an anatomy school in Edinburgh for use in dissection. Less than a month later, a second group of stolen bodies were found on a Liverpool dock headed for Scotland. In 1827, yet another case hit the headlines that shocked the citizens of Liverpool. A respected local surgeon named William Gill had been found with five dead bodies in his home.[16] Like the previous instances, he had stolen the bodies from a local graveyard and planned to dissect some of them himself and sell the others. The lucrative business of selling bodies to anatomy schools took a major turn for the worse in 1828 when two men, William Burke and William Hare, were found to have murdered 16 people in Edinburgh for the sole purpose of profiting off of the sale of their bodies.[17] Most of those murdered were paupers, prostitutes, poor laborers, and other "miserable offcasts of society, whom nobody missd because nobody wishd to see them again."[18] As one may expect, the crimes sparked outrage among the working-class population and others who felt victimized by the upper classes and the government. While Hare was spared the death penalty for cooperating with authorities, William Burke was hanged for his crimes in January 1829. His body was publicly dissected, and his skeleton was preserved as per the sentence imposed by the judge who presided over his trial. The case was so troubling and significant that it helped give rise to several new terms in the English language. The words Burking and Burker became synonymous with the murder of the poor for profit.

These cases and others like them (e.g., murders committed by Bishop and Williams in London in 1831) led to the passage of the Anatomy Act of 1832, which expanded the legal supply of bodies available to the growing number of anatomy schools.[19] While the legislation did help reduce the illegal trade of bodies in Great Britain during this time, it was widely criticized by the lower classes because most of that legal supply came from the poor who died in workhouses or on the street. In the majority of cases, the bodies were "donated" anonymously without any consent from the families of the deceased. As a result, fear of hospitals and doctors swept through working-class neighborhoods as many began to believe that the poor were being unduly targeted for hospitalization.

When cholera arrived in Great Britain in 1831, it sickened tens of thousands of people and forced many to seek out medical treatment. As increasing numbers of people entered into cholera hospitals and never left, rumors began to swirl that doctors were actively using cholera to kill the poorer patients. The situation was particularly tense in Liverpool, where cholera was spreading out of control in the slums, and people were constantly reminded of the many grave robbing and Burking episodes that occurred there in recent years. The first Liverpool cholera riot broke out on the evening of May 29, 1832, when a large group of mostly women and boys followed a sick couple as they were transported to a local cholera hospital.[20] Not believing the couple to be all that sick, the mob began shouting things like "Burker!" and "Murderer!" at the medical personnel. By the time they arrived at the hospital, the mob had grown to an estimated 1,000 people and become increasingly violent. One observer of the riot recorded some of what unfolded. "Stones and brickbats were thrown at the premises, several windows were broken, even in the room where the woman, now in a dying state, was lying, and the medical gentleman who was attending her was obliged to seek safety in flight. Several individuals were pursued and attacked by the mob and some hurt. The park constables were apparently panic struck, and incapable of acting."[21]

Although the mob dispersed later that night, they continued to assemble in front of the same hospital for the next three days. Over the course of two weeks, seven additional riots broke out near various hospitals throughout the city. Crowds destroyed palanquin carts used to transport the sick and attacked doctors, accusing them of "giving patients stuff which killed them and made them turn blue."[22] Rioters were seen chasing medical personnel and yelling, "the doctors merely want to get the poor into their clutches to Burke them."[23] This type of violence continued to erupt every few days until it finally ended on the evening of June 10, 1832. Most credit the local Catholic churches with defusing the situation and restoring peace to the city. On the Sunday after the last riot, every Catholic priest in Liverpool made a formal statement from the pulpit in which they implored their congregants to look at the epidemic rationally and behave in a manner that was in line with their faith. The priests also reassured them that they would work with local health officials to ensure that cholera victims were protected and treated with the upmost respect. Such sentiments were echoed by several local doctors who published articles in the *Liverpool Journal* during the same week.

Although the riots in Russia and Liverpool were the most prolonged and widespread of those that arose during the second cholera pandemic, they were certainly not isolated incidents. For instance, violence also exploded in Manchester, England, in 1832 after a young doctor cut off the head of a four-year-old child (John Brogan) who had died of cholera and tried to sell it.[24] When the boy's grandfather looked in the coffin and saw what had been done, he assembled a mob of over 2,000 angry neighbors and marched to the hospital. Upon arriving there, they set fire to several parts of the building and violently attacked its staff. Similar scenes unfolded in cities throughout Europe (e.g., Paris and Exeter, England) and the United States (e.g., Utica, New York) as mobs attacked gravediggers, doctors, and anyone else they believed to be disrespecting their deceased friends and family.

Once the cholera epidemic started to subside in 1833, episodes like those described above became rarer and significantly less destructive. However, when cholera reemerged later in the 19th century, so did outbreaks of violence among the underprivileged populations that were most affected by the disease. One of the most destructive and deadly of the later cholera riots took place in industrial city of Iuzovka, Ukraine, in 1892.[25] Then a part of Tsarist Russia, Iuzovka was filled with 20,000 poor laborers who worked in unsafe steel mills and coal mines that were operated by foreign businessmen. The arrival of cholera in the late summer inflamed an already volatile labor situation that had been brewing in the city for several years. On August 2, a large crowd of mostly inebriated miners came to the aid of a local woman who was being forcibly hospitalized for the treatment of cholera. After expelling the health officials from her building, the mob moved outside and began looting and destroying the local bazaar shops that for years had been taking advantage of them. The destruction was so intense that only 3 of 183 shops remained intact by the end of the riot. By the next day, the crowd of about 15,000 people turned their attention to the wealthier Jewish residents of

Iuzovka. They destroyed their businesses, burned their homes, and killed as many as 100 of them. The military was eventually called in to quell the rebellion, and peace was restored within a few days. Despite lasting only a short time, the 1892 cholera riot nearly destroyed the city of Iuzovka and severely disrupted the coal industry in the entire region. Politicians in St. Petersburg saw the shocking violence and worried about what would happen if laborers were allowed to organize into unions. As a result, they increased public forms of corporal punishment for any worker accused of promoting "lawlessness." Such state-sponsored brutality further inflamed civil unrest and later set the stage for the most significant worker uprising in history—the Communist Revolution.

Religious Freedom, Imperialism, and Public Health

The Bengal region of India was the epicenter of every cholera pandemic of the 19th century due to the ongoing presence of *V. cholerae* bacteria in the warm waters of the Ganges River. India at the time was controlled economically, politically, and militarily by Great Britain. The British first established a formal relationship with India in 1612 when the ruler of the Mughal Empire gave the British East India Company (EIC) permission to "sell, buy, and to transport into their country at their pleasure."[26] Over the next several decades, the EIC built plantations and factories in cities all over the Indian subcontinent and used them to produce valuable commodities like tea, spices, cotton, opium, and silk.[27] By the mid-18th century, the increasingly powerful EIC had pushed most of its European competitors out of India, allowing it to establish a near monopoly over the Indian economy. Such expansion created huge profits and a growing need for the EIC to protect its investments from domestic and international threats. At first, the EIC employed just a few hundred Indian soldiers as guards to watch over its trading stations in the major Indian regions of Bombay, Madras, and Calcutta. However, as EIC operations greatly expanded in the late 18th century, the private military force employed by the EIC grew to over 60,000. Those troops were trained as European soldiers and organized into large regiments called presidency armies. In addition to having cavalry and heavy artillery at their disposal, presidency armies were complemented by a relatively sizable and powerful navy.

As local Indian rulers and their subjects grew increasingly resentful of their British colonizers, armed resistance between the EIC military and various Indian groups became more commonplace.[28] The violence peaked in 1857, when a group of Indian soldiers employed by the EIC mounted a mutiny in the region of Bengal. The Indian Rebellion of 1857 lasted for over two years and resulted in very high casualties for both sides. The EIC was eventually successful in suppressing the revolt; however, the situation exposed serious flaws in how the EIC was managing India. In response, the British crown dissolved the EIC and took direct military and economic control over the Indian subcontinent and its nearly 250 million inhabitants. The British government would retain control of India for the next 89 years, eventually ending as a result of the independence movement led by Mahatma Gandhi in 1947.

The acrimonious relationship between the British and their Indian subjects was exacerbated by the six cholera pandemics that spread throughout the Indian subcontinent during the occupation. As mentioned earlier in the chapter, one of the major factors that fostered the continued dissemination of cholera was the frequent migration of millions of religious pilgrims to the Ganges during various Hindu festivals. The largest of such events, the Kumbh Melas, have been held in four different cities on a rotating basis for many centuries.[29] The two Kumbh Melas that take place along the Ganges (Haridwar and Prayag/Allahabad) typically attract enormous crowds of people from all over India. In fact, the single largest gathering of human beings in history occurred on February 10, 2013, when 30 million people assembled during the Kumbh Mela festival in Prayag. In addition to the main Kumbh Melas, there are smaller festivals called Magh Melas or Ardh Melas that are held on a more frequent basis. The duration of the festivals is not fixed nor is the length of time that each individual spends at them. Some last just a few days whereas others have continued for several months.

One of the most important events that occur during these festivals is the ritual bathing in the sacred waters of the Ganges.[30] Believed to provide a spiritual purification, holy men (*naga sadhus*) and pilgrims submerse themselves completely in the river in order to cleanse themselves from sin and help them achieve freedom from the cycle of death and rebirth (called *Moksha*). In many cases, participants will also drink the water directly or bring containers of the water back home with them. Unfortunately, exposure to the Ganges water in these ways was extremely hazardous when *V. cholerae* levels were high during a particular season and year. In addition to killing people who attended the festivals, the bacteria often traveled with returning pilgrims and established new foci of infection in cities throughout India. From there, cholera spread easily along military and trade routes to the rest of Asia, Europe, and the Americas.

Seeking to control the spread of cholera within and beyond India, representatives from 12 European countries convened in 1851 to discuss how to best limit the international spread of diseases like cholera without impacting trade.[31] Although this first international sanitation conference created discourse about the global nature of pandemics, it failed to result in any lasting policy changes. The third sanitation conference, held in Constantinople in 1866, focused entirely on cholera and how it was being propagated.[32] When discussing the role of the Hindu religious pilgrimages in triggering large-scale epidemics, the delegates concluded that pilgrims spread cholera and

that the large assembly of people at the Ganges represents "the most powerful of all the causes which conduce to the development and propagation of
cholera."[33] These conclusions created an interesting dilemma for the British.
Do they take control of the festivals and risk further outraging millions of
people that already resent their presence or do they allow the festivals to
proceed and risk future European epidemics? In the end, they initially erred
on the side of permitting the festivals to continue without interference. It was
determined that large-scale quarantines and other restrictions would be difficult to enforce, extremely expensive, and viewed as religious persecution by
Hindus.

When the British did attempt to intervene, their efforts were usually met
with the expected resistance and disdain. For instance, when cholera broke
out during the *Kumbh mela* in Hardwar in 1892, authorities forcibly dispersed over 200,000 pilgrims and prevented new ones from arriving to the
area by railway.[34] Although no violence erupted as a result, the disruption of
their holy pilgrimage enraged orthodox Hindus (and actually failed to slow
the epidemic). In 1906, British authorities attempting to clean out contaminated sacred pools near the Godavari River were physically prevented from
doing so by a crowd of Hindu priests and other holy men.[35] Later sanitary
measures, such as personal health inspections and vaccination, were similarly viewed by Hindu pilgrims as being intrusive attacks on their religion.
The British were keenly aware of the uphill battle that they faced in trying to
convince a subjugated people to willing change their ancient religious rituals, and these instances clearly demonstrate the risks of forcing such changes.
As a result, with just few exceptions, the British for the most part maintained
a "hands-off" policy when it came to controlling cholera at festival gathering
sites. Cholera was understood as a necessary evil, an ever-present trade-off
for unthinkable economic benefits.

While Hindu festivals often served as epicenters for cholera pandemics
due to their proximity to the Ganges, Islamic pilgrimages to the cities of
Mecca and Medina often played a pivotal role in spreading the disease
beyond the confines of Asia. All physically and financially able Muslims are
required to make a pilgrimage to Mecca (in Saudi Arabia) at least once in
their lifetime according to one of the five pillars of Islam. This mass migration, known as the Hajj, brings together millions of people from all over the
world for five days of rituals and prayer. Many the same pilgrims also routinely gather in the city of Medina in order to honor the site believed to be the
final burial place of the prophet Mohammed. Despite the significance placed
on these pilgrimages in the Islamic faith, most Muslims throughout history
were prevented from visiting either city due to the cost and logistics of traveling to western Saudi Arabia. As a result, most early pilgrims tended to be of
the "upper crust" of Middle Eastern society—wealthy merchants, officials,
and scholars who could afford to make the trip. This changed drastically in

the mid-19th century when trains and steam-powered ships coincided with the opening of the Suez Canal to provide an opportunity for pilgrims of more modest means to make the journey. One group that began traveling to Mecca and Medina with much greater frequency during this time period were Muslims living on the Indian subcontinent. Those pilgrims, like many of their Hindu neighbors, were often infected with cholera due to endemic nature of the disease there.

Cholera first appeared in Mecca in the spring of 1831 as roughly 50,000 Muslim pilgrims arrived to celebrate the Eid al-Adha (Sacrifice Feast) holiday.[36] A heavy rain, combined with overcrowding and a lack of clean drinking water, led to the rapid dissemination of cholera among the visiting pilgrims. By late June, it had taken the lives of 10,000–15,000 people in and around Mecca and infected tens of thousands of others. As the pilgrims departed and began their trek home, they brought cholera with them aboard ships and trains. Despite efforts by several governments to quarantine returning pilgrims, cholera outbreaks still erupted everywhere they went. Alexandria and Cairo were hit especially hard, with a combined 40,000 deaths. Beyond Egypt, cholera outbreaks were also reported in Syria, Palestine, Tunisia, Turkey, and the Balkans in the months that immediately followed the Hajj. The same pattern of spread was repeated in 1846–1848 and again in 1865. In each case, the pilgrimage to Mecca/Medina served as a critical relay point by which cholera moved from India to the rest of Asia, northern Africa, Europe, and ultimately the Americas.

The ongoing threat of cholera to Europe and the Ottoman Empire triggered a call for new sanitary regulations and quarantines. The first truly international actions against cholera came in 1831 when Egyptian authorities established the *L'Intendance Générale Sanitaire d'Égypte* (Egyptian Quarantine Board), and in 1839 when Sultan Mahmud II established a board of health in Constantinople and charged it with monitoring the movement of Muslim pilgrims in the lands and ports controlled by the Ottoman Empire.[37] Realizing that they did not have proper authority to quarantine foreigners, both boards appointed experts from other countries affected by cholera so that any measures taken would be agreed upon by the international community as a whole. Such cooperation among rival nations to combat an infectious disease was a revolutionary concept for its day since, up until this point, nations largely dealt with infectious disease without really considering the impacts on other nations. Both boards established quarantine stations in major port cities in Europe, Asia, and northern Africa, staffed them with trained medical officers, and allowed them military power.

After several additional cholera epidemics in the decades that followed (e.g., in 1865), it became clear that ineffective management and political infighting in the health boards had made them virtually impotent. It was at this point that a series of broader international sanitation conferences were convened every few years in order to address cholera and other infectious diseases that affect the entire international community. Experts from nations all over the world came together to discuss what was known about cholera and to propose fact-based measures to curb its spread. While the specifics of each conference were different, much of the tone remained the same— authorities needed to impose more stringent regulations on Muslim (and Hindu) pilgrims and pilgrimages in order to stop the spread of cholera. As one professor from the University of Paris wrote in 1873, "Europe realized that it could not remain like this, every year, at the mercy of the pilgrimage to Mecca."[38]

The result of these conferences was a series of new measures that were designed to impede traffic to and from Mecca. Quarantine stations were given greater power to block the movement of pilgrims and detain them indefinitely if they deemed them to be a health risk. They carefully inspected ships, confiscated materials and goods believed to be contaminated, and collected exorbitant taxes from pilgrims in order to offset the cost of feeding and housing them. The latter measure had the added goal of "weeding out" the poorer, less hygienic pilgrims who could not afford to pay the high taxes. In doing so, health officials hoped to simultaneously reduce the overall number of pilgrims and increase their "quality." Unfortunately, their efforts were largely in vain. Cholera continued to spread from India to the sites of Muslim pilgrimages almost every year for much of the 19th and early 20th centuries.

A number of factors contributed to this failure. First among them was that the leading authority on cholera, Great Britain, did everything in its power to block attempts at regulating the movement of pilgrims to and from Mecca and Medina.[39] Britain had much to lose by acknowledging what most experts of the day believed; mainly, that cholera was entering these holy cities as a result of Muslim pilgrims coming from India. (Islam is the second largest religion in India.) Much of Britain's wealth came from international trade generated by India, and so any attempt to quarantine people traveling into or out of India represented a major impediment to British business interests. In fact, British officials on health boards often critically derided quarantines as being outdated, overly intrusive, and unnecessary.[40] These officials, along with British representatives at the international sanitary conferences, posed strong objections for any type of internationally mandated regulations or quarantines. Instead, they argued for enforcement on the national level— allowing each nation and port to decide how to best control the movement of pilgrims. Unfortunately, they exerted a lot of influence at these venues, which allowed them to successfully block the implementation of standardized international regulations for most of the 19th century. It was not until the 1894 Paris sanitation conference that Britain finally conceded and agreed to abide by the recommendations proposed by the health experts present. The end result of this British obstructionism was 50 years of inconsistent and half-hearted measures that did little to actually stop the spread of cholera.

Another factor that negatively impacted attempts to control cholera during the Hajj was the tendency of crews and pilgrims to lie about its presence on board ships and trains. Vessels found to be carrying passengers sick with cholera were subjected to lengthy quarantines and costly disinfection procedures. Rather than being held up for weeks and potentially losing significant amounts of income, crews often falsely stated that no cases of cholera had been reported on board or hid those who were sick. In many cases, they even resorted to throwing the bodies of people who died of cholera overboard during the journey so they would not get caught with them. Such deception was extremely dangerous, as evidenced by what transpired during the 1865 epidemic. Two ships carrying pilgrims from India, Java, and Malaysia arrived in Arabian ports in February with 143 people on board suffering with cholera. When asked by port officials, the ship's crew lied and said that they had just contracted the illness after landing. The truth was that many on board were sick, and the ship was "infested" with cholera. Those who were infected but not yet showing symptoms were allowed to disembark and continue on to Mecca. Within just a few weeks, cholera levels skyrocketed in the holy city and thousands were dead. A similar situation occurred as sick pilgrims returned home along the same travel routes. For instance, most ships arriving at the Suez Canal in 1865 reported their passengers to be in perfect health despite the fact that their crews threw hundreds of dead bodies into the Red Sea after cholera had erupted on board. Those making it through the Suez checkpoints boarded crowded trains headed for Cairo and Alexandria. Not surprisingly, within weeks, cholera was spreading out of control throughout Egypt as it had in Mecca.

Even if regulations and quarantines had been properly administered and followed, chances are that cholera would have still spread to Mecca due to the religious devotion of millions of Muslims. Being that the Hajj is one of the five pillars of the Islamic faith, there is a very good chance that Muslims, sick or not, would have continued to make the pilgrimage every year no matter how stringent the international restrictions. Muslims during this time were beginning to unify under a pan-Islamic movement that was designed to collectively protect their interests against European colonialism. Those who were under the political control of Great Britain and other European powers were increasingly forming alliances with Muslims who lived in the Ottoman Empire. To them, the Hajj was a symbol of Muslim unity, a religious rite that had to be protected at all costs. Such devotion kept large numbers of Muslims traveling to Mecca even during years of famine, war, and epidemic disease. When officials tried to make travel more restrictive through the use of quarantines and high taxes, the pilgrims kept coming. Many even completed the Hajj every year with virtually no money for food or other travel expenses.

These indigent pilgrims would rely on the charity of other wealthier pilgrims for their very survival. The fact that so many were willing to risk their lives to complete the pilgrimage suggests that it would have been virtually impossible to control the Hajj at the level necessary to prevent the dissemination of cholera. Doing so would have been likely perceived as a direct attack on the Islamic faith and would have been met with extreme resistance.

In all, the role of religious pilgrimages in the spread of cholera in the 19th century is an interesting case study in the interplay between epidemiology, commerce, politics, and religion. The multinational nature of the Muslim pilgrimages and the clear role of Hindu pilgrimages in sparking cholera epidemics forced the international community to work together in order to mount a unified response against the disease.[41] Although the international health boards and conferences fell short of achieving their goal of stopping cholera, they did lay the groundwork for fostering greater collaboration between rival nations in fighting global health threats. It is a collaboration that would continue to grow over the years through various health conventions and in the establishment of multiple permanent international health agencies. The formation of the United Nations after World War II led to a consolidation of competing health agencies into a single World Health Organization (WHO) in 1948. The WHO, which has grown to include 194 member nations since its inception, has taken on the mission of protecting all of mankind from both infectious and noninfectious health threats. Its disease surveillance activities and vaccination programs have prevented epidemics and saved millions of lives.

In stark contrast to the cooperative spirit that accompanied health initiatives, the fight against cholera also exposed the ugly racism and greed that accompanied European colonialism. The British virtually ignored the presence of cholera in the 17th and 18th centuries despite the fact that it infiltrated Hindu festivals and killed tens of thousands of Indians almost every year. The first time that there was any serious push to help stop cholera among their Indian subjects was after the 1817 epidemic when cholera began to threaten the economic activities of the British EIC. It was a pattern that repeated itself later when the British government obstructed countless proposals by international sanitary conferences because they felt that prevention measures unduly interfered with free trade. Financial interests often took precedence over the well-being of human beings in large part because many Europeans blamed the colonial subjects themselves for causing cholera epidemics. Hindu and Muslim pilgrims were commonly portrayed as being filthy people that had so little regard for their own health that they would choose disease over an opportunity to be "civilized" by Europeans. As one author wrote in the 1890s, pilgrims were "unclean, utterly miserable, degraded human beings, knowing only a migratory life, in common with their camels and their vermin."[42] Such sentiments led to great resentment by

Europeans whenever cholera reached their own shores or when they were forced to pay for colonial sanitation measures with their tax dollars.

Pilgrims, in turn, viewed attempts of sanitation reform by Europeans as yet another form of control over them, an intrusion into the most personal aspects of their life and religion. They disliked being told when and how they could complete their pilgrimage by people who did not respect their religious traditions, and they resented being mistreated when aboard European-run steamships and in quarantine stations despite being required to pay excessive taxes and fees. To them, the fight against cholera was in many ways viewed as a fight against their way of life. It was one more insult among many that they were forced to bear by their European oppressors.

The Sanitation Revolution Begins

In a recent survey by the *British Medical Journal*, experts ranked sanitation as the single greatest milestone in health and medicine over the past 150 years, beating out antibiotics, vaccines, and anesthesia.[43] Why sanitation is held in such high regard is that it gives humankind the ability to control the cleanliness of its environment, food sources, and water supply. In doing so, it protects the population from exposure to dangerous toxins and pathogens that are naturally found in wastes, and it limits the propagation of vermin and vectors that can spread disease. Before effective sanitation measures were implemented in the 19th century, populations would routinely fall prey to killers like cholera, typhoid, intestinal helminths, and polio through the simple acts of getting a drink of water or taking a bath. As a result, an average person born in a city like London before the advent of modern sanitation was chronically sick and rarely lived much past their 35th birthday. Such a poor quality of life and shockingly low life expectancies prevented mankind from ever reaching its full potential. Instead of being able to focus time, energy, and creativity on developing new technologies for the betterment of our species, mankind was forced to expend much of its limited resources on simply staying alive.

The central problem with municipal sanitation prior to the Industrial Revolution was that individual citizens were largely responsible for the disposal of their own wastes. Whether one was living inside a bustling city or out in the countryside, few regulations existed to monitor how, where, and when people discarded their excrement and garbage. A common practice that was used for many centuries was to collect wastes in a chamber pot or bucket and then empty it into a yard, a street gutter, or common open pit (known as a cesspool or cesspit) nearby the home. In some cases, nicer privies were outfitted with an outlet and tube that would direct wastes out of the home without need for daily maintenance. Once outside the home, the human sewage would either soak into the soil, move down the street gutters and empty into local rivers or lakes, or be removed by professional waste workers who would dump it at sites outside of the city. The end result of such practices was the mass contamination of wells and rivers/lakes with a wide variety of dangerous gastrointestinal pathogens, including cholera and typhoid bacteria. In some cases, a city's entire supply of drinking water would become nothing more than a stagnant pool of human sewage. To make matters worse, slaughterhouses and other businesses in cities usually disposed of their waste in much the same way. It was common to see rivers of blood and animal tissue flowing down street gutters into the cesspools or local water sources.

Friedrich Engels, in his book *The Condition of the Working-Class in England*, described the sight and smell of a typical London waterway in the middle of the 19th century as being "a long string of the most disgusting, blackish-green, slime pools are left standing on this bank, from the depths of which bubbles of miasmatic gas constantly arise and give forth a stench unendurable even on the bridge forty or fifty feet above the surface of the stream."[44] Although London is often presented as the poster child for 19th-century filth, the situation was not much better in any other city in Europe, Asia, or the Americas. In some of the larger cities, the putrid smell was so intensely nauseating during the hot summer months that most city offices would close and anyone with the financial means would flee into the country. People living in such unimaginable conditions usually just accepted this as a normal part of city life. However, when the stench and recurrent mild diarrhea gave way to deadly pandemics of cholera and typhoid, health officials finally took notice and enacted changes to clean up cities and their water supplies.

The most significant improvements to public sanitation came about during the height of the second and third cholera pandemics. Ground zero of this sanitation revolution was Great Britain, which had witnessed the ravages of cholera in India for many years and experienced over 75,000 cholera deaths on its own soil from 1830 to 1860. Despite imposing strict quarantines of ships arriving from cities that had active cholera outbreaks, Great Britain fell victim to cholera in October 1831 when a ship carrying infected sailors disembarked in Sutherland (Scotland).[45] The disease spread rapidly to the south and eventually made it to London in February 1832.

Although London had experienced various epidemics throughout the centuries, the arrival of cholera that year carried with it a terror that had not been felt since the Black Death. One British doctor noted that "the cholera was something outlandish, unknown, monstrous; its tremendous ravages, so long foreseen and feared, so little to be explained, its insidious march over whole continents, its apparent defiance of all the known and conventional precautions against the spread of epidemic disease, invested it with a mystery and a terror which thoroughly took hold of the public mind, and seemed to recall the memory of the great epidemics of the middle ages."[46] Unfortunately, their fears were soon realized as cholera swept through the filthy streets of English cities and took the lives of thousands. It was particularly successful in impoverished areas of large cities like London, where overcrowding and narrow streets combined to produce extremely unsanitary environments. The cholera crisis in the poorer neighborhoods was particularly important because it led some public health officials in England to readdress how the government responded to poverty and how that affected the health of the city as a whole.

One of the first to make a push for sanitary reform in London and other filthy British cities was physician and minister Thomas Southwood Smith.[47] Upon graduating from medical school in 1816, Smith was appointed to work as a physician in the London Fever Hospital, where he witnessed firsthand the destructive capabilities of epidemic disease. Like most physicians of his day, Smith thought that these diseases were caused by a buildup of toxic miasma that permeated crowded cities. Whereas most of his contemporaries believed this miasma arose from poor climates or supernatural disturbances in the weather, Smith theorized that they came from the filth present in London's poorest neighborhoods. In an essay that he wrote for the *Westminster Review* in 1825, Smith suggested that "the air, it is certain, is often charged with noxious exhalations arising from the putrefaction of animal and vegetable matter . . . these exhalations exert a most important agency in the production of epidemic diseases."[48] This was a revolutionary idea for several reasons. For one, it placed some of the blame for epidemic diseases on bad sanitary practices; namely, the improper disposal of animal and agricultural waste and the "morbid exhalations of the human body." Although he was wrong about the exact etiology of disease (miasma), he correctly surmised that filth and its "corruption" of the environment do play some role in the spread of disease. With that being the case, Smith hypothesized that epidemic disease of many types could be prevented by "cleansing the filthy habitations of the poor"[49] and restoring the environment to its original, uncorrupted state. In other words, Smith believed that the key to controlling the health of the population was to control the health of the environment. The cholera epidemic that hit London in 1832 only further convinced Smith that his theory was correct since it seemed to do more harm in the filthier areas of the city. He continued to accumulate data in support of his sanitation ideas over the next several years and presented his findings in various reports to governmental agencies. Three such reports, written between 1838 and 1844, helped provide the foundation for some of the most important legislation in the history of Great Britain.

The first of these reports was presented to the Poor Law Commission in 1838 at the behest of his friend and fellow sanitarian, Edwin Chadwick.[50] The Poor Law Commission was a group of national leaders that was charged with determining how to best distribute relief to the poor in Great Britain. Chadwick, like Smith, believed that one of the central issues facing the poor was the ever-present filth that permeated their neighborhoods and work environments. In order to make a push for sanitation reform, Chadwick requested that Smith and two other physician friends (James Kay and Neil Arnott) describe their experiences regarding sanitation and disease to the commission. Unfortunately, Chadwick did not get along with most members of the commission and so his ideas largely fell on deaf ears. With the second cholera pandemic still raging on, Chadwick made the decision to leave his post as secretary of the commission so that he could launch his own independent inquiry into the state of sanitation in Britain's cities. With the help of Smith and a few other colleagues, Chadwick embarked on a mission to comprehensively and accurately document the devastating effects of poverty and filth on the health and well-being of the poor. He assembled data from physicians, interviewed eyewitnesses, and spoke with officials who had first-hand experience with sanitation in various cities throughout Great Britain. He made special note of examples in which improvements made to local sanitation produced concomitant improvements in the quality of life of its residents.

After years of intense research, Chadwick finally published the results of his inquiry in 1842 in the *Report on the Sanitary Condition of the Labouring Population and on the Means of Its Improvement.*[51] Understanding how important this issue could be to the future prosperity of Great Britain, Chadwick paid out of his own pocket to print and distribute thousands of copies of his report. He sent it to every member of the House of Lords, physicians, newspapers, and anyone else who would listen. A copy of the report even made it into the hands of American author Mark Twain, who, despite not fully accepting all of Chadwick's conclusions, praised him for the quality of his research. The 1842 report was wildly popular, sparking a national movement that led to the creation of the Health of Towns Association (HTA) and the publication of additional reports from Chadwick, Smith, and other sanitation reform proponents. People all over Great Britain began calling for tangible changes to be made in public health policy; however, the conservative Prime Minister Robert Peel refused to initiate any legislation on the national level. This all changed in 1848, when a new round of cholera outbreaks in London coincided with the selection of the more liberal Prime Minister John Russell. Under the advisement of Chadwick and the HTA, Russell helped push through the landmark Public Health Act of 1848, which provided a legal framework by which to improve sanitation across the country.[52]

The most important outcome of the Public Health Act was the establishment of a National Board of Health and several local boards of health in cities throughout Great Britain.[53] The National Board, which was led by Chadwick and Smith from 1848 to 1854, had oversight over all sanitation matters in the nation; however, it had little real power to enforce the recommendations contained in the Public Health Act. Instead, the power was placed into the hands of the local boards of health, which had the responsibility of maintaining sewers, regulating slaughterhouses, providing drinking water, cleaning the streets, removing nuisances, and monitoring waste disposal in newly built homes. Local health boards were also permitted to make changes to the basic infrastructure of municipal roads and sewers. They installed public bathrooms, paved roads, and even built parks and other open green spaces for people to enjoy. In all, over 300 towns petitioned to create local health boards following the passage of the Public Health Act and several hundred more were added in the decades that followed.[54] The results in those cities were dramatic. Sewage was no longer permitted to be thrown haphazardly into the streets nor was it allowed to pool in poorly constructed neighborhood pits. Public spaces were also kept free of trash, which limited the proliferation of rodents and insects, and every citizen was guaranteed to be provided with a reliable source of drinking water. People were not getting sick as much, which enabled them to live longer and more productive lives.

Although the Public Health Act of 1848 marked a monumental turning point in the history of public health and medicine, it did have some very notable flaws. Probably its most significant weakness was that its adoption was voluntary at the local level. Cities were encouraged to create municipal boards of health to oversee sanitation reform, but ultimately they were not forced to do so by the federal government or the National Board of Health.[55] Each city had autonomous control over whether it would implement the recommended policy changes, opt out of the Public Health Act completely, or adopt select measures from it. While it seems logical to think that municipal authorities would have jumped at the chance to make their cities healthier, most, unfortunately, did not. A combination of local budget shortfalls, political infighting, and pressure from the wealthy classes prevented most cities (e.g., London) from moving forward with sanitation reform. City governments either outright rejected the perceived interference from the federal government or they deemed sanitation reform too expensive or impractical for their own specific situation. Interestingly, some cities also faced fierce resistance from farmers who relied on the pooled human waste as a source of cheap fertilizer for their crops. As a result, a large number of cities in Great Britain remained mired in filth and plagued with epidemic disease for many years following the passage of the Public Health Act.

Over the next 25 years, British lawmakers and sanitation proponents worked together to expand the Public Health Act and create a more comprehensive sanitation policy for the nation as a whole. One of the major reasons for this change in policy was the ongoing nationwide struggle with epidemic diseases like cholera and typhoid. The third pandemic of cholera hit Great Britain in 1853 and took the lives of over 26,000 people, with 10,000 of those deaths in London alone. Although this pandemic was significantly less deadly than those in 1832 or 1849, it illustrated that there was still much work to do if the cities ever wanted to be free of its threat. Additionally, cities that had resisted sanitation reform in the past finally began to grow weary of constantly seeing and smelling filth everywhere. They came to realize that modest improvements to sanitation could not only improve the health and happiness of their citizens but also increase opportunities for broader economic growth for the city. For London, that moment came in 1858, when a particularly warm summer caused the sewage in the Thames to emanate a foul stench that filled the entire city.[56] Known as the Great Stink of 1858, this event pushed city officials to finally approve the release of funds to build a new, modern sewer system throughout London (headed by British engineer Joseph Bazalgette). Other local governments followed suit, and soon cities all over Great Britain began improving infrastructure and accepting greater responsibility for enforcing sanitary regulations.

In 1875, the Parliament of Great Britain passed a new Public Health Act that consolidated all previous legislation. In addition to giving the federal government increased power to force compliance, this new legislation subdivided the country into specific sanitary districts and mandated that each district establish a health board and appoint a medical official to oversee its implementation. Additionally, it set forth a standard set of uniform policies that were to be followed by all municipalities irrespective of their size, financial status, or local politics. In short, the 1875 Public Health Act finally made sanitation a national priority, a requirement rather than a suggestion. It was the culmination of 50 years of tireless work and research by unyielding sanitarians such as Smith and Chadwick. Because of them, Great Britain would never again experience widespread terror at the hands of cholera or typhoid.

Cities all over the world took notice of Britain's Sanitation Revolution and gradually began to mimic what had been accomplished there. For instance, Paris built an enormous system of underground sewage tunnels in the 1860s and 1870s and invested heavily into the construction of aqueducts to bring fresh water into the city. Other European cities like Frankfurt, Copenhagen, Rome, and Madrid also made drastic improvements to their sanitation infrastructure and passed new legislation during this time. A similar series of reforms began in the United States following the devastating cholera epidemics of 1832, 1849, and 1866. Using designs from London and Paris as models, city planners successfully built new sewers in Chicago and Brooklyn in the late 1850s and then proceeded to do the same in cities all across the country over the next several decades. By the end of the 19th century, most of the United States had successfully implemented sanitation reform to the point that waterborne diseases were no longer any real threat to the country.

The Sanitation Revolution began in large part because of cholera and its devastating effects on the inner-city poor in Great Britain. However, it ended up becoming so much more than preventing a single disease. For instance, it forever changed many of the activities of our everyday lives, including how we use the restroom, how we clean our bodies, how we discard our trash, and how we prepare our food. It also permanently altered the physical structure of almost every city on the planet and produced an overall smarter city design. Municipal (urban) engineers collaborated with architects and scientists to create expansive, structurally sound sewer systems, and water treatment facilities were built for the purpose of distributing clean drinking water over long distances. New roads were paved and fitted with gutters in order to drain water properly. In short, the sanitary movement helped create the modern city as we know it today. Finally, sanitation helped eliminate the threat of nearly all waterborne diseases in the industrialized world, and it lessened the incidence of vector-borne diseases like yellow fever, malaria, and plague. Along with improvements to nutrition and medical science, sanitation is a major reason why people are now living on average 40 years longer than they did just 200 years ago.

The Lifesaving Effects of Rehydration

When the second cholera pandemic struck Great Britain in 1831–1832, it was the first time that Western physicians were called upon to treat patients suffering from such an extreme form of diarrhea. The microbial revolution had not yet taken place and so there was relatively little information available about cholera or how to properly treat it. As a result, most physicians had no choice but to rely on tried-and-true, ancient therapies that were designed to balance out the humors or expel noxious substances from the body. These included frequent pressurized enemas with warm water or gruel in order to flush out the colon, induction of vomiting in order to purge out the harmful substance from the body, and the puncturing of blood vessels to reduce blood volume.[57] For cholera patients suffering from extreme levels of dehydration, such treatments would have only exacerbated their symptoms and hastened their death.

One of the first dissenting voices against such forms of "benevolent homicide" came from the young Irish physician and chemist William Brooke O'Shaughnessy. Fresh out of medical school, O'Shaughnessy began studying cholera in late 1831 after moving to an area of Scotland that was experiencing an outbreak. Over a period of several weeks, he closely observed patients as they rapidly progressed through the different stages of the disease. In addition to monitoring changes to their physical appearance, O'Shaughnessy carefully measured the chemical makeup of both the victims' blood and diarrhea.[58] In doing so, he repeatedly found that their blood was deficient in water and salts and had a significantly higher pH than the blood of healthy individuals. Furthermore, he found that the chemicals that were missing from the blood were now being detected in the patient's excreta. From these groundbreaking findings, O'Shaughnessy came to the revolutionary conclusion that cholera was nothing more than a chemical imbalance of the blood. The haggard eyes, the blue skin, the lifeless countenance—all were due to the loss of water and vital electrolytes. He went on to suggest that cholera could be treated by giving patients an "injection into the veins of tepid water holding a solution of the normal salts of the blood" and then demonstrated by treating dehydration in dogs with an intravenous (IV) injection of buffered saline.[59]

This was a remarkable leap forward in medicine because it represented one of the first times that an infectious disease was studied on the chemical level, and a rational plan for treatment was designed based on actual scientific analysis. O'Shaughnessy, realizing the importance of his work, successfully lobbied to have his findings published in the medical journal *The Lancet* in 1832.[60] Just a few months later, another physician named W. R. Clanny (also working in Sutherland) conducted additional experiments that confirmed the blood results of O'Shaughnessy.

The dissemination of O'Shaughnessy's cholera data did not generate as much excitement in the British medical community as one may expect when considering what cholera was doing to the population at the time. However, it did pique the interest of a Scottish physician named Thomas Latta, who, in 1832, decided to replicate O'Shaughnessy's dog experiment in humans who were dying of cholera. After initially failing in his attempts to restore blood volume and salinity through the use of enemas and oral rehydration, Latta utilized an IV needle to deliver a saline solution directly into the bloodstream of cholera victims. After testing a variety of different formulations, temperatures, volumes, and frequencies through trial and error, Latta obtained results that were shocking even to him. In his 1832 report to *The Lancet*, he recounted the amazing transformation of one patient as follows:

She had apparently reached the last moments of her earthly existence, and now nothing could injure her—indeed, so entirely was she reduced, that I feared I should he unable to get my apparatus ready ere she expired. Having inserted a tube into the basilic vein, cautiously—anxiously, I watched the effects; ounce after ounce was injected, but no visible change was produced. Still persevering, I thought she began to breathe less laboriously, soon the sharpened features, and sunken eye, and fallen jaw, pale and cold, bearing the manifest impress of death's signet, began to glow with returning animation; the pulse, which had long ceased, returned to the wrist; at first small and quick, by degrees it became more and more distinct, fuller, slower, and firmer, and in the short space of half an hour, when six pints had been injected, she expressed in firm voice that she was free from all uneasiness, actually became jocular, and fancied all she needed was a little sleep; her extremities were warm, and every feature bore the aspect of comfort and health.[61]

By simply restoring the chemical composition of the blood to its normal state, Latta was able to bring this patient back from the brink of death in just a matter of minutes. He went on to repeat the experiment with other cholera patients with varying degrees of success. Although not perfect in its design or long-term results, Latta's study was remarkable because it was the first time that anyone had ever successfully treated a person in the late stages of "malignant" cholera, and it was the first to ever use IV fluids in the treatment of any disease. One of Latta's colleagues, Dr. Robert Lewins, predicted that his method would "lead to wonderful changes and improvements in the practice of medicine."[62] Unfortunately, Latta would never see that prediction come to fruition. Just over one year after publishing his landmark study, Latta contracted cholera and died at the young age of 37.

Research on the use of IV injections as a treatment for cholera exploded during the summer of 1832 as physicians all over Great Britain began trying to replicate Latta's groundbreaking study. Many of the trials conducted early seemed to support what Latta had found. For instance, several different physicians reported in the June issue of *The Lancet* that they had been successful in using the IV rehydration therapy to treat late-stage cholera. The editor of that issue of the popular medical journal wrote the rather grandiose proclamation that it was "one of the most interesting recordings in the annals of the medical profession."[63] However, by the end of that summer, more experiments began to emerge that seemed to contradict the findings of those earlier studies (including that of Latta). One study reported a success rate of only 11 percent (89% mortality) and another described the formation of secondary blood infections as a result of the IV treatment. Some physicians even went as far as to suggest that IV therapy was hastening the decline of their patients' health.

As grumblings grew louder, many physicians returned to using bleedings, purgings, opium, or mercurous chloride as the preferred treatments for cholera. By the time the epidemic began to subside in 1833, most of the medical establishment in Great Britain had completely stopped using IV rehydration. Amazingly, in just a matter of months, IV therapy went from being hailed as a miracle to being forgotten in the vast expanse of medical literature. Unfortunately, it would remain buried there for another 60 years before finally being rediscovered in the late 19th century by German scientists studying hemorrhagic shock. During those intervening years, three more cholera pandemics would spread throughout the world and kill millions of people.

A number of factors contributed to the rejection of IV therapy by British physicians in 1832. First, most medical studies during this time were poorly designed and improperly conducted by people who rarely followed the scientific method or included proper control groups in their experiments. As a result, it was common occurrence for one study to get completely different data than another despite using similar protocols. When physicians attempted to repeat Latta's experiments, they likely failed to do so because they used IV solutions with different chemical compositions, injected different volumes for different lengths of times, or even gave patients the IV therapy in conjunction with other dangerous treatments like frequent bleedings and induced vomiting. Similarly, many studies were plagued by bad patient selection. Patients on the verge of death were usually selected to receive the IV treatment whereas those with less severe forms of the disease were given the more standard treatments. Not surprisingly, those who received IVs tended to have a much higher mortality rate as a result. Finally, the original studies were conducted by physicians who were not part of the British medical establishment. Latta was young, Scottish, and using an approach that was challenging over 2,000 years of medical practice. His peers were not generally inclined to give him or his science the benefit of the doubt as they would have had he been more well known.

Despite not being appreciated at the time, the groundbreaking work of O'Shaughnessy and Latta has finally received universal acceptance in the medical community. Intravenous rehydration therapy is currently recognized as the single most effective treatment for cholera and many other diarrheal diseases, even being preferred over antibiotics in most cases. Additionally, IV therapy is now widely used in clinics to increase a patient's blood volume, deliver medications, provide emergency nutrition, treat blood disorders, and deliver blood transfusions. It has helped drastically improve the survival rates of surgery, shock, and cancer (through its efficient delivery of chemotherapeutic agents). When looking at it comprehensively, one can make the argument that IV therapy is one of the most important techniques in all of medicine.

The Beginning of the End for Miasma

One of the most influential paradigm shifts in the history of medicine was when the Germ Therapy supplanted Miasmatic Theory as the universally accepted explanation for infectious disease etiology. As mentioned in several of the earlier chapters, Miasmatic Theory held that infectious diseases were caused by exposure to some noxious substance(s) found in "unclean," foul-smelling air. The source of miasma varied greatly throughout the centuries, with some believing it arose from stagnant bodies of water and others blaming its release on volcanoes, earthquakes, sewage, rotting vegetation, or decaying human/animal remains. If the source of infection was found in foul odors, it was logical to assume that one could avoid becoming sick by simply removing anything that smelled bad or by improving the quality of air through the use of perfumes or flowers. Because bacteria are often the cause of bad odors, avoidance of foul air sometimes serendipitously limited one's exposure to disease-causing microbes. For instance, people usually avoided eating bad-smelling meat because they were afraid of inhaling the miasma that was emanating from it. In doing so, they were unknowingly spared from being infected with *Salmonella*, *E. coli*, or other bacteria that causes food poisoning. The same situation occurred when Romans drained the smelly swamps around the city and lowered malaria deaths (was really due to stopping mosquito reproduction) and when British officials prevented the spread of cholera by cleaning up disgusting-smelling cities (was really due to cleaning drinking water supplies). While "purifying" the air did help limit the spread of disease in some very specific instances, it more often had little to no effect on preventing or stopping deadly epidemics.

The discovery of microscopic germs as causative agents of disease (also known as Germ Theory) revolutionized medicine in large part because it finally demystified why we get sick. Epidemics were no longer thought to be caused by phantom miasma, natural disasters, corrupt morality, or evil spirits. Instead, each disease was found to have a very specific cause, some bacterium, virus, fungus, or parasite that was inducing pathological changes to our body. Knowing the causes was important because it allowed for the development of novel treatments and preventatives (e.g., vaccines) based on specific structural and physiological features of the microbe. In doing so, it helped limit infection and drastically improve the length and quality of our lives.

Many medical historians have tried to identify exactly how and when the medical community came to reject miasma in favor of the Germ Theory. Such analysis has revealed that it did not occur as a result of any single scientist, experiment, or research article but rather was based on an entire body of work that was collected over the course of several decades. With that being said, the gradual shift toward acceptance of the Germ Theory did have to begin somewhere, with some experiment that first caused people to seriously question the existence of miasma. Most believe that moment came in the 1850s when British anesthesiologist John Snow decided to investigate an outbreak of cholera in the Soho neighborhood of London.

John Snow became interested in medicine early in life, beginning work as an apprentice to a surgeon-apothecary at the young age of 14.[64] During the next five years in that role, Snow gained a wealth of knowledge about how to perform surgery, synthesize and administer medications, and care for those suffering from infectious disease. In fact, Snow was working in clinics during the 1831 British cholera epidemic and treated many patients suffering from the disease. Realizing that he wanted to further his education and become a physician, Snow enrolled in medical school in 1836 and earned his degree in 1844. Snow spent the next several years working as a general practitioner in London before becoming interested in the use of ether as an anesthetic. Ether was used successfully for the first time in England in 1846, but dosage and delivery issues prevented it from being widely used for surgical or obstetric procedures. Snow, using his background as a surgeon and apothecary, developed an inhaler device that could accurately administer a set dosage of ether to patients undergoing surgery. His invention worked very well and was immediately used to dispense ether and the newer anesthetic chloroform. By 1848, Snow had arguably become the most famous and well-respected anesthesiologist in Great Britain. He assisted with anesthesia on over 5,000 medical procedures, even administering chloroform to Queen Victoria during the birth of her last two children.

Snow's career as a pioneering anesthesiologist is alone worthy of great acclaim; however, it was his work on cholera that made him one of the most famous physicians in history. When Snow first began studying cholera during the 1848 British epidemic, he approached it from the perspective of an anesthesiologist who spent his career studying the biology of inhalation.[65] In his 1849 pamphlet *On the Mode of Communication of Cholera*, Snow questioned the prevailing theory that cholera, a disease of the intestines, is acquired through the inhalation of toxic miasma from the air.[66] First of all, he found it "difficult to imagine" that a disease could spread as an airborne vapor and have such different effects on people who inhale the same air. He recorded several instances in which people continually exposed to toxic air in their workplace had no ill effects whereas those exposed to relatively little noxious miasma had high incidences of cholera. Seeing little connection between air quality and rates and severity of cholera infection, he next argued against miasma based on the improbability of a disease entering the lungs and then spreading to the digestive tract without producing any signs of pathology in the lungs, nasal cavity, blood, or other tissues. To him, it made much more sense for the cholera agent to enter the body through ingestion and then move along the digestive tract until reaching the intestine. With this being the case, Snow predicted (correctly) that the cholera contagion, what he called a "morbid material," multiplies in the intestine of those infected and is discharged from the body during bouts of diarrhea. Since raw waste was still being dumped into local water sources at this time, Snow inferred that British cholera outbreaks were being caused by sewage contamination of drinking water supplies.

Believing cholera to be a waterborne disease, Snow began to map out cholera deaths in London to see if there were any correlations between death rate and the water source of the particular neighborhood. Interestingly, he found that the South of London, which was fed by the heavily polluted lower Thames River, had more cholera deaths in 1848–1849 than all of the other districts put together. It was an interesting correlation that sparked some interest in the London medical community, but it was far from concrete proof that cholera was waterborne. In fact, some clinicians were so disgusted by the suggestion that cholera was spread by the ingestion of fecal matter that they wrote articles to *The Lancet* and strongly criticized Snow's analysis.

Snow's 1849 publication marked one of the first times that anyone had ever tried to track the location and spread of a disease in a population. Despite not being able to directly link the dirty Thames water with cholera, the study convinced Snow that he was on the right track and encouraged him to continue exploring his theory. An outbreak of cholera in London in 1854 provided Snow with that chance. An area that was hit particularly hard by cholera that year was the Soho district in the West End of London. During the first two weeks in September, more than 600 people died of cholera and 75 percent of the survivors fled for their lives. Snow arrived in Soho at the start of the epidemic and began interviewing those who had fallen ill or had family members that perished. He mapped out where they lived and worked and asked each about the water they had ingested in the days immediately preceding their illness.

In a letter that he wrote to the editor of the *Medical Times* shortly after finishing his research, Snow described what he learned during the course of his interviews. He wrote,

> I found that nearly all the deaths had taken place within a short distance of the [Broad Street] pump. There were only ten deaths in houses situated decidedly nearer to another street-pump. In five of these cases the families of the deceased persons informed me that they always sent to the pump in Broad Street, as they preferred the water to that of the pumps which were nearer. In three other cases, the deceased were children who went to school near the pump in Broad Street.[67]

He went on to further describe a number of people who lived near Broad Street and never contracted the disease. What was common to those seemingly "protected" individuals was that they all got their water (and beer) from a local brewery rather than from the well. Why this is significant is that water has to be boiled in order to be used for the brewing process so that the beer does not spoil. As a result, those who drank from the brewery instead of from the Broad Street well were never exposed to live cholera bacteria. With all of this information in hand, Snow went to the local Board of Guardians on September 7 and requested that the handle be removed from the pump that drew water out of the well on Broad Street.[68] Almost no one in the meeting believed Snow's theory was correct. One local physician later commented that "he was not believed—not a member of his own profession, not an individual in the parish believed that Snow was right."[69] However, since they saw little harm in granting his request and had no better options, the pump handle was removed on September 8. Within a few days after closing of the Broad Street pump, the cholera epidemic subsided, and the rest of the local population was spared.

Further research by Snow and his friend Reverend Henry Whitehead went on to reveal that the epidemic had begun when a mother dumped the contents of her baby's diaper into a cesspool located adjacent to the Broad Street well. That baby was suffering from severe cholera at the time, and the contents of its filthy diaper had unknowingly seeped down into the soil and into the well.

John Snow published the findings from his landmark study of the 1854 Soho epidemic in the second edition of his book *On the Mode of Communication of Cholera*.[70] Similar to the first edition, Snow included a detailed analysis of each water company that served London in an effort to link cholera cases with where those companies obtained their water along the Thames. In analyzing the sum total of his extensive data, Snow became absolutely convinced that cholera was caused by a waterborne

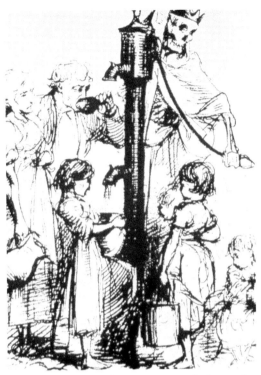

Sketch titled "Death's Dispensary," drawn by George Pinwell in 1866 around the time John Snow published his definitive studies. (Centers for Disease Control and Prevention)

contagion and not by an airborne miasma. Specifically, he concluded it was being transmitted "by the mixture of cholera evacuations with the water used for drinking and culinary purposes, either by permeating the ground, or getting into wells, or by running along channels and sewers into the rivers from which entire towns are sometimes supplied with water."[71] While his ideas were logical and his argument clearly defended, not everyone was convinced by Snow's analysis. For instance, medical statistician William Farr and sanitation reformers like Thomas Southwood Smith and Edwin Chadwick were particularly critical of his work because they felt that his data had not sufficiently ruled out miasma or other modes of transmission.[72] They pointed to the fact that Snow was never able to isolate or identify any contagion from the water that he suspected of being contaminated. Furthermore, his key piece of evidence, the Soho epidemic, was already on the decline before the Broad Street pump handle was removed on September 8. As a result, it seemed entirely plausible to them that the epidemic simply died out on its own independently of whether or not the well was in use. Snow was unmoved by such criticism and continued to fervently defend his contagion theory until his death in 1858. By that point, the second edition of his book had sold only 56 copies, and the Broad Street pump was fully back in service.

It was not until the 1866 cholera epidemic that the medical community came to accept that cholera was in fact caused by ingestion of contaminated water. Ironically, the strongest defender of Snow's theory during this time was none other than his earlier critic William Farr.[73] Farr had been investigating a cholera outbreak in the Whitechapel neighborhood of East London when he noticed an interesting anomaly in the data. Other neighborhoods around Whitechapel and elsewhere in London had very few cases of cholera despite having similar demographics and air quality. As it turns out, Whitechapel was the only densely populated area not yet serviced by the new sewer system that had been installed throughout London in the previous year. Their raw sewage was still being dumped into the streets, which allowed it to leak into the poorly protected Old Ford water reservoir that was located nearby. Farr astutely identified that this was occurring and demonstrated with mathematical certainty that the outbreak could have only been caused by the ingestion of that contaminated water. His 1867 paper made such a convincing case for a waterborne etiology that the editor of *The Lancet* proclaimed, "the elaborate array of facts which Dr. Farr has set forth with so much skill, will render irresistible the conclusions at which he has arrived in regard to the influence of the water supply in the causation of the epidemic."[74] With this one study, Farr had essentially disproven the theory that cholera is caused by miasma. In doing so, he also brought about some redemption for Snow, who died believing that his ideas were widely rejected by his peers.

The cholera studies conducted by Snow and Farr are still regarded as some of the most important in the history of medicine because they established an entirely new way of studying epidemic disease. Unlike most of their predecessors, both viewed epidemic disease as a holistic problem, one that is influenced by a large number of variables and is best examined from many different perspectives. Rather than focusing solely on disease symptoms or death rates, their research included an analysis of city infrastructure and geography, victim testimonials, weather patterns, water flow and chemistry, socioeconomic issues, and a variety of other factors that could have potentially triggered the epidemic. In doing so, they were able to gain a comprehensive understanding of how cholera was affecting the community and ultimately how the community was affecting the spread of cholera. Others saw the brilliance of their innovative approach and began to model their own studies after their work.

Over time, the concept of studying epidemic disease in a holistic way gradually morphed into an entirely new branch of medicine referred to as epidemiology. Epidemiologists of today are responsible for tracking the incidence, distribution, and spread of disease. Whenever there is a new outbreak of any disease, epidemiologists are brought in from local, national (e.g., NIH, CDC), or international (e.g., WHO) agencies in order to identify the cause and develop a plan of action. Although such experts still largely hail from a medical background, their training must now incorporate elements of advanced statistics and mathematical modeling, sociology, civil engineering, and environmental biology. Like Snow and Farr before them, each is like a Sherlock Holmes of the medical field, using evidence from many different sources and strong powers of deduction to elucidate why a disease has arisen or spread. Whether it was tracking the sudden outbreak of Ebola in the jungles of West Africa in 2014, deciphering how HIV came to arrive in California and New York in 1981, or hunting down the last few cases of smallpox in Africa in the mid-1970s, epidemiologists have helped stop existing epidemics and prevented others from beginning in the first place. They have also provided us with 150 years of experience to draw from in the likely event that we face a new threat to our survival in the future.

Another area of medicine that was impacted by the work of Snow and Farr was public sanitation. As mentioned previously, the British cholera epidemics of the mid-19th century helped usher in the Sanitation Movement and elicit major changes to city design and waste disposal policies. Since these reforms were occurring at the same time and in same place as Snow's landmark epidemiology research, it seems logical to think that the two would have complemented one another. Unfortunately, that was not the case initially.

Early sanitation reformers like Chadwick and Southwood Smith were ardent supporters of miasmatic theory who, even after the publication of Snow's book in 1854, refused to entertain the idea of a specific waterborne germ. Their insistence on cleaning up Great Britain's water supply came more from a desire to clear out noxious smells that the water produced than to remove dangerous agents from the water itself. It largely remained this way until 1868, when *The Lancet* published their acceptance of the waterborne contagion theory for cholera. From that point forward, sanitation policy moved away from miasma and became firmly rooted in the sound science of Germ Theory. Water that smelled, looked, and tasted okay was no longer assumed to be safe. As a result, many cities initiated a variety of new water treatment procedures designed to remove and kill potentially harmful microbes from all municipal drinking water sources. This included passing water through a series of sand filters, treating it with chlorine, and adding chemicals to clump up (coagulate) any foreign particles. By the start of the 20th century, such preventative measures had all but eliminated waterborne disease from much of the industrialized world. Outbreaks still occurred occasionally, especially during times of war or following natural disasters;

however, they would never again cause the widespread epidemics that were so common during the 19th century.

Knowing that cholera was caused by something specific in contaminated water fostered the next major leap in our understanding of the disease—identification of the specific microorganism responsible for it. The first clues that cholera was caused by a bacterium came from the microscope of Italian anatomist Filippo Pacini.[75] Known primarily for his discovery of the encapsulated nerve endings in our skin that detect pressure and vibration (later named Pacinian corpuscles in his honor), Pacini became interested in the pathology of cholera following its arrival in Florence in 1854. He was working in the hospital of Santa Maria Nuova at the time and had access to the bodies of people who had recently succumbed to cholera. Using a rudimentary microscope and his great skill as an anatomist, Pacini examined the feces and intestinal tissue of those victims and noticed that they all shared similar histological abnormalities that were accompanied by millions of comma-shaped bacteria.[76] These bacteria, which he named "vibrions" for their tendency to vibrate in water, seemed to be associated with the particular sections of intestine that exhibited the most signs of visible pathology. Such repeated observations led him to conclude that the bacteria were an "organic, living substance, of a parasitic nature, communicating, reproducing, and then producing a disease of special character."[77] He published this groundbreaking research in an 1854 paper entitled "Microscopical Observations and Pathological Deductions on Cholera." Unfortunately, Pacini, like John Snow, received very little support for his "vibrion" germ theory from the Italian medical community due to their dogmatic belief in miasma. Unfazed by their skepticism, Pacini spent the next 30 years of his career and most of his life savings continuing his research of cholera pathogenesis. Despite publishing five additional studies on cholera during that time, Pacini's body of work largely went unnoticed by anyone outside of Florence.

In 1884, nearly 30 years after Pacini first peered through his microscope and saw "vibrions" attached to intestinal tissue of cholera victims, microbiologist Robert Koch published a report in which he claimed to have just discovered the bacterium that causes cholera.[78] Koch first began working on cholera during his trip to Egypt in 1883 as the leader of the German Cholera Commission. His team performed autopsies on 10 cholera victims and found that their intestinal tissues were teeming with millions of small, slightly bent bacteria. Believing that he may have identified the cholera bacteria, Koch then traveled to Calcutta, India, so that he could confirm and expand upon his findings in an area experiencing an active epidemic. In the six months that they were there, Koch and his team were able to successfully isolate the new bacterium in pure culture and identify its presence in contaminated water tanks and environmental water sources. Doing so enabled them to analyze the growth characteristics and biochemistry of the individual *V. cholerae* species for the first time.

Similar to what he had done with anthrax, Koch then attempted to infect lab animals with the purified *V. cholerae* in hopes of definitively proving that it is the causative agent of cholera. Unfortunately, the animals he used were not susceptible to infection by the bacteria. Despite that setback, Koch's study had provided enough evidence to convince most of his critics that he had indeed identified and isolated the cholera bacterium. Completely unaware of Pacini's publication in 1854, the scientific community proceeded to give Koch the credit for discovering *V. cholerae*. However, the oversight was eventually rectified in 1966, when the International Committee on Nomenclature officially renamed the *Vibrio* genus of bacteria as "*Vibrio* Pacini 1854" in honor of his accomplishments.

The rediscovery of *V. cholerae* by Koch in 1884 was significant because it helped usher in the demise of Miasmatic Theory. When John Snow first presented his heretical idea of a waterborne contagion in 1849, it was universally rejected by the medical community in England and elsewhere in Europe. However, as time went on, data from other scientists working on different diseases began to add support to the growing theory that microscopic germs can and do cause disease. For instance, around the same time that Snow was first investigating cholera, another physician named Ignaz Semmelweis found a link between deadly childbirth fever (known as puerperal fever) and the filth on the hands of medical students who were delivering babies after coming from dissecting rotting cadavers in the anatomy lab. After making the connection, he recommended that all medical students in his hospital wash their hands with a chlorinated lime solution prior to treating patients and delivering babies. Cases of puerperal fever dropped precipitously and hundreds of women's lives were saved as a result. Some years later (1867), a surgeon named Joseph Lister came to similar conclusions regarding wound infections that resulted from unsanitary surgical procedures. Like Semmelweis, he recommended that all equipment, dressings, and skin be disinfected using a chemical solution in order to prevent the introduction of germs into the exposed wound. The process was extremely successful and surgery soon ceased to be the death sentence that it had always been. The groundbreaking clinical work of Semmelweis and Lister was complemented well by the lab research expertise of Pasteur and Koch. Both men spent the better part of 25 years studying infectious diseases like anthrax, silkworm disease, rabies, tuberculosis, and cholera and proving that they were caused by specific microorganisms. The sum total of this extensive research made it nearly impossible for an educated person to continue supporting the myth of miasma. By the 1890s, the Germ Theory had emerged as the dominant explanation for infectious disease, and medicine would be changed forever as a result.

Modern Cholera

Despite knowing its cause, prevention, and treatment, cholera still represents a major problem for a significant portion of the population. The reason why cholera still infects millions every single year is that nearly 2.5 billion people still lack access to sanitation facilities and a reliable source of clean drinking water.[79] Amazingly, almost a billion people still practice open defecation, using street gutters, woods, or any open water source close to their home, and as many as 750 million people eat food that is irrigated by untreated human wastewater. Considering that modern sanitation practices were developed 150 years ago, it is a sad commentary on our society that nearly one-third of the Earth's human population lives in conditions that closely resemble those of the Middle Ages.

Modern cholera thrives in areas that lack basic municipal infrastructure and governmental oversight. This includes most of the impoverished countries of sub-Saharan Africa—many of which have per capita GDP (PPP) of less than $2,000—and much of rural Asia and Latin America. Additionally, any areas ravaged by violence, political unrest, and natural disaster are highly susceptible to experiencing a significant cholera outbreak. Despite widespread poverty in much of the world and countless wars, revolutions, and natural disasters, there have been only four significant cholera outbreaks in the past three decades.

The first took place in Latin America in the early 1990s when a new strain of cholera appeared on the Peruvian coast and spread to 21 countries in the Americas.[80] The bacteria flourished in the warm tropical waters there and ended up infecting over 1 million people over a six-year period (killing 11,875). The fatality rate was especially high in poverty-stricken rural areas, where access to clean water and medical treatment were often nonexistent. At about the same time cholera was ravaging Latin America, it also appeared in eastern Africa following the Rwandan genocide.[81] The mass slaughter of the Tutsi by the Hutu and the subsequent war between the two groups created over 2.1 million refugees. By August 1994, most had fled into neighboring countries like Zaire (now the Democratic Republic of Congo), Tanzania, and Uganda and settled into one of the 35 refugee camps established there. The unprecedented size and speed of the exodus created a logistical nightmare for those managing the ill-prepared camps. As one refugee who moved west into Zaire noted, "We have no water, no toilets. We are suffering here. No food. The Government has brought us nothing. Nobody is helping us."[82] Unfortunately, the conditions described so vividly by this young man are a perfect breeding ground for diseases like cholera and dysentery. In July 1994, a deadly cholera outbreak erupted in the refugee camp located in Goma, Zaire. In just a couple of weeks, cholera claimed the lives of an estimated 12,000 people.[83] The fatality rate in the first few days of the outbreak was exceptionally high (about 20%) due to a lack of available intravenous fluids and other medical resources. International relief agencies were eventually mobilized, and the number of new cases gradually declined by August.

Another major outbreak of cholera occurred in Africa in 2008. Unlike the one in 1994, which occurred as a result of war and displacement, the 2008–2009 outbreak in Zimbabwe was due to a comprehensive breakdown of nationwide resources.[84] An economic crisis brought on by a declining agriculture industry and political mismanagement led to a litany of domestic issues that included widespread food shortages, unusually high HIV incidence, collapse of the national healthcare system, and the destruction of municipal water supplies. The population was poor, malnourished, and improperly educated about the dangers of poor sanitation. Not surprisingly, a cholera outbreak exploded in August and promptly swept through the entire nation. By the time it finally subsided in June 2009, it had infected almost 100,000 people and killed 4,288.

Cholera reappeared just one year later in the Americas following the devastating 7.0-magnitude Haiti earthquake that took the lives of roughly 100,000–150,000 people and left over 3 million homeless.[85] Haiti, already one of the poorest nations on Earth prior to the earthquake, was left in utter ruin. Most homes and businesses in the capital city of Port-Au-Prince were reduced to rubble as were most governmental buildings (including the National Palace). The sheer devastation of national infrastructure left the government grossly unable to care for the massive numbers of victims in the wake of the disaster. As a result, most survivors were forced to move to makeshift tent cities where violence against women and children, disease, and hunger were commonplace. One disease that was initially not a concern was cholera since it had never reached Haiti throughout its entire history. Unfortunately, that changed in October 2010, just three months after the earthquake.

Cholera erupted along the banks of the Artibonite River and quickly spread across the ravaged country.[86] Despite attempts by UN peacekeeping forces and the WHO to control the epidemic, it infected over 750,000 people and killed over 9,000. Soon after the epidemic began, many began to wonder how the disease made it to the isolated island in the Caribbean. Years of epidemiological and genetic research has revealed that the cholera was brought to Haiti by a UN peacekeeper from Nepal. The outhouses on the Nepal base were found to be improperly emptied, which allowed untreated human waste to spill directly into the nearby Artibonite River. Once inside the warm water of the river, the bacteria replicated to a high level and spread to most other natural water sources on the island. Amazingly, UN officials strongly denied this account and refused to accept responsibility for the epidemic despite overwhelming empirical evidence to the contrary. Genetic tests on the *V. cholerae* strain in Haiti showed that it very closely resembled strains commonly found on the Indian subcontinent while being very different from strains normally present in South America (which is much closer to Haiti). Additionally, investigators uncovered interviews in which the sanitation company that serviced the Nepal base admitted to dumping the waste directly into the river near where the epidemic first began. The stubborn refusal of the UN to accept such convincing evidence was highlighted by scholar Philip Alston in his scathing 2016 report to the UN General Assembly about the epidemic. In the introduction, Alston called the UN's behavior during and after the cholera epidemic "morally unconscionable, legally indefensible, and politically self-defeating."[87] In response to this report, Ban Ki-moon, the Secretary General of the UN, finally relented and admitted that the UN played a role in initiating the cholera epidemic in Haiti.

Cholera has undergone a major transformation over the past 50 years. Once the most significant and feared epidemic disease in the world, cholera is now a disease with a relatively low mortality rate that is mostly confined to isolated pockets in a handful of countries. It will always be an ever-present danger in times of war and disaster; however, cholera no longer poses a threat to the population globally. The main reason for this change is that the innovations it gave rise to—most notably sanitation, oral rehydration therapy, and epidemiology—ultimately succeeded in helping us control it. This has been complemented by the recent development of multiple effective oral vaccines against cholera and greater worldwide education about waterborne diseases. Hopefully, with enough monetary investment in infrastructure and sanitation, the world will see an end to cholera as we know it.

CHAPTER NINE

Influenza

If the epidemic continues its mathematical rate of acceleration, civilization could easily disappear from the face of the earth within a few weeks.
—Dr. Victor Vaughan, Surgeon General of the U.S. Army, 1918[1]

When considering the most common symptoms of modern-day influenza (a.k.a. the flu), one may question its inclusion in a book about the 10 worst epidemic diseases in human history. People who contract the flu typically experience an acute upper respiratory illness that is accompanied by muscle aches, cough, general malaise, and fever. Symptoms usually begin about two days after first exposure and last for only one to two weeks. Although flu sufferers will feel awful and might be bedridden for most of the infection, they usually recover without requiring any hospitalization or other medical intervention. For most of the population, the flu is nothing more than a nuisance, a disease that causes us to miss work or ruins our vacation. However, for anyone who has preexisting lung condition (e.g., COPD, asthma) or is very young, elderly, pregnant, malnourished, or immunocompromised in any way, influenza can be extremely dangerous and even fatal. In fact, flu is believed to be responsible for over 300,000 deaths every year, with most of those resulting from more serious complications of flu-like pneumonia and heart failure. Such high mortality rates are frightening considering that effective vaccines have been available for some time as have several antiflu drugs (e.g., Tamiflu, amantadine). Despite the control efforts, many epidemiologists believe that influenza still represents the single greatest microbial threat to our species. As the quote at the beginning of the chapter alluded to, history has proven that their fears are justified.

The single worst epidemic of any disease to ever hit the human population in terms of deadliness and speed was the 1918 influenza pandemic, often referred to as the Spanish flu. Despite its name, the 1918 pandemic very likely originated in the United States (Kansas) and moved across the Atlantic Ocean as a result of the mass movement of American troops to France during World War I. Upon gaining a foothold in war-torn Europe, the disease spread rapidly to the rest of the world and killed millions in a matter of a few months. In total, it is believed to have infected one-third of the world's human population, killing about 50 million during the course of a single year. Some later estimates have the number of deaths closer to 100 million. To put these numbers into perspective, that is more deaths than occurred in 100 years of the Black Death and in the first 25 years of HIV. Unbelievably, the 1918 flu killed almost 5 percent of the global population and lowered the overall life expectancy by over 10 years. It claimed three times as many casualties as from World War I, which came to a close in that very same year. When adjusted for modern population numbers, the total fatalities resulting from 1918 flu would be equivalent to about 400 million people in today's world. What makes that even more staggering is that the pandemic occurred after the advent of Germ Theory, vaccines, and modern medicine.

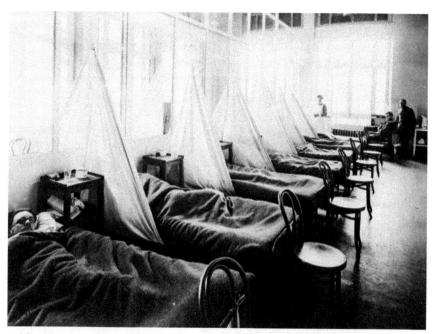

Soldiers are treated in the influenza ward at a U.S. Army camp hospital in France during World War I. (National Library of Medicine)

In addition to having abnormally high mortality rates, the 1918 flu pandemic was unlike any other in history in terms of how it killed and who it targeted. Early clinical reports of the 1918 flu describe a disease that was unusually violent in terms of the pathology it produced in its victims. Within just a few hours after the onset of standard flulike symptoms, many of those infected developed a fatal pneumonia, widespread cyanosis, and hemorrhaging out of the nose, mouth, eyes, ears, and anus. The disease progression was so abnormal that doctors who had treated thousands of cases of flu in their career were having trouble diagnosing it. Never before had flu killed so quickly or with such ferocity. There were countless reports of people waking up in the morning feeling healthy and then dying before nightfall with lungs full of bloody mucus. One physician working in Boston in September 1918 described seeing

> men start with what appears to be an ordinary attack of LaGrippe or Influenza, and when brought to the hosp. they very rapidly develop the most viscous type of pneumonia that has ever been seen. Two hours after admission they have the Mahogany spots over the cheek bones, and a few hours later you can begin to see the cyanosis extending from their ears and spreading all over the face, until it is hard to distinguish the coloured men from the white. It is only a matter of a few hours then until death comes, and it is simply a struggle for air until they suffocate. It is horrible.[2]

The question as to why the 1918 flu produced such uncharacteristic pathology remained a mystery for the next 90 years. It was not until 2005 that experiments began to reveal what made the 1918 flu unique. (The details of these experiments will be discussed later in the chapter.)[3] Surprisingly, those studies found that most of the worst damage was caused by an explosive immune response to the pathogen rather than the pathogen itself. In particular, the 1918 flu triggered host immune cells in the lungs to release massive quantities of toxic inflammatory chemicals. Cytokines normally help immune cells activate and communicate with one another; however, when too many of them are released in a short period of time (called a cytokine storm), widespread tissue death and excessive fluid accumulation can result. Since excessive inflammation caused most of the morbidity and mortality associated with the 1918 epidemic, it stands to reason that individuals with stronger immune systems should have had a more violent response to the infection. Interestingly, that is precisely what was observed. Unlike other seasonal flu strains, which primarily kill just the very young, elderly, and those with weak immune systems, the 1918 flu claimed the lives of millions of young, healthy adults with no preexisting conditions. In fact, about half of all flu deaths in 1918 occurred in people who were 20–40 years old, and those that were younger than 65 years old had an overall greater risk of dying from flu than those older than 65. It was the only flu epidemic in history in which being physically and immunologically strong was of very little advantage to the host. It was indiscriminately deadly, killing the young and the old, the healthy and the sick, and people on every continent.

While the 1918 pandemic of flu was the most well-known and deadly, it was not the only one to strike the population over the last few centuries. The first time that influenza became a worldwide threat was in 1889, when an outbreak started in Russia and spread rapidly across Asia, Europe, and the Americas aboard newly built railways and metal steamships.[4] Similar to other diseases during this time period, increases in population density and improvements to transportation provided a perfect situation for a contagious respiratory disease like influenza to infect a large number of people in a short amount of time. It reappeared in three successive waves over a period of three years and killed a total of about 1 million people. Newspapers all over the world provided daily updates about the movement of the Russian flu and how it was negatively impacting communities everywhere it went. In many cases, these accounts reached readers weeks before the arrival of the disease itself. The media coverage of the 1889 flu was unprecedentedly intense in large part because of the rise of the global newspaper industry and the invention of the telegraph in the decades that immediately preceded the pandemic.[5]

For the first time in history, the public was able to track an epidemic disease in real time, independent of its geography. A person living in Savannah, Georgia, for instance, could read about influenza in Chicago, Kansas, and even Paris just days after its arrival in those far-off locations. The public was hungry for news about the pandemic, and the media was more than happy to oblige. The media frenzy that ensued helped shape public perception about the 1889 pandemic, which, in turn, drastically influenced the narrative of future outbreaks of the disease.

Of the many pandemics that followed the 1918 Spanish flu, the Asian flu of 1957 and Hong Kong flu of 1968 were the most significant and deadly. Starting in Southeast Asia, the 1957 pandemic spread rapidly around the world and caused between 1 and 2 million deaths.[6] It was the first large-scale flu outbreak that occurred during the age of modern medical research. Fearing a repeat of the 1918 pandemic, influenza experts had collaboratively established a World Influenza Research Centre in 1948 with the hopes of closely monitoring flu in humans and in animal hosts. The Centre utilized the concept of crowdsourcing; it established a network of national and regional influenza labs in countries all over the world to independently study and track flu in their specific regions. In doing so, scientists were able rapidly share their findings about any new strains of flu that had appeared and report any abnormal clinical manifestations of the disease. The development of several new biotechnologies also allowed them to learn a great deal about the genetics and pathogenesis of flu during this time.

Despite having all this new knowledge and modern epidemiological tools, flu made a deadly comeback in Asia in 1957 and moved throughout the world in just six months. It was a shocking failure at a time when many believed that epidemic diseases would soon be conquered by our intellect and technology. One public health official expressed his disappointment over what had transpired when, in 1957, he wrote, "Although we have had 30 years to prepare for what should be done in the event of an influenza pandemic, I think we have all been rushing around trying to improvise investigations with insufficient time to do it properly. We can only hope that people will have taken advantage of their opportunities and at the end it may be possible to construct an adequate explanation of what happened."[7] Unfortunately, no explanations were given and no improvements were made prior to the start of another serious pandemic in 1968. Although it was somewhat less deadly than the previous three pandemics, the 1968 Hong Kong flu infected tens of millions of people as it marched rapidly through Southeast Asia prior to spreading to Europe and the Americas.

A vaccine was created shortly after flu's reappearance in 1968; however, the vaccine did not become broadly available until months after the pandemic had already peaked in most locations (including the United States). It was yet another ineffective response to a disease that seemed to be capable of moving and mutating faster than health officials could contain it. Fortunately, our ability to monitor flu in the population, contain it, treat it, and create vaccines in advance of flu season has improved drastically since the late 1960s. While there have been a few scares in recent years with "bird flu" and "swine flu" (e.g., 2009), there have been none as deadly as the one that began in Hong Kong in 1968.

A Virus and Its Hosts

Human influenza is caused by infection with one of three types of influenza virus. Human influenza A and B viruses are responsible for the vast majority of seasonal flu cases that crop up each winter, whereas the influenza C virus only causes an uncommon minor respiratory illness. Influenza A viruses were responsible for every pandemic of the 19th and 20th centuries and is the type that elicits the most concern from epidemiologists each year.

Influenza viruses have several unique genetic features that make them effective human pathogens. First of all, influenza viruses have a genome that is composed of RNA rather than DNA. As mentioned in chapter 1, all living things (e.g., bacteria, fungi, humans) use DNA as the genetic material because it is more chemically stable and less prone to being altered or mutated. Many viruses also use DNA as their genome; however, some, like influenza virus, have evolved to use RNA as their genetic material. One of the major issues facing viruses that use RNA as their genome is that host cells do not contain the enzymes that are needed to copy the viral genome. As a result, all RNA viruses must make their own genome-copying enzymes. For the influenza viruses, that enzyme is unusually error prone. In other words, every time influenza viruses invade new cells and begin to replicate, the new genomes that are made often contain small mutations. This is important because as influenza viruses continue to mutate little by little in hosts all over the world, it increases the chances that a brand-new and deadly strain will emerge and ravage the population. This process by which influenza viruses mutate gradually due to an accumulation of small mutations in its genome is commonly referred to as antigenic drift. It is one of the main reasons why we must be inoculated with the flu vaccine annually: the flu strain present during one flu season may mutate enough by the following year so that our immune system no longer effectively recognizes it.

One other aspect of influenza virus genetics that make it particularly dangerous is that its genome is collectively made up of seven or eight different pieces of RNA rather than one continuous strand of RNA. While having a split-up (segmented) genome is not in of itself harmful, it can cause serious problems in cases when two different viral strains happen to infect the exact same cell. When this situation occurs, both strains of influenza virus will replicate their genomic pieces in the same exact location within the cell. When those viruses go to package their newly made genomes into new virus particles, mistakes could be made, and some genomic RNAs could end up in the wrong virus. For instance, imagine that a dangerous bird flu strain happens to infect the same cell as a harmless human strain. When new viruses start assembling together, some of the human flu RNA pieces could accidentally end up in the same virus particle as RNA pieces from the bird strain. What would result is a brand-new hybrid strain that is genetically distinct from the two "parental" viruses. In other words, it could produce a strain that is both dangerous and able to infect humans. This genetic reshuffling, known as antigenic shift, can quickly create new pandemic strains that have never been seen before by the human immune system. Like antigenic drift, antigenic shift is random and impossible to predict or control. As a result, our population is always one mutation or genetic-reshuffling event away from potential disaster.

Influenza A and B viruses infect humans and a variety of other animal hosts, including many types of birds, pigs, horses, seals, and dogs. In general, a strain of flu virus that has affinity for one species will usually not infect other species that well. The major reason for this has to do with the specific nature by which flu viruses adhere to the surface of cells in host tissues. The attachment process involves an interaction between the hemagglutinin (HA) protein found on all flu viruses and a common sugar called sialic acid that coats the surface of lung cells and several other animal tissues. Each flu strain has a unique version of the HA protein that folds in a slightly different manner than HA proteins found on other flu viruses. Similarly, each animal species has a somewhat unique form of sialic acid on its cells. Thus you can have a bird flu strain with an HA protein that is folded in such a way that it will only recognize the bird version of sialic acid. That strain would likely not infect humans well because the virus would poorly adhere to human cells. This seemingly logical relationship between influenza HA and sialic acid is complicated by the fact that some animals produce multiple types of sialic acid on their cells. For instance, pig cells contain sialic acid that resembles what is found in both birds and humans. As a result, pigs can be infected by many different strains of flu simultaneously and serve as a living mixing vessel for the creation of new hybrid strains of flu through antigenic shift. The 2009 swine flu pandemic arose when bird flu, human flu, and pig flu strains all infected the same pig and reassorted into a brand-new flu strain with properties of all three.

HA is not the only influenza protein that interacts with host sialic acid residues. The surface of the virus also contains a protein called neuraminidase (NA or N), which functions to cut sialic acid when newly made flu viruses are attempting to exit the cell they just replicated in. Sialic acid, while serving as a great target for flu viruses when they attach to cells initially, become a hindrance for viruses trying to leave those same cells and spread to new ones. The flu NA protein solves this problem by working like a machete to enzymatically cleave any sialic acid that is holding up any new flu viruses wanting to leave that cell. Like HA, the NA protein is very specific for the type of sialic acid it can cut. Some forms of NA preferentially cut bird sialic acid, whereas others cut sialic acid from humans or other animals. Thus, if you have a version of NA that best cuts sialic acid from one species (e.g., birds) and the virus goes into a different species (e.g., human), newly made flu viruses would never make it off the cell surface and the infection would essentially stop. Both HA and NA must "match" the particular species they are infecting. For this reason, scientists typically focus on those two proteins when they are classifying a new strain of the virus (e.g., H1N1).

The Quiet Catastrophe

Any pandemic that spread to every corner of the planet and killed more than 50 million people would be expected to have enormous impacts on various social, political, health, and economic issues for many decades afterward. Interestingly, when one closely examines the 1918 flu pandemic and the years that immediately followed, it is often difficult to find any type of lasting footprint of its existence. There was almost no rioting, political upheavals, scapegoating, or long-term economic impacts. Furthermore, it did not have any significant effect on any battle during World War I nor did it noticeably impact the Russian Civil War that followed. Despite exposing the massive failures of public health policy in the face of a deadly crowd disease, the 1918 flu pandemic also did not provoke any sweeping reform of how cities or nations handled epidemic threats. It was almost as if the world was so weary from years of war and disease that it just decided to put the whole ordeal behind it and move on. In this way, the 1918 flu is unique in the pantheon of epidemic diseases mentioned in this book. It is almost paradoxical that the worst killer of humans had almost no long-term impact on those humans.

In order to better understand why this happened, one must first consider how governments, media outlets, and the public responded to the pandemic while it was occurring. When flu appeared in January 1918, most initially thought that it was just another seasonal flu outbreak that would have to run its course.[8] However, by September, it became clear to public health officials that this flu epidemic was so uniquely virulent and fast that standard control measures were not working. In response, cities all over the world began to quarantine the sick and propose restrictions on public gatherings, personal hygiene, and business practices. The extent to which these restrictions were mandated depended heavily on the individual local board of health in a given city and how much power it held with respect to local businesses. Some cities changed relatively little during the pandemic for fear of disrupting the local economy or inciting panic among the public. For instance, the New York City Health Commissioner Royal Copeland erred on the side of not imposing any outright ban on public gatherings.[9] Instead, he initiated less intrusive measures such as asking businesses to stagger their hours to reduce crowds, increasing surveillance and disease reporting by city physicians, and educating the public about the dangers of coughing and spitting in public. As Copeland stated in a paper in the following year, "my aim was to prevent panic, hysteria, mental disturbance, and thus to protect the public from the condition of mind that in itself predisposes to physical ills."[10]

On the opposite end of the spectrum, some cities virtually shut down all municipal activities during the height of the pandemic. They closed schools, libraries, movie theaters, saloons, stadiums, shopping centers, dance halls, and any other place where people gather in large numbers. Some cities closed churches in order to minimize exposure between congregants, and many others banned public funerals. A few cities, like San Francisco and San Diego, even required its citizens to wear surgical (gauze) masks when going out in public.[11] Collectively, it was the most widespread and comprehensive public health response ever executed. Unfortunately, the fact that 50 million died from the disease suggests that it was still inadequate.

Cities that instituted stringent public health measures did not necessarily fare much better than those with more lax policies. For instance, Boston, Philadelphia, and New Orleans, all of which had outright bans of most

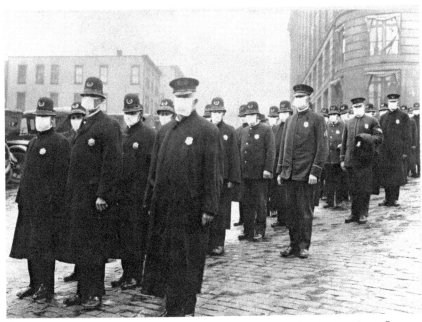

Members of the Seattle police force wear protective masks during the influenza pandemic of 1918. (American Red Cross)

public gatherings, had significantly higher mortality rates than New York City and St. Louis had, which had similar or less rigorous sanctions. Epidemiologists and medical historians spent decades trying to understand this unexpected disparity. Finally, in 2007, several studies published in the prestigious journal *Proceedings of the National Academy of Sciences* shed new light on this mystery.[12] Researchers identified two key factors that may have played a significant role in determining how well a city fared during the 1918 pandemic. The first was the timing of when the measures were implemented. Cities that took action before the pandemic hit or within the first few days following the first cases had much lower overall mortality rates than those that delayed enforcement. Philadelphia, which had one of the highest mortality rates of large U.S. cities, took over two weeks after flu arrived to limit public gatherings in any way. In fact, they even held a large parade during that lag period. In contrast, St. Louis initiated its public health response almost immediately after exposure and had mortality rates that were eight times lower than Philadelphia as a result.

The second factor that was uncovered in these studies was the timing of when cities lifted their restrictions. A number of cities eased their public health measures just after the pandemic peaked rather than when it was over. In doing so, they gave people a false sense of security at a time when the pandemic was still raging and killing large numbers of people. Such false security increased risky "crowd" behaviors (e.g., riding public transportation), which allowed flu to cause much damage when it came back around in its second wave. Making matters worse, local health boards often fought with one another and with larger (state/regional/national) boards. This produced unnecessary delays and created confusion in populations who often were getting mixed messages.

The extreme measures taken by many cities during this time were tolerated fairly well by the public. While disagreements did arise between officials, politicians, and business owners, the general public for the most part accepted the restrictions placed upon them. Riots and large protests were uncommon as were instances of organized subversion of sanitation rules (other than the occasional illegal saloon). It is an interesting reaction that is quite different from what was observed for most other epidemics throughout history. Some believe that the public saw the exceptional danger posed by the 1918 flu and accepted the fact that extreme measures were required to combat it. Most people had been negatively affected by the pandemic in some way, either through reading about it in the newspaper on a daily basis or by knowing someone who had become ill or died from it. Whether one was living in the city, in a small town, or in relative isolation, everyone knew how awful this particular flu was. While it is true that some never knew the full extent of the enormity of the pandemic, it is hard to imagine that anyone living in 1918 would have taken the flu lightly.

A second possibility is that people had grown accustomed to greater governmental control as a result of the awful situation created by World War I. "Sacrificing for the greater good" became a common attitude as citizens were called upon to ration their food, go to work in factories, and even offer their own lives for the sake of the nation. Recognizing the extraordinary circumstances of the situation, most people readily gave up certain rights in order to ultimately win the war. When flu arrived near the end of the war and cities began to impose quarantines and regulations, most likely viewed the measures as just another sacrifice needed in a time of emergency. It was a conditioned response of submission ingrained in them from four continuous years of war and death. In the end, their willingness to obey authorities likely saved millions of lives and prevented the pandemic from escalating further.

Bridging the gap between local health boards and the public was the newspaper industry, which served as primary source of information about the 1918 pandemic and how communities were responding to it. Newspapers not only reported daily statistics about infections and deaths in their local area, they were also usually responsible for alerting the public any time the health board had imposed new regulations. In many cases, newspapers would go a step further and editorialize these announcements by giving them their full endorsement. For instance, a day after Charlotte,

North Carolina, imposed a strict ban on all public gatherings, a writer for the *Charlotte Observer* wrote, "The only way influenza can be stopped is the way in which Charlotte stopped paralysis, and that is by an all-embracing quarantine . . . Wisdom has again guided the hand of the Charlotte administration."[13] In supporting the actions of health officials in this way, newspapers often served as the mouthpiece of the local government during the pandemic.

While such reporting generally had a positive impact on citywide responses, there were many instances when newspaper coverage of the 1918 flu had more deleterious effects. For instance, in many places, newspapers downplayed the seriousness of the pandemic in its early stages, thus reassuring the public that the flu was under control in their city or by discussing how much worse it was elsewhere. Such reporting created a false sense of security during the time when intervention was most critical. Some of the newspapers also printed advertisements for false tonics and potions that sellers claimed would cure the flu. Desperate victims who were watching family members die or were dying themselves were duped into spending money on useless cures that in some cases even hastened their lung damage. The ads also had the secondary effect of dangerously misleading the public into thinking that a cure existed. Diseases that have cures tend to be viewed in a less serious light than those that do not. If their illness could be fixed by taking a pill or gargling a miracle tonic solution, why should they fear passing it on to others? Furthermore, why should they inconvenience themselves by obeying overly restrictive public health recommendations? It was an unethical abuse of the media that was allowed because of the revenue it generated. A number of papers realized that it was a mistake and printed apologies to their readers.

Many newspapers also reported on the pandemic in a way that minimized the true human cost of the disease. Articles about World War I were usually vivid descriptions of suffering and heroism that were prominently displayed on the front page with huge headlines. They were written to evoke an emotional response in the reader, which would make them more likely to support the war effort. In contrast, early articles about the 1918 flu tended to be nothing more than short technical blurbs about death statistics and policy. They rarely contained specific details about individuals or the struggles they were facing. Because of their superficial nature, these reports were usually buried in the middle of the paper with small headings and little "fanfare." Some have argued that this was done by design in order to keep the public from overreacting to the pandemic. There was a real fear that oversensationalization of the flu could trigger "panic, hysteria, mental disturbance," which many felt was more dangerous than the flu itself. Unfortunately, minimizing flu in this way hid how dangerous the pandemic really was, which ultimately negatively impacted the behavior of the people most at risk.

The previous discussion of how the world responded to the 1918 pandemic while it was occurring provides some clues as to why it failed to induce the same type of long-term changes as other epidemics. First of all, the timing of the pandemic was unique. It occurred during one of the deadliest and most widespread wars in history. This led many to view the flu as a by-product of the war rather than as a separate entity with independent causes and effects. The fact that the deadly second wave of the pandemic peaked and ended around the same time as the signing of the armistice (winter 1918–1919) further reinforced in people's minds that flu was just another awful extension of the war. When the war ended, people were eager to put it behind them and return to some sense of normalcy. Since the pandemic and war were psychologically intertwined in many people's minds, moving on from one meant moving on from the other.

A second factor that affected the "legacy" of the 1918 flu was its duration. No other major epidemic in history began and ended in such a short period of time. By the time people were able to process what was happening to them, the flu was gone. It did not last for many years like the Black Death or HIV, it did not keep coming back sporadically every few years like yellow fever or cholera, and it was not endemic like TB or smallpox. This pandemic lasted just over one year and it was never heard from again (at least with that level of intensity). People were not forced to permanently alter their way of life to deal with it because they were not constantly being harassed by it. In this sense, the 1918 flu acted more like a natural disaster than a plague.

Maybe one of the most surprising observations in the post-1918 era was that the pandemic failed to cause any significant change in how we approach public health. By any qualitative or quantitative measure one uses, the public health response in 1918 failed miserably. Influenza seemed to go wherever it wanted, whenever it wanted, no matter what control measures were in place. Public health officials who were armed with a vast knowledge of infectious disease, epidemiology, and medicine were no more able to control the 1918 flu than plague doctors were able to control the Black Death in the 14th century. This is an interesting part of the flu story because the public health sector actually had a rational and scientifically sound plan for stopping the disease. In fact, if a similar flu were to arise today, we would likely also respond with quarantines, public gathering bans, and educational initiatives (the flu vaccine and antiflu drugs like Tamiflu would also be employed).

Public health policies did not change all that much following the 1918 flu because they were not inherently wrong. As mentioned above, the timing of when they were implemented and lifted and the consistency by which they were followed in different cities was somewhat poor. Also, the inability of local, regional, and national boards of health to communicate effectively was an obvious failure of the response. Indeed, both of these aspects of public health planning were improved in the years that followed. However, at the basic level, the theory behind what was done demonstrated a modern understanding of infectious disease transmission. So why did the measures not work? The answer lies in the fact that we still have seasonal flu outbreaks in 2017. The influenza virus is highly contagious and difficult to control because people are naturally drawn to crowded places and are reluctant to follow basic hygienic practices even when they know of the dangers involved. For this reason, no amount of planning or implementation could have totally prevented or stopped the 1918 pandemic.

The Real-Life Jurassic Park

The 1918 influenza pandemic ravaged our population for over 16 months before mostly dying out during the summer of 1919. Almost immediately after the pandemic ended, scientists from all over the world began studying the disease in order to determine its etiology and to understand why it was so virulent when compared to other strains. Unfortunately, they had limited technological tools at their disposal at the time and were hampered by an inability to properly store samples from 1918 flu victims. The influenza virus carries a genome that is composed of RNA, which is unstable and prone to rapid degradation if not stored at ultracold temperatures (e.g., $-80°C$). Since modern-day cryopreservation techniques and freezers did not become widely available until the late 1940s, the majority of clinical specimens isolated from 1918 flu victims were rendered useless within a few years after being stored in suboptimal conditions. Without a supply of intact samples or advanced technology, scientists had no way of ascertaining what was unique about the 1918 strain. As a result, they had no ability to generate a vaccine or determine whether another similar deadly strain was developing somewhere around the world in bird or pig populations. We were sitting ducks, completely in the dark about the worst strain of any virus to ever hit the human population.

The advent of the molecular biology age of microbiology in the 1960s and 1970s gave scientists a variety of new tools with which to understand and alter pathogens at the genetic level. One of the most significant techniques developed during this time was one that enabled us to obtain the specific sequence of every nucleotide in the genomes of viruses, bacteria, and nearly any other living thing. All genomes are composed of four types of nucleotides—adenine (A), thymine (T), guanine (G), and cytosine (C). Although all organisms have the same four nucleotides in their genome, the specific order of these nucleotides is unique for each species. That order is what determines exactly what proteins are made by each individual species and is ultimately what makes all living things unique. In other words, the genome is a detailed blueprint of sorts. Knowing every component of that blueprint is vitally important when scientists are trying to ascertain how a given microbial pathogen is causing disease or what makes one strain of a pathogen different from another.

The first genomes ever sequenced were that of two small viruses that infect bacteria. Although modest in scope by today's standards, the sequencing of these small phage virus genomes in 1976 was a monumental achievement because it demonstrated that it was possible to obtain a complete picture of how microbes are constructed. A number of other viral genomes were sequenced in the next several years, including that of the human influenza virus in 1982. Genome sequencing took a huge step forward in 1995 when scientists at the Institute for Genomic Research used a new "shotgun" sequencing method to obtain the first complete sequence of a bacterium, a human pathogen known as *Haemophilus influenzae*.[14] Its genome is over 1.8 million nucleotides long and is significantly larger and more complex than any of the viral genomes that had been examined previously. Rapid improvements to shotgun sequencing followed and soon genomes from virtually every other human pathogen were sequenced. Amazingly, sequencing technology has now progressed to the point that genomes of viruses and small bacteria can be sequenced in a matter of hours.

Despite major advancements in genome sequencing in the latter part of the 20th century, the sequence of 1918 strain of the influenza virus remained elusive due to the lack of properly preserved specimens from that time. However, in 1997, scientists at the U.S. Armed Forces Institute of Pathology (AFIP) began looking into the possibility of retrieving 1918 flu genome from tissues that were preserved in formalin and paraffin wax. Led by Dr. Jeffrey Taubenberger, scientists purified genetic material from 28 separate tissue specimen and attempted to sequence the small portions of the 1918 flu genome that remained after nearly 80 years.[15] In doing so, they were able to get bits and pieces of the 1918 flu genome sequenced. While not entirely successful, it demonstrated that it might be possible to get a complete 1918 flu genome sequence if a slightly better preserved specimen could be located.

In just the following year, a scientist named Johan Hultin informed the AFIP team that he had just exhumed a body of an Inuit woman in western Alaska who was buried under seven feet of permafrost after dying of flu in 1918. Being kept nearly frozen for 80 years, the lung tissue contained enough preserved flu virus for the AFIP team to obtain a complete sequence of the 1918 flu genome in 2005.[16] While this was regarded as one of the most significant moments in the history of microbial genetics, it was not without controversy. The researchers who completed the study published the complete 1918 flu genomic sequence in the scientific journal *Nature*. Some members of the public were extremely concerned that people with bad intentions could use the sequence to potentially create a new bioweapon that was capable of killing millions of people. After extensive discussion between members of the U.S. National Science Advisory Board for Biosecurity and the Centers for Disease Control and Prevention (CDC), all agreed that the sequence should be published in the interest of proper scientific protocol.

Concerns about the 1918 genomic sequencing being made available were intensified by news that scientists at the CDC were successful in using the sequence to recreate the 1918 flu virus.[17] They employed reverse genetics technology to first reconstruct the 1918 genome piece by piece from fresh nucleotide building blocks (using their sequence as a map), and then they added the newly made genome to human cells. After a few additional steps, influenza viruses emerged from cells that were genetically and structurally identical to the strain that killed over 50 million people and disappeared from the Earth in the early 1920s. A collaborative group of scientists from several universities and research centers then began testing the resurrected 1918 strain on various animal

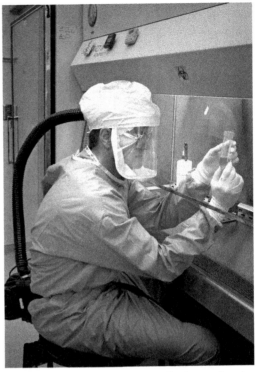

Dr. Terrence Tumpey, a microbiologist for the Centers for Disease Control and Prevention, examines the reconstructed version of the 1918 pandemic influenza virus. (Centers for Disease Control and Prevention)

models in order to gain clues as to why it was so incredibly pathogenic to humans. As hoped, this work was extremely productive. It not only identified the exact mutations in the 1918 genome that were responsible for most of its deadly effects on the lungs, it also enabled scientists to observe how the strain works on a cellular level. Equally important, it allowed scientists to finally produce a specific vaccine that would protect the population in the event that a similar strain develops naturally or is somehow created as a bioterrorism agent. After eight decades of fearing the unknown, mankind was finally able to rest a little easier.

Despite the scientific merit and novelty of bringing an extinct disease back to life in order to better understand it, not everyone celebrated the recreation of the extinct 1918 flu.[18] Many believed that the enormous risk associated with making such a deadly agent far outweighed its benefits. In particular, people worried that the 1918 virus could possibly escape from secured facilities that harbored it and enter back into the population.

Examples of other deadly pathogens escaping secured laboratories include the accidental release of the SARS virus in 2003 and 2004 from multiple labs in Asia and the illegal removal of weaponized anthrax from labs in 2001 (which was famously used in the mail terrorist attacks that year).

Many also feared that terrorists or enemy nations could use the information found in the published articles to recreate 1918 flu themselves or even make something worse (e.g., a hybrid of 1918 flu and another pathogen). Two prominent bioethicists, Arthur Caplan and Glenn McGee, published the following joint statement related to this concern: "A decade ago, the manipulation of deadly viruses could be restricted to a high-security vault . . . Today, however, the super-secret stores of deadly viruses have been reduced to a set of instructions, which might at some point become a cookbook for terrorists and other malcontents or amateurs."[19] To them, the dangerous and irresponsible aspect of the 1918 flu project was the publication of the step-by-step instructions and sequences needed to make the deadly virus. It was a roadmap that others could easily follow if given basic training in genetics and some pieces of molecular biology equipment. The success of bioweapons programs of the United States, Soviet Union/Russia, Japan, and many other countries over the past 40 years supports such fears. In saying that, it has been nearly 12 years since the 1918 flu genome was sequenced and recreated, and no reports have come forward of its attempted use for harm. It does not mean that safety concerns were unwarranted; however, mechanisms put in place to protect the public have so far been quite effective.

The re-creation of the 1918 flu came at a time when scientists were increasingly using technology to genetically alter microbes and other, larger species. Such genetically modified organisms, also known as GMOs, have become a hot button issue throughout much of the developed world over the past two decades. In addition to concerns over GMO safety and effects on the environment, many believe that unnaturally altering the genetic material of a living thing and interfering with the natural process of evolution is ethically akin to "playing God." Considering that the 1918 flu re-creation went a step further and brought an extinct disease back to life in a manner similar to what was fictionally illustrated in the movie *Jurassic Park*, many feel that scientists went too far and may have opened up Pandora's box. These are issues that will need to be addressed in the near future as our scientific ability and understanding continue to advance at an exponential rate.

A New Paradigm in Vaccine Programs

People who are suffering from the flu often develop secondary infections caused by other bacteria and viruses. For instance, the initial damage and inflammation that result from influenza virus replication often makes the host more susceptible to being infected with bacterial pathogens like *Strepto-coccus pneumoniae*, *Staphylococcus aureus*, or *Haemophilus influenzae*.

In fact, a great deal of morbidity and mortality associated with flu is actually caused by these other pathogens rather than by anything the influenza virus itself is doing to the lungs. For this reason, many physicians will prescribe antibiotics for people with the flu even though antibiotics have absolutely no effect on viruses. Although it is a dangerous practice in terms of the creation of new antibiotic resistant strains, prophylactically giving antibiotics to flu patients does save countless lives every year.

The high prevalence of co-infecting pathogens was problematic for scientists who were initially trying to identify and purify the causative agent of the flu in the early 20th century. Such studies led many to incorrectly identify *Haemophilus influenzae* as the cause of flu (hence its name); however, when Koch's postulates were applied, pure *H. influenzae* failed to produce the flu when given to test subjects or animals.[20] It was not until 1931 that it was finally discovered that the flu was caused by a virus rather than a bacterium. Just two years later, British scientists were able to successfully purify the influenza virus for the first time, which allowed for the development of a vaccine.[21]

The first flu vaccine that was tested was a live, attenuated vaccine created by the Soviet scientist Anatoly Smorodintsev in 1936.[22] He grew the flu virus in chicken eggs for 30 separate replication cycles in order to select for weakened (attenuated) variants of the virus that had lost the ability to cause significant disease in people. After injecting his vaccine into human subjects, he found that those who developed antibodies in response to the vaccine were generally protected from being infected by flu. However, modern analyses of his study design reveal that it contained several significant flaws, which now suggest his vaccine was only minimally effective overall.

Around the same time, an American physician named Thomas Francis also began working on an influenza vaccine with a team of extremely talented junior scientists that included Jonas Salk (who would go on to develop the first polio vaccine). The Francis vaccine was different from that of Smorodintsev in that it was treated with the chemical formalin in order to destroy the virus so that it could no longer cause disease.[23] Such an inactivated virus vaccine was completely safe and could still spark an immune response in its recipients as long as enough of it was injected. The Francis team was working on this vaccine during the early 1940s when Francis was serving as the director of the U.S. Army Commission on Influenza. When the United States entered into World War II in late 1941, Francis was charged with protecting the millions of U.S. troops who would be deployed to areas where flu routinely caused mass casualties. The U.S. military was extremely concerned about the possibility of a repeat of the 1918 flu epidemic, which claimed the lives of over 46,000 U.S. servicemen who were stationed in Europe. Such worry prompted the military to give Francis and his team free rein to use large numbers of U.S. servicemen in their clinical trials. The end result of their massive clinical trials was the development of flu vaccine that was scientifically proven to be both safe and effective. Following the publication of their findings in 1943, their vaccine was mass produced and eventually distributed widely to the public.[24]

One of the most important developments in the search for the ideal flu vaccine was the realization that there were different types of influenza viruses that could further mutate into different strains. The first flu type isolated in 1933 was an influenza A virus that belonged to the H1N1 strain/subtype (A/H1N1). In 1940, a new type of flu virus was discovered, named influenza B, that had significant protein differences than A/H1N1.[25] Those working on the A/H1N1 vaccine soon realized that it failed to protect subjects from infection with the new influenza B type. As a result, they were forced to develop a new vaccine, a bivalent one that contained both inactivated A/H1N1 and B.[26]

The bivalent vaccine was mass administered for over a decade and seemingly worked to reduce flu-related infections and deaths. However, the reemergence of a deadly flu pandemic in 1958 made it obvious that flu would not be defeated without a fight. The flu strain that caused the 1958 pandemic was an influenza A that had mutated into a subtype that had never been seen in the population before (H2N2). With this information in hand, vaccine companies began producing a new bivalent vaccine that included just the A/H2N2 and B subtypes.[27] This was the most common flu vaccine given for about a decade. When the 1968 flu pandemic was shown to be caused by yet another new subtype (H3N2), vaccine companies were again forced to switch to producing a different bivalent vaccine. Since that time, the occasional reemergence of the H1N1 and various B subtypes led to matching changes in the composition of the yearly flu vaccine. In each case, flu vaccine development was reactionary, only changing after new strains had already emerged and began infecting large numbers of people. In fact, the lag time between strain identification and vaccine development was often so great that many flu outbreaks were long over before the vaccine was available to the public. It was an inefficient and ineffective approach to vaccine development that was in need of a major overhaul.

The creation of the World Health Organization (WHO) Influenza Surveillance Program in 1952 provided the right opportunity for the development of a smarter flu vaccine.[28] The program worked by establishing national surveillance centers in countries around the world that would monitor what flu strains had emerged in their area. Starting as a loose collection of laboratories in influenza "hot zones," the surveillance program has since grown to include 136 centers located in 106 countries. These local centers are responsible for regularly testing samples from both humans and animals and then reporting what they find to one of five regional WHO centers. When all of the data from the world are finally processed and the most common flu strains in the population have been identified for that specific year, the WHO issues its recommendations to companies that manufacture the seasonal flu vaccine. The vaccine is usually trivalent, which means it contains the three most significant flu strains for that year (usually A/H1N1, A/H3N2, and B). However, since 2012, the vaccine has contained a fourth strain (quadravalent) due to the widespread presence of multiple B strains of flu in the population.[29] Each year's vaccine is an educated guess, a well-informed prediction about which flu strains are most likely to appear and cause problems during the upcoming flu season. Despite the occasional mistake, creating the flu vaccine in this way has been infinitely more effective than waiting for flu to strike before starting the production of the vaccine.

The seasonal flu vaccine has pushed the boundaries for what is deemed acceptable in vaccine production industry. Never before has a vaccine been changed and mass distributed to the population on a yearly basis, and never before has one been based on a prediction. It was previously unthinkable to make a vaccine that only protected recipients for a single year because the cost of doing so would be prohibitive when compared to its long-term benefits. However, considering that the seasonal flu still leads to 200,000 hospitalizations and $87 billion in economic losses in the United States every year, it is clear that altering the composition of the vaccine every year is necessary to keep up with a virus that mutates as well as influenza does. Not doing so puts the entire human population at risk for a pandemic even worse than what was experienced in 1918.

CHAPTER TEN

Polio

It was the robber of hope for a generation, several generations of children. There were diseases, and scientists will chart them, that were more devastating, affecting more children, more deadly than polio. But polio left kids crippled, and that was an image that this big strong postwar country simply couldn't abide. We had children lining up in wheelchairs, in iron lungs, whose very vitality and everyone's hope for their future was allayed right at the most critical time in their childhoods.
—Polio survivor Mark Sauer, in *A Paralyzing Fear: The Triumph over Polio in America*[1]

Imagine that you are a young married couple living in 1932. You have a beautiful young daughter who is your pride and joy. One morning, while on vacation, your family decides to go for a swim in the lake near the cabin where you are staying. The water is cold but very refreshing on a hot summer's day. After you are finished, you go home and have a relatively uneventful rest of your day. About a week later, your daughter begins to complain that she does not feel well. She has a slight fever and her muscles are a little stiff and achy. Believing that she must have picked up a cold that was aggravated by swimming in the frigid lake days earlier, you give her some warm soup and put her to bed early. When you awake on the following morning, you are startled by the screams coming from your daughter's room. You run in to find her crying. To your horror, you realize that she cannot move her legs and is having difficulty lifting her arms. You immediately pick up her lifeless body and rush her to the nearest hospital. When the doctor comes into your room after conducting some tests, she confirms what you already know. Your daughter has contracted polio. She tells you that your daughter will survive; however, she will likely be confined to a wheelchair for the rest of her life. Your heart sinks as you realize what this means for her. She will not be able to finish school or will she likely get married or have any semblance of a normal life.

The fictional account described above attempts to illustrate the horrifying nature of the 20th-century polio epidemic. Although it did occasionally affect teens and adults (around 25–30% of the cases), children under the age of 10 were more commonly the targets of polio. It spread in a seemingly random fashion, sparing one child while killing or paralyzing another. The vast majority of children (around 70%) who were exposed to the causative agent of polio, the human poliovirus, showed no signs or symptoms that they were infected. Their immune systems fought off the infection, and they recovered with no ill effects. Some children (around 25%) did not fare quite as well and developed flu-like symptoms as their bodies battled with the virus. Like the asymptomatic group, they ultimately recovered after about a week with no long-term damage. Unfortunately, there were about 5 percent of children that had more severe complications from their infection. As illustrated in the story above, some developed muscle stiffness and fever after exposure, which was then followed by meningitis (3–4%) and/or flaccid (relaxed) muscle paralysis in the limbs (1%). In extreme cases, paralysis also spread to the muscles involved in breathing, swallowing, and speaking. This was the deadliest form of polio. The few who managed to survive such widespread paralysis were often confined to artificial respirators for the remainder of their lives.

Although evidence suggests that polio had been around since ancient times, it did not appear in any type of medical literature until finally being described in 1789 as a "debility of the lower extremities in children."[2] A landmark report by German orthopedist Jacob von Heine in 1840 was the first to describe the different clinical forms of polio and differentiate them from other similar paralytic diseases.[3] It was also the first time the disease was referred to as infantile spinal paralysis. Over the next three decades, several researchers from France uncovered the cellular basis of the paralytic symptoms. They found that the infection invades the central nervous system and kills nerve cell bodies (grey matter) in the spinal cord and brainstem. Dead motor neurons are unable to transmit signals from the brain to the body's muscles, which results in a state of paralysis.

At this point in the history of polio, it was still an extremely rare disease. It would arise sporadically in the United States or Europe, infect a small number of people, and then disappear after a short time. However, by the 1890s, larger clusters of infection started to appear in places like Boston, Vermont, and Sweden.[4] The size and severity of these localized polio outbreaks only grew worse as the 20th century began. There was an epidemic in the Swedish countryside in 1905 that affected over 1,000 people and one in

New York City in 1907 that involved 2,500 victims. The first widespread epidemic of polio occurred in the United States in the summer of 1916. First appearing in an Italian community in Brooklyn, New York, the disease spread in a radial pattern through the Northeast and infected 27,000 people (mostly children) and killed 6,000 of them. It was the first time that the world really took notice of the little known poliovirus; the targeting of children, visually shocking symptoms, and extremely high fatality rate had parents all over the country scrambling to protect their kids.

It is a fear that would reemerge every summer for the next four decades. Yearly polio epidemics only continued to get worse in the 1930s–1950s, peaking in 1952 with 58,000 cases of paralytic polio in the United States alone. In all, the 20th-century polio epidemic is believed to have killed about 1 million people and left as many as 20 million with some form of physical disability. It was not nearly as deadly as the other epidemic diseases described in this book, but it was horrifying and extremely influential.

Polio, also known as poliomyelitis, is caused by infection with one of several human polioviruses. These viruses belong to the picornavirus family, which is a group of exceptionally small, sturdy viruses that use RNA as their genome. Other picornaviruses include those that cause the common cold (rhinoviruses), hepatitis A virus, and the foot and mouth disease virus that commonly affects livestock. In the case of poliovirus, exposure is primarily through the ingestion of food or water that is contaminated with feces; however, some evidence suggests it can also be transmitted directly between people through saliva. Once the virus enters the gastrointestinal tract, it replicates in the intestinal cells for about a week prior to moving to local lymphoid tissues like lymph nodes and tonsils. It replicates there and eventually spills into the bloodstream. The presence of large amounts of poliovirus in the blood (known as viremia) is what usually causes the flu-like symptoms seen in nearly all symptomatic individuals.

Depending on the immune system and age of the host, the virus may move from the blood into the spinal cord, where it can cause meningitis and damage to the motor neurons. If the virus stays localized to the lower spinal cord, it will ultimately cause varying degrees of asymmetrical paralysis in the limbs. This form of the disease, called spinal polio, makes up about 80 percent of the paralysis cases. In some people, the virus will leave the lower spinal cord after a short time and move up toward the brain. As it kills neurons in the brainstem, the person can develop an abnormal heartbeat and difficulty with breathing and swallowing. This most deadly form, called bulbar polio, accounts for about 2 percent of the paralysis cases. Finally, the virus will sometimes simultaneously replicate in both the lower spinal cord and brainstem. Spinobulbar polio, as this third type is known, is an intermediate of the other two in terms of severity and prevalence (around 18%). In general, older kids, teens, and adults tend to develop the bulbar and spinobulbar forms of polio at a higher rate than younger children, making their prognosis much worse on average. Furthermore, many of those who developed any level of paralysis also experienced extreme muscular pain and weakness during their recovery and for many years afterward. In some extreme cases, survivors develop a condition called post-polio syndrome (PPS) in which they experience muscle pain and loss of function decades after they seemingly recovered from the disease.

Psychological Damage to a Generation

If one were to rank epidemic diseases by mortality rates or persistence in the human population, polio would likely not be found in the top 50. It is a disease that only spread to epidemic proportions for about 50 total years, and it killed significantly fewer people than many diseases not included in this book (e.g., measles, typhoid, syphilis). Despite not being statistically as severe as other diseases, polio is worthy to be included on any list of destructive epidemics due the intense psychological damage that it caused to the population. Polio terrorized vulnerable children. It maimed them. It destroyed their hope for a future and isolated them from everything they loved. It attacked what adults hold most dear and it did so in ways that were far worse than what is seen in nightmares. Polio may not have killed hundreds of millions of people, but it still managed to affect the population as if it had.

One of the most significant by-products of the polio scare was that it fundamentally changed how many parents raised their children. Before polio, kids typically played outdoors during the summertime, enjoying activities such as swimming, riding bikes, and playing sports with their friends from the neighborhood. Most parents did not think twice about letting their kids leave the house for long periods of time as long as they made it home for dinner or before it got dark. This changed dramatically when polio arrived, and it became clear that it was attacking kids while they played outside away from their parents. In response, many parents began taking a more active role in deciding where, when, and who their children could play with. More often than not, this meant keeping them isolated indoors where it was safe.

In his book *A Hole in the World*, Richard Rhodes recounts how his own feelings of social isolation during this period when he wrote, "The city closed the swimming pools and we all stayed home, cooped indoors, shunning other children. Summer seemed like winter then."[5] Millions of kids who were never even exposed to polio lived under this cloud of foreboding for much of their childhood. It was a time in which socialization took a back seat to safety and freedom gave way to control. Polio forced parents to shift their attention to their children in ways that no other disease had or has since. Although "helicopter parenting" did not become into vogue until the 1980s, one can trace some of its origins to what transpired during these polio years.

Ironically, the very same generation of kids who felt sheltered by their parents due to polio eventually became the generation of parents who ushered in the "helicopter parent" movement three decades later. The fear had changed (from polio to child predators), but the response was eerily similar.

For those who were directly affected by polio, the psychological impacts were much more harmful and long lasting. In the hours following a polio diagnosis, the infected individual was usually whisked away to a special ward in the hospital where family and friends were not permitted to enter for several days, weeks, or even months. Their toys, clothes, and other possessions were immediately collected into a pile and burned so that the disease would not spread to their siblings. When family members were finally allowed to visit, it was usually only for a few minutes and was separated by a glass or curtain partition. Leaving behind everything and everyone that was familiar to them often produced intense feelings of abandonment and isolation, which were compounded by a real fear that they may die or be permanently paralyzed.

The families of those affected no doubt experienced similar emotions during those first few weeks. In many cases, they additionally had to deal with being ostracized by their community. People were afraid of polio and anyone that had any connection to it, including the families of the victim. Their homes were marked with large yellow quarantine signs, and they were treated as though they themselves were dangerous. One polio survivor once recalled, "My mother said that when she and Dad would go to the beach in town, people would grab their blankets and umbrellas and move. At the grocery store, my mother said she could hear people whispering and staring. No one wanted to be near my family."[6] Polio had forever marked them as being tainted; they were outcasts that served as a constant reminder to everyone around them that polio was present and their kids could be next. It was an unfortunate response that only became more common as polio continued to spread in the 1940s and 1950s.

A number of studies have addressed how polio affected the long-term psychological well-being of those who faced long recoveries or were permanently disabled by the disease. While data do vary depending on the specific focus of the study, most researchers agree that polio survivors suffer from higher levels of depression and anxiety on average than those who did not have polio.[7] Survivors often went through an extended period of mourning for the life they lost and the uncertainty they now faced. How would they support themselves? Would they ever walk again? Who would marry them? Questions like these permeated the minds of millions of polio survivors as they struggled to reacclimate to a world that was now somewhat foreign and hostile to them. Other survivors battled constant anxiety that they would get sick and be institutionalized again. Such feelings are triggered by vivid memories of being mistreated or even abused by hospital workers during their

recovery. Many remember being left unattended for hours as they lay helpless sitting in their own urine and feces or being hit for accidentally wetting
themselves despite having no control over their body functions. Some even
reported being sexually abused by their caretakers. These experiences were
unfortunately not uncommon during a time when most hospitals were overwhelmed and understaffed. As polio survivors continue to age, many have
begun to suffer from PPS. Symptoms include pain, muscle weakening, and
loss of mobility in limbs that had seemingly recovered from polio 50 years
previously. The thought that this dreaded disease is still capable of harming
them has reignited old fears and new feelings of depression in a great number
of survivors. It is an awful postscript to a terrifying epidemic.

The Sanitation Paradox

An examination of epidemiological data from the 20th-century polio epidemic reveals an interesting paradox that baffled scientists for many years.
Polio, a mostly waterborne gastrointestinal disease, emerged and caused its
worst epidemics at a time when sanitation was drastically improving. Cholera, typhoid, and almost every other diarrheal disease declined precipitously
when modern sanitation measures were implemented in the late 19th century. In fact, some studies have estimated that as high as 12 percent of our
overall improvement in life expectancy over the past 100 years is directly
attributable to the reduction of these waterborne illnesses by sanitation. In
contrast, polio seemed to thrive most in places that had cleaned up their
water supply and improved food-handling practices. For instance, it caused
its worst epidemics in the wealthier areas of the United States and Western
Europe at a time when those populations were living virtually free of waterborne epidemics. Furthermore, epidemics seemed to only worsen in frequency and intensity as cities attempted to implement more stringent
sanitation measures in response to the disease. It was almost as if the very
response designed to stop polio was actually responsible for it.

Several theories have been put forth to explain this apparent paradox. The
first, and most accepted, is that the advent of sanitation in the late 19th century did not increase one's exposure; it only delayed it.[8] Modern research has
shown that the human poliovirus was relatively common in environmental
water sources in the 19th century and earlier. Due to the nearly ubiquitous
nature of the virus during this time, a person would have likely been exposed
to polio in the first few months of life. While this may seem more dangerous
than getting polio as an older child or adult, it was actually not the case. The
primary reason is that very young children (0–12 months) still have high
levels of maternal antibodies in their bloodstream that protect them from a
wide variety of diseases. These antibodies, called maternal IgG, are obtained
when a fetus is developing inside of the mother's womb. In the last trimester

of pregnancy, massive quantities of IgG antibodies are transferred across the placenta from the mother's blood into that of her developing fetus. The antibodies that are transferred are a sampling of what the mother has made in the course of her lifetime based on what diseases she has been exposed or vaccines she has received. If she was exposed to polio at any point, she will have antibodies in her system that are protective against polio and pass them onto her fetus. When her child is born and is eventually exposed to the poliovirus, the maternal IgG still in the child's system attacks the virus and prevents it from entering the spinal cord. As a result, the baby is able to recover with almost no symptoms or complications. This is the situation that occurred in most children prior to the 20th century.

As environmental water sources began to be cleaned up through modern sanitation practices, children were no longer being exposed to the poliovirus in the first few months of life when they still harbored high levels of maternal IgG. Instead, they were being exposed a few years later when they had no protective IgG left over from their mother. (Maternal antibodies degrade gradually over the first year of life.)[9] Without any protection, the poliovirus is able to replicate to high levels and spread to the spinal cord. Thus it is not that children were first being exposed to poliovirus in the early 20th century as many thought at the time. The issue was that they were actually being exposed to it less, which negatively altered the timing of their first infection.

While the above description helps explain why paralytic polio first appeared in the early 20th century, it does not reveal why epidemics grew worse in the 1940s and 1950s. Scientists have examined factors like water sanitation, seasonal patterns, childhood behaviors, and government responses to see if anything changed dramatically enough to explain the escalation of polio in the 1940s. After five decades of not making much progress toward answering this question, a study published in 2015 in the journal *PLOS Biology* finally shed some light.[10] Complex mathematical modeling and advanced statistics were used to analyze historical polio data. At the completion of their extensive analysis, the researchers came to a rather mundane conclusion—polio epidemics expanded in the 1940s and 1950s simply because there were more children born in the years that followed World War II than before it. The postwar "baby boom" effect produced millions of new young hosts for the poliovirus to infect. More children meant that there were greater opportunities for polio to spread in the population and cause paralysis and death.

The 20th-century polio epidemic is an anomaly in the history of infectious diseases. No other major epidemic disease actually grew worse because the population became healthier and more prosperous. People were dying of polio because the disease preyed on our ongoing quest for cleanliness, the very quest that had saved us from so many other waterborne diseases. It was an inevitable situation that was almost a self-fulfilling prophecy. Fear of waterborne disease changed our behavior, which ultimately caused the fear to be realized.

An Explosion of Medical Innovations

The polio epidemic left as many as 20 million people with chronic health problems such as paralysis, disfigurement, and respiratory deficiency. This put an enormous strain on the healthcare industry as polio survivors often required intensive medical care for many years after they first contracted the disease. The stress of the dramatic increase in demand revealed glaring deficiencies in how hospitals were caring for both critically ill patients in the acute phase of the disease and those requiring long-term care. What resulted were sweeping changes in how hospitals treated patients with life-threatening illnesses.

One of the most immediate concerns facing patients with advanced polio is the paralysis of the muscles involved in breathing. In order to pull air into the lungs (inhalation) and expel it out (exhalation), a combination of inter-costal muscles, abdominal muscles, and the diaphragm must all work together to move the rib cage and change the volume of the lungs. Paralysis of any of these muscles can make it extremely difficult to breathe, which can lead to suffocation and death if left untreated. The current treatment for respiratory arrest is to provide artificial ventilation either through mouth-to-mouth resuscitation or with some mechanical device. Unfortunately, when polio cases began to increase in the 1910s, there was no such device available for those who were at risk of respiratory arrest. Kids who entered hospitals gasping for every breath often died as the poliovirus gradually weakened their chest muscles. After watching thousands of young polio victims suffo-cate to death in this manner, it became clear to healthcare professionals that someone needed to develop a mechanical device that could act as an artificial lung to keep these kids alive. In doing so, they hoped to give them enough time to heal so that they could eventually breathe on their own again.

The first successful mechanical ventilator was invented by Drs. Philip Drinker and Louis Agassiz Shaw in 1928 in direct response to the polio epi-demic.[11] Their device, later called the "Drinker ventilator" or "iron lung," consisted of a large, airtight cylindrical metal tank that was hooked up to several air pumps. The person in need of breathing assistance entered the tank so that only their head remained outside. When the air pumps were turned on, a negative pressure vacuum was created inside of the tank that helped lift the rib cage and allowed air to enter into their expanded lungs. After a few moments, air pumps reversed the pressure inside of the tank, which allowed the air to be expelled out of the lungs. Although this may seem like a complicated way to move air into and out of a person's lungs, this negative pressure system of artificial ventilation closely mimics the natural

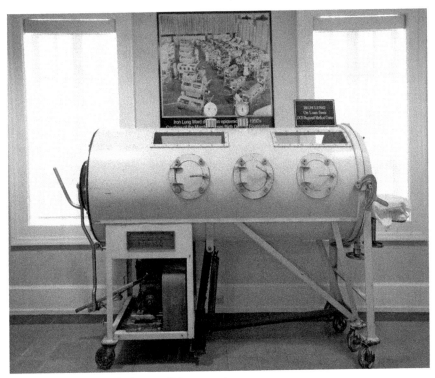

Iron lung, ca. 1933. (Library of Congress)

respiration process. The pressure changes essentially do the work in place of the paralyzed chest muscles.

The Drinker ventilator was first used clinically in 1928 when it was employed to save the life of an eight-year-old girl who was on the brink of total respiratory failure from polio.[12] Although it was fairly large, noisy, clunky, and expensive, the Drinker iron lung machine became an overnight sensation for its lifesaving capabilities. In the 1930s, several individuals in Europe and Australia (e.g., Emerson, Henderson, and Both) made improvements to the Drinker iron lung design and increased production efficiency.[13] By cutting costs by over 90 percent and making the design more user friendly and less cumbersome, these new iron lungs became available to hospitals everywhere in the world. Children who formerly would have likely died of polio were now being saved by this amazing invention, and the fatality rate of polio plummeted as a result.

The iron lung is still one of the most enduring images of the polio era. Those living during that time will never forget the heartbreaking scenes of expansive hospital wards filled with hundreds of little children encased in these large metal tubes. For those who only needed the iron lung temporarily

(1–2 weeks), the machine was viewed as a miraculous lifesaver. As one man recalls his short time in an iron lung, "There was a tremendous psychological element at work in all of us in our relationship to the lung. The metal respirator assumed an almost animate personality and became a symbol of protection and security. . . . We were incomplete embryos in a metal womb."[14] The iron lung, for as grotesque as it was, served as a symbol of life and hope for many in the polio generation. However, to others, the iron lung represented a metal tomb more than it did a womb. Some had such extensive paralysis that they were forced to stay inside of the machine for months, years, or even the rest of their life. In fact, there are several people who stayed inside of an iron lung for over 50 years, with one even surpassing 60 years. While some adjusted and went onto live productive and fulfilling lives despite their limitations, there many were others who suffered immense psychological harm by being permanently confined to a metal tube. The iron lung to them was a symbol of a life lost, a permanent extension of their broken bodies, and a constant reminder of their illness.

The revolutionary invention of the iron lung went beyond polio in that it forever changed how the medical profession approached advanced life support. For one, it served as a model for the development of more sophisticated forms of mechanical ventilators. Positive pressure ventilators, which forcibly push air into the lungs in order to inflate them, appeared for the first time near the end of the polio epidemic. They were found to be much more efficient at oxygenating the blood than negative pressure systems were (like the iron lung), and they did not require the recipient to remain completely immobilized in any type of device. Before long, they replaced their negative pressure predecessors and became an important piece of equipment in every hospital and urgent care clinic in the world. Patients once at risk of respiratory arrest from a traumatic brain or spinal cord injury, heart failure, drug overdose, infectious disease, or genetic disease (e.g., Parkinson's) could now be kept alive long enough for other lifesaving measures to be implemented. Additionally, surgeries could now be performed in a more controlled manner with less worry of respiratory failure as a result of anesthesia.

Although mechanical ventilation alone drastically improved the prognosis of polio and these other serious medical conditions, it was not initially complemented by other necessary components of an advanced life support system. In the first 35 years of the polio epidemic, hospitals were ill equipped to deal with the volume of critically ill polio patients and their around-the-clock medical needs. Polio patients required constant monitoring of their blood pressure, respiration, nutrition, heart rate, medication, and a multitude of other medical issues. Care was often inconsistent, insufficient, and disorganized, and people were dying as a result. It was at this point that a pioneering anesthetist from Denmark named Bjorn Ibsen had an idea for a better system of care.[15] In response to the devastating 1952 polio epidemic in

Copenhagen, he helped create a special unit in his hospital that provided focused, intensive care for its polio patients. Each patient was assigned their own nurse and a team of doctors and medical students to monitor every aspect of their care every minute of the day (which included hand-powered mechanical ventilators 24 hours a day). This unit, the world's first intensive care unit (ICU), helped drop polio mortality in his hospital by half in 1953. News of the Copenhagen (Blegdam Hospital) ICU spread rapidly, and soon the ICU concept was modeled in hospitals all over Europe and eventually in the United States. With time, ICUs benefited from improvements to technology and increased funding. Modern ICUs now care for over 4 million patients per year in the United States alone. These are people who would very likely die if left to be treated in a traditional medical setting.

In addition to laying the foundation for modern advanced life support, the polio epidemic also forever changed how we rehabilitate people following a serious incapacitating illness, injury, or surgery. During the early stages of the epidemic, patients recovering from paralytic polio were instructed to rest as much as possible. In many cases, doctors immobilized paralyzed limbs in splints, leg braces, or plaster casts because they incorrectly believed that rest prevented weakened muscles from being damaged by the stronger muscles nearby. Children were often bedridden for months or even years during this recovery period. Famous director and producer Francis Ford Coppola, who contracted polio when he was eight and spent nearly a year in bed, recalls, "When you had polio then, nobody brought their friends around; I was kept in a room by myself, and I used to read and occupy myself with puppets and mechanical things and gadgets; we had a tape recorder, a TV set and things like that."[16] He later credited this extended bedrest with sparking his interest in storytelling, an interest that would culminate in writing, directing, and producing movies such as *Apocalypse Now* and *The Godfather.*

A similar instance of extended bedrest also helped to revolutionize the candy industry. Frank Mars contracted polio as a young child and was bedridden for months while he recovered. Seeing her son becoming lonely and withdrawn, Elva Mars brought Frank into the kitchen and taught him how to cook and hand dip chocolate.[17] Throughout the years, his interest in chocolate continued to grow and he eventually founded the Mars Chocolate Company, maker of M&Ms, Snickers, and the Milky Way bar. He never fully recovered from polio and walked with a cane the rest of his life.

The board game Candyland also came about because of forced bedrest from polio.[18] A woman named Eleanor Abbott was convalescing in a polio ward in 1948 when she had the idea for a fun game that could entertain the many children who were in beds around her. What she developed was a wonderfully simplistic game that young kids could learn and enjoy without much help from adults. This was important since kids were often isolated away from most adults during these long periods in recovery. Interestingly, early versions of her game had cartoon graphics depicting children with braces on their legs. Those images were removed by Milton Bradley after they bought the rights to the game; they likely did not want it to be associated with polio. It went on to become immensely popular in the 1950s due to the large number of children that were now being forced to play indoors because of the threat of polio outdoors.

Despite little evidence to support its efficacy, most physicians during this time vehemently defended immobilization as the only viable treatment option for paralytic polio. One of the first people to challenge this orthodoxy was a young Australian woman named Elizabeth Kenny, who had little formal medical training.[19] Kenny first became fascinated with the human body as a child when she broke her wrist and received treatment from a local physician named Aeneas McDonnell. Seeing her interest in medicine, Dr. McDonnell lent Kenny some of his anatomy books and took her under his wing. After receiving some informal nursing training, Kenny began working as a "bush nurse" in a remote area of Queensland, Australia. It was during this time (1911) that Kenny was first exposed to the awful aftereffects of polio. A little girl who was in constant excruciating pain because her deformed leg muscles were perpetually contracted was receiving little help from local physicians. Kenny, seeing no benefit to immobilization, felt compelled to try alternative treatments to help alleviate the girl's pain. She experimented with the application of warm compresses and gently moving the child's legs every day in order to "remind" them how to properly contract. Amazingly, her unconventional treatment worked and the child regained use of both legs. Kenny then successfully repeated the new motion therapy with five other hopeless cases of paralytic polio. She continued her work with polio victims locally until joining the Australian army as a nurse during World War I. During her service, Kenny was promoted to the rank of "Sister," which was a common British term to denote a lead nurse. Sister Kenny finished her service and eventually returned to Australia to resume her polio work.

With all the successes she had in treating polio cases that no one else wanted, one may expect that the medical community would have taken notice and embraced her new type of treatment. Unfortunately, that was largely not the case. Most physicians in Australia either ignored her new approach outright or accused her of falsifying data in order to deceive the public. Sister Kenny herself perfectly summed up the cold response from the medical community when she wrote in her autobiography, "I was wholly unprepared for extraordinary attitude of the medical men in its readiness to condemn anything that smacked of reform or that ran contrary to approved methods of practice."[20] She was shocked by the dogmatic support of methodologies that had never been proven to work in the first place. Although discouraged by her inability to make her case, Sister Kenny continued her work and eventually moved her operation to the United States in search of more opportunities for research. Unfortunately, most physicians in the United States initially shared the same skepticism as their Australian counterparts. Major funding agencies like the National Foundation for Infantile Paralysis and the American Medical Association (AMA) still remained unconvinced and refused to finance her investigations. Despite these limitations, her movement therapy continued to grow in popularity among the public.

By 1941, Sister Kenny started to gain support from a few local doctors in Minnesota. Their research into her methods was eventually published in an article in the prestigious *Journal of the American Medical Association* (*JAMA*).[21] Although she still faced resistance from much of the medical community, the publication of that article and a subsequent book in 1943 helped legitimize her life's work.[22] From then on, more and more hospitals came to realize that the Kenny method was vastly superior to immobilization in the treatment of polio. Sister Kenny eventually shifted her focus to training other nurses and physical therapists in how to properly exercise paralyzed muscles, offering educational literature and courses at the newly established Elizabeth Kenny Institute in Minneapolis. As success stories continued to appear in newspapers all over the country, Sister Kenny's popularity soared, and she became one of the most beloved women in the world. In fact, she was voted by Americans as the most admired woman in the world in 1951, beating out Eleanor Roosevelt. It was an amazing transformation for a woman who spent the bulk of her career defending herself against the male-dominated medical establishment.

The pioneering work of Sister Kenny impacted medicine well beyond the field of polio. Her belief that injured and diseased muscles need frequent movement for optimal healing was a heretical idea that has now become the standard of care among physical therapists. From strokes and spinal cord injuries to surgeries and neurodegenerative diseases, conditions that were once worsened by prescribed inactivity are now rehabilitated using a similar methodology as that developed by Sister Kenny in 1911. Conservative and one-size-fits-all approaches for treating neuromuscular disorders have been largely replaced by more aggressive and personalized treatment regimens. Her work helped initiate a major shift in philosophy that forever changed how physical therapy is practiced. In doing so, she cemented her legacy as one who was not afraid to push boundaries and rattle cages for the sake of her patients. It is a legacy that has and continues to improve the quality of life for millions across the world.

Polio and the March of Dimes

One of the most important moments in the history of polio came in July 1921 when a wealthy politician and lawyer contracted polio while visiting a Boy Scout camp in New York. Two weeks later, he was vacationing with his

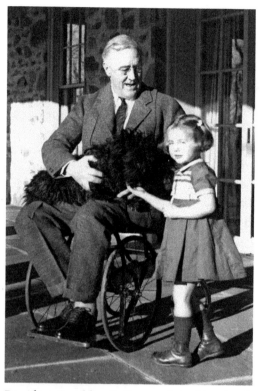

President Franklin D. Roosevelt in his wheelchair on the porch at Top Cottage in Hyde Park, NY, ca. 1941. (Franklin D. Roosevelt Presidential Library)

family in Canada when he felt nauseous and feverish following a swim. His condition continued to worsen over the next three days as he developed severe leg pain, numbness, weakness, and paralysis from the chest down. These symptoms were then followed by blurred vision, facial paralysis, and an inability to control his bladder or bowels. Examinations and tests (e.g., lumbar puncture) performed by several doctors over the next two weeks confirmed that the man had contracted polio. His condition gradually improved over the course of many years with the help of intense physical therapy and time spent convalescing at Warm Springs, Georgia; however, he would never regain the use of his legs and was confined to a wheelchair for the rest of his life. This man, future president of the United States Franklin Delano Roosevelt (FDR), became the voice for a generation of polio survivors and forever changed its history as a result.[23]

Roosevelt was a rising star in politics when he contracted polio in 1921. Born into the prominent Roosevelt family, which included his distant (fifth) cousin Teddy Roosevelt and a number of very wealthy businessmen, FDR began his political career in 1911 after unexpectedly winning a New York State Senate seat. He served in that role for just over two years before being appointed as the Assistant Secretary of the Navy by President Woodrow Wilson in 1913. (Interestingly, Teddy Roosevelt held the exact same job 15 years earlier.) FDR remained in that post throughout the entirety of World War I, resigning in 1920. He was then selected to be the vice presidential candidate of the Democratic Party. Although the Democrats lost that election by a landslide, FDR seemed destined to follow in his famous cousin's footsteps. However, just eight months later, that plan took a major detour when FDR made the trip to the Boy Scout camp and contracted polio. In one instant, it seemed as if his political career was over.[24] Who would ever elect someone who was unable to walk or even stand on his own? Who would elect someone who has the appearance of being feeble and chronically ill? Who would elect someone who had been out of politics for almost a decade in order to recover?

After spending eight painful years in recovery and out of the public eye, FDR did the improbable and won the governorship of New York in 1928. He was in office for less than a year when the country was plunged into the Great Depression. It was his leadership and innovative social works programs during these trying times that eventually led him to be chosen as the Democratic nominee for president in 1932. FDR would go on to win that election and three others that followed, becoming the first and only president to have ever been elected four times. The fact that he had overcome polio actually helped boost his popularity because it served as a testament to his relentless strength and willpower in the face of adversity.[25] Most Americans in 1932 could relate to FDR because they too were facing unprecedented hardships as a result of the Depression. They saw in him a leader who had refused to be broken by polio, a symbol of hope for their own difficult situation. It was this fighting spirit shaped by polio that many believe gave FDR the resilience he needed to lead the country through the Great Depression and World War II.

In addition to serving as a voice for millions of polio survivors, FDR used his position as president to directly attack the disease. One of his initial areas of focus was the creation of a national therapeutic center where polio victims could go to recuperate outside the confines of a hospital ward. The location he chose was a resort in Warm Springs, Georgia, where he spent many months during his own recovery in the 1920s. He was a firm believer in the healing power of the relaxing, warm mineral water and credits it with helping him regain his strength. When the resort fell on hard economic times in 1926, FDR purchased the property and attempted to transform it into a place where polio patients from all over the country could go and heal. Unfortunately, his contributions and that of his close friends were not enough to keep Warm Springs in business. By the early 1930s, it was on the verge of closing its doors.

It was at this point that a businessman named Henry Doherty had an idea to save Warm Springs (and hopefully earn favor with the president). He organized a series of celebration dances in cities all over the country that coincided with the president's 54th birthday on January 30, 1934.[26] Each of these more than 600 President's Birthday Balls acted as fundraisers, with all proceeds going to the Warm Springs facility. Amazingly, in just one night, these dances raised a total of over $1 million. FDR was so touched by the gesture that he went on the airwaves and said, "As the representative of hundreds of thousands of crippled children, I accept this tribute. I thank you and bid you goodnight on what to me is the happiest birthday I have ever known."[27] The first Birthday Ball was so successful that they continued to hold them every year on FDR's birthday. Over the next several years, millions of dollars were raised for Warm Springs and various other local polio treatment facilities.

Realizing that Warm Springs was not having the national impact on polio as he had hoped, FDR decided to establish a new national organization whose sole focus would be to help existing polio victims and prevent others from contracting the disease. This National Foundation for Infantile Paralysis (NFIP) came into being on January 3, 1938, and included a diverse group of scientists, healthcare workers, volunteers, and people focused on fundraising. Initially, funding for the new NFIP came from the President's Balls and large donations from wealthy philanthropists and companies. After only a short time, however, it became clear that the costs of running the NFIP were going to far exceed what was being brought in by these few funding sources. As a result, FDR reached out to his friend and radio personality Eddie Cantor for help in raising public awareness for the NFIP.[28] Cantor went on the air shortly thereafter and asked the public to send whatever donations they could spare. Every penny, nickel, and dime would make a big difference in the fight against polio. Jokingly, Cantor stated that he wanted the "march of dimes to reach all the way to the White House."[29]

It was the first nationwide call for monetary support for fighting a disease. The response from the public even shocked FDR. In the weeks that followed the broadcast, tens of thousands of letters arrived at the White House on a daily basis, most of which contained dimes. In his birthday message of 1938, Roosevelt told the nation, "Yesterday between forty and fifty thousand letters came to the mail room of the White House. Today an even greater number—how many I cannot tell you—for we can only estimate the actual count by counting the mail bags. In all the envelopes are dimes and quarters and even dollar bills—gifts from grown-ups and children—mostly from children who want to help other children get well."[30] When it was all finally counted, the public had sent over 2.68 million dimes to the White House. It was an amazing example of crowdfunding. By asking ask lots of people to donate just a single dime, the burden of fundraising transferred from a few wealthy individuals to the entire nation.

The "march of dimes" fundraising campaign was repeated in 1939 and every year that followed. Celebrities like Elvis Presley and Marilyn Monroe enthusiastically appeared at fundraising events and lent their fame to the cause of curing polio. So much money came into the NFIP (later renamed the March of Dimes) that they were able to begin funding research efforts aimed at finding a cure for polio. That investment paid off in 1955 when Jonas Salk and the NFIP announced that they had successfully tested a polio vaccine (see later section). Unfortunately, it was a victory that FDR did not live to see. He died in 1945 as a result of a massive cerebral hemorrhage.

After his death, the government and public alike wanted to memorialize him by placing his image on a piece of U.S. currency. In the end, the choice of currency was an obvious one: on January 30, 1946, the U.S. Mint debuted the Roosevelt dime.

In addition to fighting polio, the NFIP/March of Dimes has funded research projects in a variety of different scientific disciplines.[31] For instance, the organization has funded eight Nobel laureates, including James Watson (discovered the structure of DNA), Max Delbrück (characterized how viruses replicate), Linus Pauling (characterized the basic structure of proteins), and Joseph Goldstein (described how cholesterol is metabolized by the human body). In addition, once polio was largely under control because of the vaccine, the NFIP/March of Dimes diverted much of its resources to fighting causes of birth defects and premature births. They have organized mass vaccinations against rubella (which causes significant birth defects) and initiated campaigns to promote better prenatal screenings and maternal health. Such work has led to significant improvements in child mortality rates and better education for those responsible for caring for children. It is an amazing legacy that began with one epidemic disease and has now grown to encompass all that puts the lives at children at risk.

Arguably one of the most significant impacts made by the NFIP/March of Dimes had nothing to do with polio or other childhood disease. Before the NFIP, it was unusual for an organization dedicated to a disease to raise money through national fundraising. Although some charitably organizations like the Red Cross and YMCA flourished in the years that followed World War I, large-scale medical philanthropy had not yet been attempted. When the March of Dimes succeeded in raising enough money to actually cure the disease it was targeting, similar charities took notice and started to follow their blueprint. By the 1950s and 1960s, nonprofit organizations dedicated to other diseases began initiating their own year-round fundraising campaigns. Charities like the American Cancer Society, American Heart Association, and Muscular Dystrophy Association appealed to the public through mass mailing, phone calls, and television ads. Many held national fundraisers like community walks/runs (e.g., Heart Walk) or telethons (e.g., Jerry Lewis MDA telethon) to raise awareness and money.

Finding cures for diseases was no longer just the concern of health officials or wealthy philanthropists. The general public had joined the fight and the results were mind boggling. For instance, the MDA telethon, which was held every Labor Day for 43 consecutive years, brought in a total of $2.45 billion; the American Cancer Society raised a staggering $812 million in 2015 alone; and the American Heart Association raised $650 million in that same year.[32] While some have questioned whether the money raised every year by these charities is being used appropriately, there is no doubt that the fundraising has resulted in significant improvements to our health and has saved millions of lives. Medical philanthropy, with its humble beginnings of envelopes filled with dimes, has morphed into something that has forever changed how we fight disease. It has given scientists almost endless resources with which to develop new vaccines and treatments. It has given doctors new tools to diagnose diseases earlier and shorten recovery times. Finally, it has given patients a much better quality of life and hope that the cure is possible.

Disability Rights

The combination of polio and the two world wars left tens of millions with some permanent physical disability. In the middle of the 20th century, having a serious disability usually meant that a person was restricted from going to school, getting a job, and having access to public gathering places. In the most serious cases, the disabled were removed from their family and communities and forcibly institutionalized for the remainder of their lives. The impact of such social isolation was absolutely crushing for the spirit and mental health of the millions who were treated in this way. One particularly eloquent polio survivor named Mark O'Brien aptly described this feeling when he wrote, "For centuries, disabled people had been locked up in state-owned or state-subsidized institutions. We will never know how many lives were wasted, how many intellects dulled, how many souls murdered, through that system. The people who began and ran this system were good people who thought of themselves as reformers helping the helpless. But they never asked us what we wanted."[33] After graduating from the University of California, Berkeley, O'Brien published several books of poems and an essay that later served as the subject of an Academy Award–winning film named *The Sessions*. He accomplished all of this while confined to an iron lung for over 44 years.

Millions of disabled polio survivors like Mark O'Brien began demanding that improvements be made to how they were being treated. Mimicking the civil, gay, and women's rights movements of the 1960s and 1970s, the disability rights movement organized around the premise that the disabled deserve equal protection under the law. Specifically, activists fought for greater access to independent living facilities, laws that forbade discrimination of the disabled at school or in the workplace, and guaranteed access to all public buildings. They were tired of being segregated from the rest of the world who viewed them as being helpless. They were tired of being rejected from universities who refused to accommodate their wheelchairs or sensory impairments. They were tired of being denied employment. The disabled only wanted the opportunity to prove their worth.

Although people with all different forms of disability joined the movement, much of its core leadership initially was composed of polio survivors.

People like Justin Dart Jr., Ed Roberts, and Judy Heumann founded organizations like Disabled in Action and World Institute on Disability and organized grassroots lobbying campaigns that put pressure on lawmakers to pass new legislation protecting the disabled. They additionally filed lawsuits on behalf of those who were being discriminated against and organized nationwide marches and sit-ins to demand equal rights. Their hard work paid off in 1973 when the U.S. Congress passed the Rehabilitation Act. Section 504 of the new law stated, "No otherwise qualified individual with a disability in the United States, as defined in section 705(20) of this title, shall, solely by reason of her or his disability, be excluded from the participation in, be denied the benefits of, or be subjected to discrimination under any program or activity receiving federal financial assistance."[34] It went on to say that any agency that accepted federal funding had to make "reasonable accommodations" for persons with disabilities. This included providing access to all public buildings, transportation services, and housing.

For the first time, people with disabilities had some measure of protection under the law. However, the law failed to address several key issues, including how it would be enforced, when it would be implemented, and how to deal with private businesses that were independent of federal money. These concerns proved to be justified, as many organizations and services dragged their feet in formally approving Section 504. In response, the American Coalition of Citizens with Disabilities organized a national sit-in in government buildings throughout the country in 1977.[35] Hundreds of people with all different types of disabilities flooded municipal buildings and refused to leave until Section 504 was signed by local governmental leaders. Although they were successful in some cities, they were not in most. What followed was an additional 13 years of sit-ins, protests, and legal battles over enforcement of the Rehabilitation Act.

Finally, in 1990, the U.S. government passed the Americans with Disabilities Act (ADA), which gave comprehensive protection to the disabled in both public and private sectors as it pertained to employment, transportation, communication, recreation, and education. Unlike the Rehabilitation Act, this law provided a specific timetable for implementation and imposed much harsher penalties for those businesses and services that refused to make the necessary changes. When President George H. W. Bush signed the law, he said, "Let the shameful wall of exclusion finally come tumbling down."[36] It was a victorious moment that was a long time coming for those affected by the more than 20 mental and physical disabilities covered under the ADA. It was truly a turning point in history for the disabled, one that has since improved the lives of millions in our country and other countries (e.g., United Kingdom) that have followed our lead.

Race to the Vaccine

When people are asked about the polio vaccine, most tend to recall that it appeared in the 1950s and involved two different scientists, Jonas Salk and Albert Sabin. Those who are old enough may even remember receiving the shots in school or reading headlines like "Salk's Vaccine Works," "Vaccine Triumph Ends Polio Threat," and "Polio Routed" in the months that followed mass vaccinations. It was a time of national celebration and sober reflection on all that had been accomplished in the previous two decades. While these memories paint a nice picture of polio's ultimate demise, they fail to accurately represent what actually occurred during those years. Most know little about the disasters and near disasters that occurred during vaccine development, the groundbreaking science that made the vaccine possible, or the global political crisis that resulted from testing the vaccine. It is story of intrigue and brilliance that is perhaps unrivaled in the history of vaccines.

Two independent research groups began working on a polio vaccine in the mid-1930s.[37] The first, which was headed up by New York University physician Maurice Brodie, attempted to create a "killed" polio vaccine by taking virus samples from monkey tissues and treating them with formalin. In doing so, he hoped to destroy the structure of the virus so that it would not cause the disease, but at the same time not destroy it so that the immune system would no longer recognize it. He first tested his new vaccine on a few chimpanzees, himself, and a handful of local children. When no ill effects were observed in this small test group, he expanded his trial to include thousands of children (some of which were orphans). Unfortunately, when the data were examined in 1935, it became clear that the Brodie vaccine provided virtually no protection against polio. Children receiving the vaccine ended up contracting polio at the same rate as children who received a placebo vaccine. To make matters worse, some of the children developed severe allergic reactions to the chemicals in the vaccine.

Around about the same time, a second research team was in the process of developing a live, attenuated polio vaccine.[38] Led by Dr. John Kolmer from Temple University, this group aimed to induce a more robust immune response by giving patients a weakened version of polio that was capable of replicating at low levels. After being tested in a few primates, the experimental attenuated vaccine was given to Kolmer, his own children, and 23 other children in the Philadelphia area. The results showed that there seemed to be little, if any, adverse effects of the vaccine on recipients in this small group. Encouraged by these findings, Kolmer enrolled several thousand additional children to take part in a larger clinical trial. Unlike the Brodie vaccine, which simply just didn't work, Kolmer's live vaccine was found to be actively harming many of its recipients. Nine children ended up dying of polio, and many others were paralyzed as a direct result of the vaccine. The problem was later revealed to be due to an error in the attenuation process during production. Rather than giving test subjects an extremely weakened version of the poliovirus, Kolmer had unknowingly injected a nearly full-strength virus into their bodies. Such disastrous early results led Kolmer to permanently discontinue the use of his vaccine in September 1935.

The failure of these two well-publicized polio trials sent shockwaves through both the research community and general public. In particular, people were bothered by the sloppy manner in which thousands of unsuspecting children were exposed to harmful chemicals and a deadly pathogen. Despite denials from both researchers, evidence has since shown that many of the children recruited into these trials were orphans who were "volunteered" by their caregivers. The other children who took part similarly had little choice to refuse treatment once their ill-informed parents signed the consent forms. A group of antivivisection activists responded by mobilizing a mass letter-writing campaign aimed at trying to convince Eleanor Roosevelt to protect at-risk children from medical experimentation.[39] Their efforts did not go unnoticed. Soon after receiving their letters, Eleanor Roosevelt met with the Surgeon General of the United States and asked that he investigate the allegations that orphans were being used improperly during these studies.

While no immediate legal action was taken nor were any lawsuits filed, the public outcry that resulted forever changed how researchers approached clinical trials that involved children. Gone were the days of using children as human guinea pigs in the preliminary stages of testing. Researchers could no longer rely on the public inherently trusting them simply because of their position or the worthiness of their goals. They now had to prove that their methods were safe before employing the use of children. Unfortunately, subsequent human studies like the horrific Tuskegee syphilis experiment revealed that these apparent new checks-and-balances were ineffective without laws to back them up. The U.S. Congress responded by passing the National Research Act (1974) and establishing the Office for Human Research Protection to oversee and regulate all medical trials involving human subjects. Similar laws were also enacted in most Western European nations around the same time. Collectively, such legislation helped ensure that at-risk populations (children, disabled, prisoners, impoverished, military personnel) would no longer be coerced into becoming test subjects for agents that could harm them. It was change that was desperately needed to finally usher in a new, more responsible era in human clinical trials.

One of the major limitations that slowed the development of a safe and effective polio vaccine was the inability to produce large amounts of the virus. The human poliovirus initially could only be grown in primates (i.e., chimpanzees). Housing, feeding, and providing medical care for hundreds of primates is so expensive that very few labs were able to afford to work with polio in the 1940s. Those that could afford it spent months laboring to isolate a small amount of virus. This led researchers to begin actively searching for alternative ways to grow the virus so that sufficient quantities could be isolated for better vaccine studies.

The first breakthrough came in 1936 when two scientists working at the Rockefeller Institute developed a way to grow poliovirus in human embryonic brain tissue that was being cultured in petri dishes.[40] Albert Sabin and Peter Olitsky, two colleagues of Max Theiler (who created the yellow fever vaccine in that same year at the same location), discovered the exact composition of growth media required to keep humans cells alive for long periods outside of the body (*in vitro*). Although others had grown viruses *in vitro* before, their new methodology was especially groundbreaking in its efficiency and productivity. They were able generate large batches of poliovirus using relatively few reagents in a short period of time.

Despite its potential, Sabin and Olitsky never attempted to use their new system for vaccine development because they feared that poliovirus grown in brain tissue would develop an affinity for the nervous system in human hosts. In other words, they did not want to see a repeat of the disastrous early yellow fever vaccine trials in which virus grown in nervous tissue *in vitro* began attacking the central nervous system of people receiving the vaccine (see chapter 7). Instead, they erred on the side of safety and only used their system to learn more about the poliovirus itself. In 1948, another group, led by John Enders, Thomas Weller, and Frederick Robbins, solved the potential neurotropism problem by developing a new *in vitro* growth system for poliovirus using only skin and muscle tissue.[41] Polioviruses grown in those cells replicated to very high levels and did not develop any increased ability to cause disease in animals. It was a high throughput system for growing poliovirus that helped jumpstart a renewed search for a safe and effective vaccine. Furthermore, researchers working on other viruses saw the low cost and amazing efficiency of this new growth system and soon began using it as well. The entire field of virology expanded exponentially as a result, leading to the development of vaccines for dozens of different viruses in the years that followed. For their incredibly innovative work, Enders, Weller, and Robbins were jointly awarded the Nobel Prize for Medicine in 1954.

The race for the polio vaccine had officially begun. Scientists from all over the world started working to develop either a live attenuated or an inactivated polio vaccine using this new growth system. One such scientist was a young physician by the name of Jonas Salk. As mentioned in the previous chapter, Salk was a virologist who was a member of the research team that developed the first effective flu vaccine in the 1940s. Salk moved to the University of Pittsburgh in 1947 and began working on a polio vaccine in his own laboratory as the Dean of Medicine. His experiences with the flu vaccine led him to favor inactivated vaccines over live attenuated ones due to their higher level of safety. With significant funding from the NFIP, he grew large amounts of all three strains of human poliovirus *in vitro* and carefully inactivated them using a dilute formalin solution.[42] By 1952, he was ready to test his vaccine on a small group of subjects to see if it were safe and could induce their immune system to produce antibodies against the virus (which is something the Brodie inactivated vaccine failed to do). About 15,000 adults and children were recruited from the Pittsburgh area to take part in his initial study.

After accumulating and analyzing his data, Salk went on national radio to announce that his vaccine had induced a significant protective antibody response against several strains of the human poliovirus while showing no measurable toxicity in its recipients. He published the findings of his pilot study in the next issue of *JAMA* and began planning the next phase of testing.[43] What followed was the largest clinical trial in human history—a multinational, double-blind study involving 1.8 million children and 325,000 volunteer workers.[44] With the 1954 polio season quickly approaching, fearful parents lined up to enroll their children in the experimental study. Dr. Thomas Francis, Salk's former mentor and developer of the flu vaccine, was selected to design and manage the enormous undertaking. He primarily chose children in grades one through three who had not been previously exposed to polio and separated them into three groups—one that received three shots of the real vaccine, one that received shots of a placebo vaccine, and one that received nothing. Their health and antibody levels were then monitored over the course of the next year. For their part, the kids were given a metal pin and certificate that celebrated them as Polio Pioneers. When all of the data were finally collected and analyzed, Salk's team planned a press conference to announce their findings publically.

On April 12, 1955, the 10th anniversary of FDR's death, Thomas Francis stood in front an international audience and succinctly proclaimed, "The vaccine works. It is safe, effective, and potent."[45] Specifically, it was found to be as safe as the placebo and provided protection against paralytic polio 72 percent of the time. Despite such promising results, Salk was visibly unhappy during much of the press conference. He had hoped that his vaccine would be 100 percent effective at preventing polio and anything short of that was viewed as a disappointment to him. When he stood up to speak, he shockingly (and incorrectly) declared that his next batch of vaccine would be absolutely protective. Although he never did achieve that level of success, his vaccine became an immediate international sensation. The developed world collectively rejoiced as the destroyer of their children was defeated and four decades of fear were now over. It was a celebration that was reminiscent of scenes that followed the end of the World War II. For weeks, newspapers and radio stations ran stories about Salk, his vaccine, and the wonderful work of the NFIP. Salk became an instant celebrity and national hero as a result. He appeared in *Time* magazine several times within the next several months and was even honored by President Eisenhower at the White House on April 22 of that year. His popularity soared even higher when it was revealed that he refused to patent the vaccine so that it would be more readily available to everyone. When asked why he refused to profit from the life-giving vaccine, Salk replied, "Could you patent the sun?"[46]

In the days that followed the historic press conference, Salk's vaccine started being mass produced by five different companies. Mobile polio vaccination clinics were initially set up in schools so that most children would have access to the vaccine no matter their location or socioeconomic background. The NFIP organized vaccination campaigns in every community. Over the next several years, hospitals and doctors' offices gradually took over the role of vaccine administration. Millions of children worldwide received the vaccine and the results were startling. In 1955, there were 28,985 cases of polio in the United States. After the vaccine started being used, that number had dropped to 5,894 by 1957 and to only 161 by 1961. Such staggering declines clearly show that the fanfare surrounding the Salk vaccine was warranted. In only a decade, it succeeded in virtually eliminating polio as an epidemic disease in much of the world.

Despite its amazing success, the Salk vaccine was not without controversy. The first major area of concern was related to the safety of the vaccine. Theoretically, inactivated vaccines should be absolutely safe since there is no

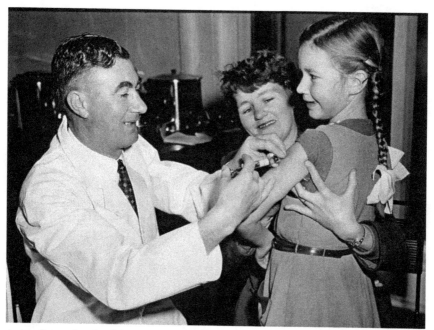

Australian schoolgirl receives Jonas Salk's polio vaccine. (National Institutes of Health)

live virus left to cause disease in its recipients. Unfortunately, sometimes errors cause normally safe vaccines to become dangerous. This occurred in April 1955 when two pharmaceutical companies, Cutter and Wyeth, improperly inactivated the Salk vaccine with formalin.[47] Over 100,000 doses of vaccine were shipped out of their facilities with live poliovirus inside. The lack of oversight and proper quality control led to hundreds of cases of paralytic polio and several deaths. It was a massive blow to the reputation of the beloved vaccine at a time when health officials were trying to convince the population that the vaccine was safe. A temporary lull in vaccination rates resulted, which led state health boards to launch a new public relation campaign to restore trust in the vaccine. It worked and vaccinations continued at rates similar to that before the scandal.

A much more widespread and potentially dangerous safety scandal hit the polio vaccination effort in 1960. In November, a report came out detailing a newly discovered virus that may have contaminated as much as 30 percent of all polio vaccines.[48] In the mid-1950s, Salk and others (e.g., Sabin) began using special monkey kidney cells to grow the poliovirus because they divided faster than their human counterparts and were cheaper to maintain. Unfortunately, none of the researchers using those cells realized that they were silently harboring another virus called Simian Virus 40 (SV40). When poliovirus was isolated from the monkey cells, SV40 was often brought with it. Since almost nothing was known about SV40 at the time, scientists began studying it to see if it had potential to cause harm in humans. Their worst fears were realized when several studies came out indicating that SV40 had a propensity to induce tumor formation when injected into monkeys, mice, and other mammalian species. It is impossible to overstate the horror that resulted when health officials realized that they unknowingly exposed over 100 million people to a virus that may cause human cancer. Thankfully, evidence collected over the past 40 years has indicated that SV40 does not cause human cells to form tumors.[49] Additionally, those who were exposed to SV40 during the early years of vaccination were found to have no greater chance of developing cancer than those who did not receive the vaccine. Despite public outrage over the entire incident, it appears that the medical community dodged a huge bullet.

Interestingly, scientists went on to characterize how SV40 causes tumors and learned a great deal about human cancer as a result. For instance, their work on SV40 led to the discovery of a new protein in our cells that functions to protect our genome from mutation. This protein, called p53, is believed to be one of the most important factors that normally prevent tumors from forming in humans. When the protein is lost for any reason, our cells begin to divide out of control and become cancerous. Knowing this about p53 has enabled physicians to better screen patients for their risk of cancer and has provided potential targets for future cancer therapies.

In addition to safety issues, Salk's vaccine was also a frequent target of criticism from the scientific community for its design and long-term effectiveness. His vaccine, being composed of inactivated viral parts rather than live virus, induced a relatively weak immune response after one injection. As a result, recipients had to receive two additional booster shots in order to achieve antibody levels that were high enough to be protective against polio. While this may seem like no big deal in developed countries, it is a significant issue in parts of the world where people have little access to health care. First of all, a vaccine that must be injected requires trained medical personnel to administer it and expensive equipment like needles and syringes. Secondly, what often happens when multiple boosters are required is that patients will get one shot of the vaccine and never return for the others due to forgetting or not having the resources to travel back to the clinic. In doing so, they will be under the false impression that they are protected from the disease when in fact they are not. It is a problem that has been frequently observed with other vaccines that require a series of administrations (e.g., MMR, Hepatitis B, Varicella, Tetanus).

Even with multiple injections, the Salk vaccine was shown to produce poor long-term immune protection. Antibodies made in response to the vaccine protected children from polio in the short term; however, within a couple of years, antibody levels drop to the point that the recipient is almost as susceptible to polio as before receiving the vaccine. It is an issue that led many in research circles to criticize Salk for mass distributing a less-than-ideal vaccine prematurely. They felt that he should have waited for a better vaccine to be developed, one that involved only a single administration, required no needles, and induced stronger long-term immunity. In Salk's defense, although his vaccine was not perfect, it was an effective bandage that succeeded in slowing the epidemic, which saved hundreds of thousands of children in the process. The idea of waiting for a perfect vaccine while children continue to die is absurd and inhumane.

One person who thought a better polio vaccine was possible was Polish-American researcher and physician Albert Sabin. Upon graduating from New York University School of Medicine in 1931 and subsequently moving to the Rockefeller Institute, Sabin began working on trying to better understand how the poliovirus causes disease.[50] As mentioned previously in the chapter, his early work on polio was focused on growing the virus in isolated human nervous tissue *in vitro*. After successfully accomplishing that goal in 1936, he moved onto examining different tissues from polio patients to determine where the virus infects and how it spreads. This work paid off in 1941 when Sabin, along with his colleague Robert Ward, demonstrated that poliovirus enters the body through the digestive tract and later spreads into the blood before moving into the central nervous system.[51] Not only did this result help epidemiologists better control the spread of polio by targeting contaminated water sources, it gave Sabin hope that an oral vaccine could be developed. If native poliovirus could survive the harsh environment of the stomach and small intestine, an oral poliovirus vaccine should be able to do the same. Furthermore, if he could somehow stop the virus from spreading from the digestive tract to the central nervous system, he could create a vaccine that was both safe and effective.

After serving in the U.S. war effort abroad for the next several years, Sabin returned to working on a polio vaccine at the Children's Hospital Research Foundation in Cincinnati, Ohio.[52] For the next decade, Sabin searched diligently for a natural mutant variant of the virus that was incapable of spreading to the spinal cord. He eventually did succeed in isolating such a mutant, which was later used as the foundation for his oral, live vaccine. By 1957, Sabin was ready to test his new vaccine for its ability to induce an immune response and protect recipients from developing paralytic polio. Like Salk before him, he initially tested his vaccine on a small group of young adults (local federal prisoners), himself, his neighbors, and his family. After this phase of testing showed that his vaccine worked and was safe, Sabin started preparing for a much larger clinical trial. Unfortunately, he would soon learn that several very serious factors threatened to derail his lofty plans.

One of the most significant hurdles facing Sabin in 1957 was the widespread use of the Salk vaccine. Millions of children had been receiving the Salk vaccine for over two years before the Sabin vaccine was ready for testing. In that time, the media had declared polio defeated, Salk a hero, and the matter essentially closed. As a result, funding agencies like the NFIP and the U.S. Public Health Service were hesitant to pour more money into a cause that they felt had already been won. Additionally, so many American children had already received the Salk vaccine that getting enough nonexposed kids to test the new vaccine would have been extremely difficult. These factors, combined with a bitter rivalry that was festering between Sabin and Salk, led Sabin to look elsewhere for an opportunity to test what he believed to be the superior vaccine. That opportunity came when three Soviet scientists visited with Sabin in January 1956 to inquire about how they may slow the polio epidemic in their own country.

The Salk vaccine, though widely available throughout the United States and Western Europe, had not yet effectively been distributed in any of the countries of the communist Eastern bloc. As a result, polio had continued to rage out of control there despite almost being eradicated in the United States. Sabin, who was of Russian Jewish heritage, became friends with one of the Soviet scientists, Mikhail P. Chumakov. Just six months later, Sabin accepted an invitation from Chumakov to go to Moscow to discuss how his vaccine might be tested using Soviet citizens.[53] When Chumakov approached the Soviet Ministry of Health about the possibility of conducting a large-scale trial with an untested American-made vaccine, they refused. They trusted the Salk vaccine because it had already been used on the American population. Some in the Soviet government believed that Sabin was secretly trying to use his vaccine as a weapon to harm the Soviets. Chumakov refused to accept their decision and went above their heads to a member of the Politburo. That leader, Anastas Mikoyan, trusted Chumakov and gave him permission to proceed with the study.

The first Soviet test of the live oral polio vaccine (OPV) involved about 20,000 children and was an enormous success.[54] Encouraged by these findings, Chumakov contacted Sabin and let him know that he was planning on giving the OPV to several million Soviets in a final, decisive test of its efficacy. Amazingly, over 10 million children and young adults received the vaccine in just a few months in late 1959. Because it was an oral vaccine that required no needles, health officials were able to efficiently administer it by dripping it directly into the mouths of children or by applying onto pieces of candy. The results of the study showed that one dose of Sabin's OPV provided both immediate and long-term protection against paralytic polio. The antibody response was significantly higher than that seen with the Salk vaccine and lasted for a much longer period of time. Some recent estimates suggest that antibodies induced from the OPV have been detected as many as 40 years later. Furthermore, being a live vaccine, the mutant poliovirus variant was able to replicate and spread from those who were vaccinated to the many others who were not. This amplified the beneficial impacts of the vaccine in the population as whole.

It was an amazing outcome that led the Soviets and their allies to vaccinate almost every individual under the age of 20 (about 100 million people).[55] In just a matter of a few years, polio levels in the Soviet Union and Eastern Europe plummeted. For his role in saving the lives of countless children, Sabin, an American, received high praise and a medal of gratitude from Soviet leadership. It was one of the few examples (along with the Smallpox Eradication Program) in which Americans and Soviets chose diplomacy and collaboration over politics in order to defeat a common enemy during the Cold War.

Sabin returned to the United States feeling vindicated that his years of hard work had paid off. He had succeeded in creating a vaccine that was more effective, cheaper, easier to administer, and nearly as safe as the Salk vaccine. Unfortunately, both the public and U.S. government initially viewed his results and vaccine with suspicion rather than acclaim. His was seen as the "communist" vaccine, one that could not be trusted because the Soviets were prone to use propaganda to spread falsehoods about the relative successes of their system. Realizing that the West would never be convinced on his word alone, Sabin requested and received help from the World Health Organization (WHO).[56] They sent representatives to Russia to directly observe how the trials were being conducted and to verify the veracity of their findings. The reports were favorable enough that many scientists around the world generally began to accept Sabin's vaccine. By 1960, the mounting evidence in support of the OPV eventually led to the WHO to give the vaccine its seal of approval. The United States followed by allowing Sabin to license his vaccine in 1961. After only two years of mainstream use, the superior OPV officially supplanted the Salk vaccine as the vaccine of choice in the United States and the rest of the world. The Salk vaccine was eventually phased out completely in favor of the OPV.

The race was now on to rid the world of this dreaded disease once and for all. The first countries in the world to eradicate polio were Czechoslovakia in 1960 and Cuba soon thereafter. The United States officially eradicated polio in 1979, joining many other developed nations who already accomplished the feat. Realizing that total global eradication was possible, the WHO, CDC, UNICEF, and Rotary International joined forces in 1988 and announced the formation of a Global Polio Eradication Initiative.[57] Their goal was to immunize every at-risk child in the world so that by the year 2000, the virus would have no host left to infect and would be eliminated. Although the initiative did not achieve that goal, it succeeded in reducing the total number of infections in the world to only 719 in 2000 and less than 40 in 2016. Polio is now only found naturally in three countries in the world—Afghanistan, Nigeria, and Pakistan. Poor health infrastructure and interference from groups like the Taliban have prevented international health officials from vaccinating children in the more remote areas. However, with renewed funding from organizations like the Gates Foundation, many hope that 2017 will be the year that polio is wiped off the Earth.

CHAPTER ELEVEN

HIV/AIDS

We may take refuge in our stereotypes, but we cannot hide there long, because HIV asks only one thing of those it attacks. Are you human? And this is the right question. Are you human? Because people with HIV have not entered some alien state of being. They are human. They have not earned cruelty, and they do not deserve meanness. They don't benefit from being isolated or treated as outcasts. Each of them is exactly what God made: a person; not evil, deserving of our judgment; not victims, longing for our pity—people, ready for support and worthy of compassion.

—Mary Fisher, HIV-positive mother and activist, at the
1992 U.S. Republican National Convention[1]

On June 5, 1981, a group of doctors from UCLA and Cedars-Sinai Hospital published a paper in the *Morbidity and Mortality Weekly Report* (MMWR) that described a cluster of five young healthy men in Los Angeles who had developed a rare form of pneumonia around the same time.[2] What was particularly striking about their condition was that in addition to pneumonia, the men developed several other diseases that are normally only seen in people with severely weakened immune systems (e.g., organ transplant recipients, cancer victims, elderly). Besides all being homosexual, the men had no connection to one another and did not share any common friends. Examination of blood from three of the men revealed that they had dangerously low counts of an important cell of the immune system called a T cell. Furthermore, the T cells that they did have were relatively unresponsive to stimulation and useless for fighting off infections. The editor of the journal went on to suggest that the men had contracted some new infectious disease that weakens the immune system and is possibly spread by sex. Although they had no idea at the time, these doctors had just become the first to describe a pandemic disease that has since claimed the lives of about 40 million people. That disease, Acquired Immune Deficiency Syndrome (AIDS), continues to kill about 1.2 million people every year. Along with tuberculosis, it is still one of the two leading causes of death from an infectious agent in the world. (Some years TB tops the list; some years it is AIDS.)

AIDS is caused by infection with one of two types of viruses—Human Immunodeficiency Virus Type 1 (HIV-1) or HIV-2. Both types of HIV can spread directly between humans through the transfer of certain body fluids like semen, vaginal fluid, anal fluid, blood, and breast milk. The most common way that HIV is transmitted in the population is through sexual intercourse. Despite the fact that HIV was historically associated with homosexuals, it is much more commonly acquired through heterosexual sex. Additionally, it can be spread from a mother to her child during pregnancy or childbirth or while breastfeeding. In places like southern Africa, where HIV prevalence is high and availability of anti-HIV medications is low, breastfeeding represents a major mode by which the virus moves into the next generation. Other routes of transmission include the shared use of needles during intravenous drug use, blood transfusions, and exposure to improperly disinfected medical equipment. In rare cases, HIV has also been reported to be acquired following an accidental blood exposure in the workplace (e.g., needle stick by a nurse). HIV is not spread through casual contact, kissing, or respiratory secretions since there is very little virus present in saliva, sweat, mucus, or tears.

Once the virus enters the body, it initially infects one of two types of cells. The first is a special type of T cell called a helper T cell, which normally functions to help chemically stimulate the other immune cells around it. HIV infects these cells and very effectively replicates in them until they burst open and release new virus particles. The new viruses can then find and infect more helper T cells and begin spreading around the body. At the same time that it is killing T cells, HIV will also begin infecting local tissue macrophages. As was discussed in the chapter on tuberculosis, macrophages normally function to ingest and destroy any foreign entity (e.g., bacteria, viruses) that happens to come near them. Unfortunately for the human host, HIV has mechanisms by which it enters, takes over, and inactivates the powerful macrophages. Unlike its effect on helper T cells, HIV normally does not kill its macrophage host. Instead, it uses it like a safe sanctuary, a place where it can remain undetected by the rest of the immune system for long periods of time. While the host is actively fighting off HIV particles that are floating in the blood or inside of T cells, those that are in macrophages remain silently hidden away from the immunological war going on outside of it. Macrophages thus serve as a stable reservoir for HIV, holding the virus long term until the time is right for it to reemerge. In addition to T cells and macrophages, evidence suggests that HIV can also infect bone marrow stem cells, neurons, and dendritic cells. The exact role of these other cell types in the pathogenesis of HIV/AIDS has yet to be fully explained.

When HIV first infects a person, the rapid death of large numbers of T cells causes a temporary suppression of the immune system and general flu-like symptoms for several weeks. However, the person's immune response eventually recovers and clears most of the virus from the blood. HIV then enters into what is called a clinically latent phase. The virus is still replicating at low levels during this time, but it does not kill enough T cells to produce any noticeable symptoms. This period can last from 1 year to more than 20 years, depending on the strain of the HIV, the health of the victim, and whether any anti-HIV medication is taken. Going unnoticed for so long is what makes HIV such a successful human pathogen. For instance, someone harboring the virus could infect 100 other people before it is detected.

As the virus continues to replicate over time, it gradually picks up mutations that make it more effective at evading the host immune response. Eventually HIV starts to win the battle and large numbers of helper T cells die in a short period of time. As this occurs, the person will become infected with various other fungal, bacterial, and viral diseases because their immune response is severely weakened by the loss of T cells. It is at this moment when the person is said to have AIDS. They will often come down with pneumocystis pneumonia (as the men in 1981 did), oral and vaginal yeast infections (known as thrush), reactivated herpes and TB infections, and various gastrointestinal illnesses. Since the immune system plays a pivotal role in killing precancerous cells that develop in the human body, AIDS patients will usually develop one or more types of cancers (e.g., Kaposi's sarcoma, brain cancer, lymphomas). The almost constant state of being sick causes the person to lose weight precipitously, and HIV replication in neurons in the brain can lead to the rapid onset of dementia. The medications eventually stop working, and the person succumbs to one of these opportunistic infections or cancer. While no single AIDS patient acquires every one of the secondary diseases described above, they usually have enough of them to make the last few years of life increasingly painful and debilitating. It is an extended death filled with pain, constant hospitalization, and horrifying changes to the person's appearance and personality.

HIV Origins—A Long Road to the Truth

The origin of HIV as a human pathogen has been the subject of many different conspiracy theories since it was first described in the early 1980s. The most prevalent theory centers around a belief that the U.S. government created the virus as a weapon in a military laboratory with the purpose of killing off some specific group of people.[3] "Communists," homosexuals, and

African Americans have been most commonly suggested to be the targets of this secret military program. As one looks at each group carefully, the false logic behind the accusations becomes pretty clear.

First, AIDS was initially described in the United States during the height of the Cold War arms race, which stoked long-standing rumors that the U.S. government was actively engaged in an offensive biological warfare research program during these years. Soviet intelligence pounced on this allegation and used it as opportunity to mount a comprehensive smear campaign against the United States and its allies. Manufactured scientists employed by the KGB utilized fake data to construct a narrative that suggested that the U.S. government created HIV as a weapon in 1977.[4] According to these "reports," government scientists at Fort Detrick, Maryland, engineered HIV by combining two other retroviruses and then released it into unsuspecting populations in the developing world in an effort to stop the spread of communism. Operation INFEKTION, as the propaganda campaign was called, used left-leaning newspapers in Soviet-friendly countries to disseminate the conspiracy theory in over 80 different countries. Some poorer countries like India and Ghana were even paid by the Soviet Union to run the propaganda stories in their own local papers. Even though such lies have been universally condemned by scientists throughout the world, Operation INFEKTION was amazingly effective at damaging U.S. credibility abroad and at home. For instance, studies conducted in 2005 suggest that 25 percent of U.S. citizens still believed that HIV was created in a lab by the U.S. military, and over 10 percent believed they purposely released it on the population.[5] It is a conspiracy theory that has persisted for several decades despite strong evidence that suggests HIV arose naturally in Africa sometime in the 1920s (see below).

The homosexual community is another group that previously accused the U.S. government of using HIV as a weapon to harm them. Much of their suspicion is based on epidemiological and historical data that show they were the first major group to have the virus in the United States. The Gay Rights Movement was picking up steam in the late 1970s with the passage of several antidiscrimination ordinances, gay pride marches, and election of openly gay politicians (e.g., Harvey Milk). Many in the United States were openly hostile to their movement, including several leaders in the intelligence community who associated their liberal ideals with that of communism. It was thus fairly logical to believe that the government may have released HIV onto the gay community in an effort to weaken their growing movement.

Some have speculated that this occurred during a hepatitis B vaccine trial that was conducted in 1978–1981.[6] In this study, researchers recruited 1,083 homosexual men living in major cities like New York and San Francisco and injected them with either a placebo or a new HBV vaccine. Homosexual men were recruited for the study because at the time, they were at a much higher risk for contracting HBV than was the general population. Having a focused group of at-risk individuals allowed researchers to use a much smaller sample size than they would normally be able to. The results, which were published in the *New England Journal of Medicine*, demonstrated that the vaccine was efficacious, reducing HBV transmission by over 96 percent.[7] Despite the success of the vaccine and trial, many in the gay community believed it was a ruse designed to expose them to HIV. However, subsequent testing of the HBV vaccine and men who received it revealed little evidence to support this theory. The vaccine was later shown to be free of HIV, and the 1,083 men who participated did not have any higher rate of HIV than gay men not enrolled in the study.

Similar to theories about homosexuals, there are many African Americans who feel that HIV was created as a means of eradicating the black community. In fact, several recent studies show that about 50 percent of African Americans polled still believe the government created HIV in a lab and are purposely withholding a vaccine from the population.[8] On first glance, such widespread distrust seems to have no basis in reality. However, the fact that the government had unethically tested a deadly disease (syphilis) on the black community just a decade before the arrival of HIV suggests they may have good reason for their suspicion. The Tuskegee syphilis experiments were so shocking because poor and uneducated black men were purposely allowed to suffer with syphilis for 40 years simply to see what would happen to them, even though penicillin was readily available for about 30 of those years. To the black community, this clearly showed that the government and medical community were willing to use them as human guinea pigs: if they did it once, it makes sense to believe that they could be doing so again with HIV. It is an assertion that some feel is supported by data that show HIV is more prevalent in young African Americans than in other races.

Another common conspiracy theory related to HIV is that it came about as a result of contamination of the polio vaccines that were grown in chimpanzee cells. Similar to the very real SV40 scandal, some believe that the simian cells used to make the polio vaccine were cross-contaminated with the simian version of HIV. This virus, called simian immunodeficiency virus or SIV, is genetically very similar to HIV and is widely accepted by scientists as the virus that gave rise to HIV. The fact that this idea was somewhat plausible led a team of scientists to analyze old samples of the polio vaccine to see if they contained any remnants of either SIV or HIV. Their findings, which were published in the journal *Nature* in 2004, conclusively showed that the vaccines were completely free of any retroviral DNA sequences, indicating that HIV did not enter the population as a result of any vaccine.[9]

With so much speculation, innuendo, and flat-out lies being told about the origin of HIV, it became clear that science would have to provide persuasive evidence to convince people that HIV was not a manmade weapon.

Several key experiments performed in the 1990s and early 2000s provided such data and finally put the matter to rest. One of the most significant was the discovery of HIV in the preserved remains of a central African man who died in 1959.[10] This was important because it demonstrated HIV existed in the mid-1950s, long before geneticists had the ability to manipulate DNA in a lab. In fact, HIV was probably in that person's body before Watson and Crick had even described what DNA looked like. This conclusively showed that HIV had to have come about due to natural evolutionary processes rather than some evil plot by the U.S. government.

Such findings were confirmed when scientists began to analyze the sequence of HIV and other retroviruses. Construction of the evolutionary tree of these viruses revealed that HIV-1 and HIV-2 were only distantly related to each another.[11] Each was found to be more related to a different SIV strain than to each other. The major cause of the AIDS pandemic, HIV-1, appeared to have evolved from an SIV strain that infects chimpanzees in the Democratic Republic of Congo (DRC), whereas the less prominent HIV-2 strain came from an SIV strain that infects sooty mangabeys. This was groundbreaking because it suggested that HIV evolved from SIV on multiple separate occasions in central and western Africa. In 2009, scientists found a new strain of SIV that has some sequence similarity to other SIV strains and some similarity to HIV. They believe that this represents the long sought-after evolutionary missing link between the two viruses, proving that pandemic HIV-1 did in fact evolve from SIV. Most genetic studies suggest that event occurred some time in the first two decades of the 20th century between southern Cameroon and the Kinshasa region of the DRC.

Spread of HIV in Africa and to the World

One of the central questions surrounding the HIV/AIDS pandemic is how the virus spread from a small isolated group of Africans to over 80 million people worldwide within just a few decades. As one traces its initial jump to humans and early spread in Africa, it becomes clear that the pandemic was born as a direct consequence of the widespread colonization of Africa by Europeans in the late 19th century. As described in chapter 4 (malaria), the discovery and distribution of protective quinine enabled Europeans to travel deeper into African territory and remain there for longer periods of time without fear of dying from malaria. As more Europeans began exploring the African interior, they discovered a wealth of natural resources. What followed was one of the largest land grabs in history, a period of 30 years during which Europeans systematically invaded the heart of Africa and stole its resources, enslaved its people, and forever altered its culture.

In the Congo region of central Africa, two of the most sought-after products were ivory and rubber. Both required an enormous amount of time and manpower to harvest and transport. To maximize their profits, Europeans used millions of African slaves to work as harvesters, transporters (referred to as porters), and construction workers for the many new roads and railways that were needed. The end result of this mass enslavement was a total destruction of the traditional tribal systems that had existed for centuries. More and more Africans were taken out of their small, isolated villages, where behavior was strongly influenced by local customs, and forcibly moved into overcrowded cities where drug use, promiscuity, and prostitution were much more commonplace. Such a migration provided the ideal environment for HIV to transition from a local, rural disease to one that had potential to spread worldwide. In their 2012 book *Tinderbox: How the West Sparked the AIDS Epidemic and How the World Can Finally Overcome It*, authors Craig Timberg and Daniel Halperin argue, "To fulfill its grim destiny, HIV needed a kind of place never before seen in central Africa but one that now was rising in the heart of the region: a big, thriving, hectic place jammed with people and energy, where old rules were cast aside amid the tumult of new commerce."[12] The place that fit this description perfectly was the large colonial city of Kinshasa, which was established by the Belgians in 1881 and grew to become the largest city in central Africa. It was in Kinshasa that pandemic HIV was born.

The pathogenic strain of SIV that later gave rise to pandemic HIV-1 is believed to have originated in a chimpanzee in southern Cameroon in the 1910s or even earlier.[13] What epidemiologists think occurred was that hunters killed the SIV-infected chimp for its meat. Eating primate bushmeat was a practice that grew to be more common during the colonial era due to the loss of traditional food sources. During either the butchering or consumption process, SIV infected the hunters and began to replicate inside their bodies. The infected hunters are believed to have then traveled south along trade routes (possibly as porters) to Kinshasa. It was there the virus acquired additional mutations and began to spread among humans at an epidemic rate.

Most researchers cite the increased levels of high-risk sexual activity occurring in Kinshasa at the time as the primary mode of initial spread. However, some have argued that it was also fostered by the increased use of injectable medications during the early and middle parts of the century. Colonial authorities not only mass distributed vaccines against smallpox, yaws, and polio, they also regularly injected the population with penicillin and antimalarial drugs. Studies done in the 1960s found that injections were so common in Africa at the time that 75 percent of households reported receiving some injection within the previous two weeks.[14] Unfortunately, the widespread availability and use of injectable medications led to a common practice of sharing syringes in order to save on costs. In some cases, a single syringe was used to deliver vaccines to an entire community. The end result of such poor sanitary practice was that HIV, a blood-borne virus, began to spread rapidly among the population in central Africa. Over the next several decades, the virus gradually migrated with people along trade routes and entered into villages and cities throughout sub-Saharan Africa. What started as a small isolated outbreak in the 1910s slowly emerged into a continent-wide epidemic by the 1970s. It was at this point that scientists believe HIV made the jump to other parts of the world and evolved into a pandemic disease.

Ironically, one of the most significant factors that facilitated the pandemic spread of HIV was the end of European colonial rule in Africa. The African independence movement began in earnest following the end of World War II and continued through the late 1970s. During the extended decolonization process, European administrators turned over control to 58 new independent countries. Unfortunately, several centuries of systematic oppression, violence, and slavery had left most regions devoid of leaders who were trained in running a government. As a result, many of the newly sovereign nations reached out to experts in other countries to help them successfully transition into independence. Economists, doctors, teachers, politicians, and other intellectuals from all over the world flooded into Africa. One country that was particularly generous with its support was Haiti. In 1960, Haiti sent 4,500 of its best and brightest to the new African nation of Zaire (now the DRC) to help it organize its government and jump-start its economy.[15]

At some point during their extended stay in the Congo, one or more Haitian experts are believed to have contracted HIV from locals.[16] Upon returning to Haiti in 1966, the infected carrier(s) gave the virus to others on Hispaniola, thus establishing a small focus of infection on the island. Three factors that increased transmission rates in Haiti at the time were poverty, dangerously poor healthcare infrastructure, and popular blood donation centers that reused needles. The virus spread rapidly there for a few years before eventually moving into the United States in 1969–1970. Although no one knows exactly how HIV entered the United States from Haiti, most genetic studies agree that it was due to a single infected person. Some have speculated that an infected Haitian traveler brought the virus to the United States, whereas others believe that an American picked up the virus while visiting Haiti for its illicit sex tourism trade that was common there during the time. In the end, we only know that HIV first arrived in New York City from Haiti at the start of the 1970s and that it primarily infected members of the homosexual community upon its arrival. This jump to the United States was significant epidemiologically because it was from there that HIV eventually spread to the rest of the Americas during the 1970s and 1980s. Around the same time, HIV also spread to Asia and established itself in both developed and developing nations.

It is amazing to consider that within a matter of a single century, HIV went from nonexistence to infecting tens of millions of people worldwide.

The rapid progression of the pandemic reveals the power of a pathogen that has a long asymptomatic period and spreads through sexual contact. It also demonstrates how destructive human decisions can be when new diseases are developing. HIV was not created in a laboratory, but its pandemic was surely manmade. Without the invasion and subsequent destruction of African culture by European imperialism, HIV in all likelihood would have remained a disease localized to the jungles that burned itself out. Instead, HIV was able to enter into newly built cities where rampant sex and widespread use of injectable medications allowed it to find an enormous number of new hosts in a relatively short period of time. The atrocities of colonialism created the spark and chance fanned the flames to create a nearly unstoppable inferno.

The "4-H Club" and Its Effect on Haiti

After the initial clinical identification of AIDS in June 1981, ever-increasing numbers of gay men began showing signs of AIDS in hospitals in New York City, Los Angeles, and San Francisco. By early 1982, health officials realized that a new epidemic had arrived and for some reason was only targeting homosexuals. As a result, some called the new disease gay-related immunodeficiency disorder or GRID, and a few others in the media began referring to it as a gay cancer (due to the inordinate amount of cancers seen in affected patients). However, by the middle of 1982, it started to become clear that other groups could also contract the new disease. In particular, IV drug users and hemophiliacs who had recently received blood transfusions were at high risk of getting the new disease. Additionally, a significant number of people who had emigrated from Haiti in the early 1980s were also showing characteristic signs of the illness.

A meeting of health experts, gay-community leaders, and federal authorities convened in July 1982 to discuss what to call the disease that clearly affected groups other than homosexuals. They decided on "acquired immunodeficiency syndrome" (AIDS). From then on, a furious search began to identify how the new disease was being spread and what risk factors increased one's chances of contracting it. In March 1983, the Centers for Disease Control and Prevention (CDC) released a statement in the MMWR that summarized who was most at risk for AIDS. They wrote, "For the above reasons, persons who may be considered at increased risk of AIDS include those with symptoms and signs suggestive of AIDS; sexual partners of AIDS patients; sexually active homosexual or bisexual men with multiple partners; Haitian entrants to the United States; present or past abusers of IV drugs; patients with hemophilia; and sexual partners of individuals at increased risk for AIDS."[17] In sifting through the list, four groups stand out as being identified as major carriers of AIDS: homosexuals, hemophiliacs, Haitians, and heroin (IV) drug users. These groups, colloquially known as the "4-H Club," soon became targets by those who felt that they represented a major threat to the health and safety of the nation.

For Haiti, being included on the CDC list was catastrophic for its reputation and economy.[18] Once one of the most profitable Caribbean islands and a popular tourist destination, Haiti suffered a long period of decline following a series of military coups, dictatorships (e.g., "Papa Doc" Duvalier), and corruption scandals in the 1940s–1970s. However, by the mid-1970s, tourism was again on the rise, and the island nation appeared to be poised for a small economic revival. This came to a crashing halt in 1982 when AIDS hit the newspapers in the United States and Haiti was being mentioned as its source. The disease that was nearly universally feared and despised by the American people was now also associated with Haiti.

The immediate effects of being singled out by the CDC were dramatic. Between 1982 and 1983, the number of visitors from the United States dropped from 70,000 to 10,000 (an 86% decline).[19] People canceled their vacation plans to Haiti's many beach resorts, business trips and international conferences were moved, and cruise ships refused to dock in its ports. Investors and their millions of dollars withdrew, and shipments of products bearing the label "Made in Haiti" were often sent back without payment or explanation. It was a devastating blow to a country that already had an unemployment rate of over 50 percent at that time. Although the CDC removed Haiti from its at-risk list just two years later, the damage was already done. Haiti's economy collapsed precipitously in the years that followed, which contributed to plunging the nation into three decades of chaos. Haiti currently ranks as the poorest nation in the Western hemisphere and the 20th poorest in the world.

In addition to damaging Haiti as a nation, the inclusion of Haitian ethnicity as a risk factor for AIDS caused Haitians living in the United States to be discriminated against irrespective of their HIV status. They were often fired from their jobs, denied housing and educational opportunities, and quarantined whenever they traveled simply because they were Haitian. In February 1990, the FDA imposed regulations that prevented anyone of Haitian descent from donating blood to blood banks or hospitals.[20] Even though the ban was overturned only a few months later because of widespread protests, the action taken by the federal government demonstrated its distrust of Haitians. It is a stigma that has followed a generation of Haitian Americans and caused many to feel a sense of shame over who they are. The situation has progressively improved in the 21st century; however, the wounds are occasionally reopened by renewed forms of discrimination. For instance, in October 2015, a help wanted ad for a female nursing position appeared in a New York *Pennysaver* that stated "no Haitians" should apply.[21] While it is possible that the racist undertones of the ad had nothing to do with AIDS, members of the Haitian community were rightfully outraged by once again being openly targeted.

A Modern Leprosy

The 1993 film *Philadelphia* tells the story of a young, successful lawyer named Andrew Beckett (played by Tom Hanks) who is fired from one of the top law firms in Philadelphia after his bosses find out that he has AIDS. Believing that he was wrongfully terminated because of his disease, Beckett hires a personal injury attorney named Joe Miller (played by Denzel Washington) to sue his former employer for discrimination. Through the course of the ensuing trial, it is revealed that the partners in his firm discovered Beckett had AIDS after seeing characteristic Kaposi's sarcoma lesions on his forehead during a game of racquetball. They are shocked and disgusted by the thought that Beckett had hid his homosexuality from them, that he brought AIDS in their offices, locker rooms, and homes. Rather than confront him directly, they secretly conspire to make him look incompetent at work so that they could fire him with "just cause." Beckett's attorney, who himself was homophobic and scared of AIDS at the start of the film, successfully reveals what they had done and wins the case and nearly $5 million for Beckett. Sadly, the movie ends with Beckett's loved ones attending his memorial service only days after his court victory.

What made *Philadelphia* so powerful was its raw and accurate depiction of the real-life struggles faced by those living with HIV during the height of the epidemic. It helped shine a light on the rampant discrimination and social stigmatization that they faced at school, in the workplace, at church, in their neighborhood, and even in their own home. Not since the days of leprosy had an epidemic disease so isolated its sufferers from physical and social contact and made them feel like permanent outcasts by those around them. In doing so, AIDS helped create a new social class that was defined not by income, ethnicity, or educational level but rather by HIV status alone. It was a class that was subjected to unimaginable ugliness from people who feared them and oftentimes despised their very existence. It was a class that felt abandoned and even targeted by governments that should have been protecting them. It was a class that bore a great deal of internal shame and sorrow for a life that was slowly slipping away from them. AIDS in a sense had become a modern-day incarnation of leprosy. It left its victims emotionally defeated, socially alienated, and highly vulnerable to different forms of discrimination and abuse in the years leading up to their actual physical death.

Many have attempted to explain exactly why AIDS was stigmatized so much more than other deadly epidemic diseases. Such analysis has revealed that a variety of interrelated factors contributed to the creation of the AIDS stigma. Perhaps the most significant of these factors was that the disease

If You're Dabbling In Drugs...
You Could Be Dabbling
With Your Life.

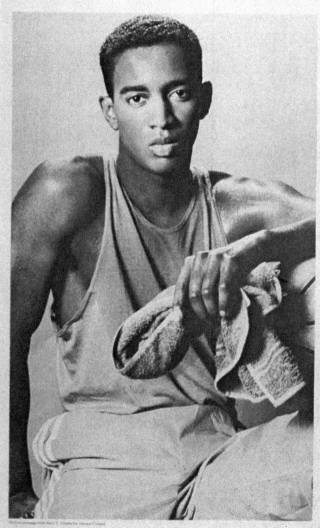

Skin popping, on occasion, seems a lot safer than mainlining. Right? You ask yourself: What can happen? Well, a lot can happen. That's because there's a new game in town. It's called AIDS. So far there are no winners. If you share needles, you're at risk. All it takes is one exposure to the AIDS virus and you've just dabbled your life away.

For more information about AIDS, call 1-800-342-AIDS.

AIDS Awareness poster from 1989. (National Institutes of Health, Public Health Library)

appeared to be initially targeting specific groups of people. Unlike respiratory, waterborne, or vector-borne diseases, which tend to spread "randomly" due to chance encounters with pathogens, AIDS was killing people selectively. In doing so, it marked them as being inherently different from the rest of the population and increased the odds that they would be singled out and stigmatized. Those odds increased dramatically when it was determined that over 86 percent of adults diagnosed with AIDS in the United States were homosexual, IV drug users, or prostitutes (as of 1988). Since these groups were engaging in behaviors that many considered to be sinful and immoral, people with AIDS were often blamed for contracting the disease because of their "poor decisions." In fact, two separate Gallup polls conducted in 1987 found that over half of Americans agreed that "most people with AIDS have only themselves to blame" and "in general, it's people's own fault if they get AIDS."[22] Their AIDS was thus seen as a by-product of their own risky lifestyle, a form of punishment that they had brought upon themselves. Blaming victims in this way was instrumental in shaping how society treated those with AIDS, even if they were not necessarily homosexual or drug addicts. Rather than looking upon the sick as suffering victims in need of compassion and support, many instead viewed them as deserving of contempt and disdain. It is an attitude that fueled the widespread discrimination against people living with HIV for much of the 1980s and 1990s.

Another factor that played a significant role in influencing public perception about AIDS was the inherent seriousness of the disease itself. AIDS is a deadly, transmissible, and incurable illness that slowly kills its victims in a visibly grotesque way. In the first decade that we were aware of it (before antiretroviral therapy), AIDS had a mortality rate close to 80 percent. It was essentially a death sentence that a person was forced to live with for many years without any hope of a reprieve. Such an extreme prognosis was terrifying because it preyed on our fundamental fear of death. In the past with other diseases, that fear was eased by the establishment of a strict quarantine in order to temporarily separate the infected from the rest of the population. Unfortunately, since AIDS is a chronic condition that can take over a decade to develop, no such quarantine protections were possible unless one considers the establishment of a leper colony–type facility. That was obviously not deemed an acceptable option in the late 20th century and so people were left with an uneasy feeling that AIDS was an ever-present threat to their lives. This led to a concerted effort by some to avoid any situation where they might be forced to be near anyone who had AIDS. When avoidance was not possible, many resorted to using threats or violence to actively remove an "AIDS threat" from their community. It was an appalling response that was not unlike the Jewish pogroms during the Black Death or the persecution of Christians during the smallpox epidemic of 166 CE.

Up to this point, the discussion has largely focused on what factors contributed to the creation of the AIDS stigma. While understanding its causes is clearly important, it is also essential to identify how the stigma has tangibly impacted people living with HIV and any group believed to be associated with the disease. In doing so, it may be possible to finally eliminate the vilification of the HIV community and undo some of the damage caused over the last three decades.

One of the most overlooked aspects of the AIDS stigma is the destructive impact that it has on the mental health of its victims.[23] Guilt, shame, hopelessness, and feelings of isolation so often accompany an HIV diagnosis that many feel it is imperative for victims to receive counseling as part of their normal treatment protocol. Studies have shown that people with HIV suffer from significantly higher levels of depression, PTSD, drug/alcohol abuse, and suicidal thoughts than the rest of the population. In fact, in the years before antiretroviral therapy, suicide rates were about three times higher and suicide risk nine times higher in people with HIV. These numbers have gradually declined as people have learned to better manage their illness and obtain counseling services; however, numbers are still much higher than the average. In addition to suicide, people who suffer from HIV often have lower levels of adherence to antiretroviral treatment programs and other forms of preventative measures. This is a very serious problem that can lead to a much more rapid progression of the disease in those individuals and increase the chances that they will transmit the virus to others. Thus, through its negative effects on the emotional well-being of its victims, the AIDS stigma can have much broader implications for the spread of the disease in the population as a whole.

The negative reactions that one faces in the home and local community are often a major cause of emotional distress for those with HIV. For instance, many have expressed concern that their HIV status would impact current or future relationships or that they would actually lose family and friends if their HIV status were ever revealed. Such fear, as it turns out, is firmly grounded in the real-life experiences of people living with HIV, many thousands of whom have been kicked out of their homes or hidden away by family members who are ashamed of them, ashamed that they are now themselves associated with a deadly disease that is commonly associated with homosexuals, drug users, and promiscuous individuals.

Unfortunately, many respond to a threat of community rejection by either disowning their family member or completely isolating them so that no one in the community discovers that they are sick. The person living with HIV, in turn, can feel an immense pressure to save family "face" by willingly leaving or staying out of the public eye. They often feel responsible for harming their family's reputation, social status, and livelihood. As one 30-year-old, HIV-positive woman living in China explained,

It was my family who told me not to tell [my brother], because he is now over 30 years old and not married yet, and he does not have a good job, either—no achievement. They were afraid that if I told him my serostatus, it would affect his job and his life. So they told me not to tell him. Yes, because he is not married yet. If he finds out, or if some of his friends find out—if he wants to have a girlfriend, I think it will certainly affect him.[24]

It is an enormous burden that carries with it grave consequences for the person living with HIV. Feelings of rejection, guilt, and loneliness commonly lead to depression, and the actual isolation typically causes what is tantamount to social death for most people. Those living in smaller, more traditional communities are especially susceptible to this type of stigma as are members of already marginalized groups like ethnic minorities, homosexuals, and transgender individuals.

Discrimination against people with HIV in the workplace is also a serious problem that has taken on many forms and has been justified in many different ways. As described in the synopsis of *Philadelphia* earlier, one of the most common and damaging forms of workplace discrimination is the termination of employment. Several studies conducted abroad in the 2000s indicate that about 15–20 percent of HIV-positive employees had been fired from their job because of their status, and about the same number of employers reported that they would or have already fired someone with HIV.[25] An even greater number of employers (50–65%) indicated that they would never hire someone with HIV because of health risks it poses to other employees, higher potential for missed work, increased costs for their insurance premiums, disruption of workplace harmony, and potential loss of profits if customers were to find out that someone with HIV was working there.

Since antiretroviral drugs have enabled people to more effectively hide their status from potential employers, some countries and professions began requiring applicants to submit to a full health assessment as part of the hiring process. This provides the perfect ammunition for employers who wish to keep their workplaces free from HIV. The systematic denial of employment has helped create a new challenge for those living with HIV—poverty. While poverty has been long recognized as a risk factor for contracting HIV, there is now strong evidence to suggest that it can also result from it. This is a serious problem because without money for housing, insurance, or proper health care (medication), a chronically unemployed person living with HIV can see their health decline rapidly. As they grow sicker, their chances of finding new employment also decline precipitously. They thus enter into devastating cycle of illness and poverty that few are ever able to escape.

Those who are able to remain employed following their diagnosis often experience other forms of discrimination in the workplace. For instance, in a 2009 survey conducted by UNAIDS, about 20 percent of people reported either being forced to change jobs in their company or passed over for promotion because of their HIV status. Many others experience anxiety and loneliness as a result of being socially and sometimes physically isolated from coworkers who are afraid of becoming infected. The only recourse that HIV-positive employees have in these situations is to either voluntarily quit or file a lawsuit against their employer. Since both options risk a significant loss of income, most people who experience discrimination at work do nothing about it.

One of the places where one least expects to see discrimination against people with HIV is in a healthcare setting like a hospital or clinic. It is there where the sick go for compassion, healing, and understanding at perhaps the most difficult time in their lives, and it is there where they are most vulnerable and exposed. Medical facilities are supposed to be safe places where patients can let down their guard and not worry about being judged or harmed in any way by those treating them. Workers in these settings are expected to be knowledgeable experts who understand the biology and epidemiology of their illness. As a result, they should in theory be less prone to the irrational fear mongering and bigotry that is so often seen in the general population during a new epidemic. However, healthcare workers are human, and humans sometimes experience fear and make bad decisions based on that fear.

When AIDS patients first began appearing in clinics in the early and mid-1980s, there was a general concern among healthcare professionals about treating HIV-positive patients.[26] At the beginning of the epidemic, this fear was fully understandable, especially considering that healthcare workers were routinely exposed to infected bodily fluids and universal precautions were not yet widely practiced. (Universal precautions of wearing gloves and eye protection when working with body fluids actually began in 1985 as a result of HIV.) Studies conducted in clinics throughout the United States, Canada, France, and Great Britain during this time revealed that healthcare workers often feared infection to the point that it affected how they cared for HIV-positive patients. For example, there were instances of workers refusing to treat HIV-positive patients altogether or doing so with such care that it negated the treatment. Some patients reported workers utilizing unnecessary amounts of protective gear to do routine exams that had no inherent risk of infection. Additionally, there were other cases in which workers posted insensitive warning notices on the doors of rooms housing HIV-positive patients, made those patients use special toilets not accessible to others, or placed them in complete isolation.

While such precautions may seem reasonable in the early years when we did not know how HIV was being spread, they are wholly inappropriate in the 21st century. Not only do they dehumanize and embarrass people with HIV, measures such as these often lead to major breaches in confidentiality (which amplifies the damage of the stigma). A study conducted in March 2017 found that 60 percent of European countries examined still had significant levels of AIDS discrimination in their healthcare systems.[27] Similar data have also been observed in the United States and in many other nations throughout the world. In particular, marginalized groups like homosexuals, prostitutes, and drug users reported the highest levels of perceived discrimination while being treated in clinical settings. The end result is a general distrust for healthcare professionals and a reduced likelihood that patients will willingly seek out treatment.

Over 60 percent of nations that report data to the UNAIDS program have some antidiscrimination laws in place to protect people with HIV/AIDS.[28] These laws are designed to ensure that one cannot be denied employment, access to health and social services, housing, or education simply because they are HIV-positive. Despite having protections, rights violations still commonly occur without any financial or legal ramifications for those breaking the law. A recent survey conducted in countries that have antidiscrimination laws revealed that on average, only about 30 percent of people who experience discrimination because of their HIV status ever report the crime. Major reasons for such shockingly low report rates include poor access to legal counsel and fear that lawsuits will prompt even greater levels of discrimination and abuse in their communities. Much of this fear is based on a fundamental belief that governments are powerless to protect them, do not care, or are themselves complicit in encouraging discrimination.

The AIDS community has a long history with government agencies either neglecting them when they needed their help or actively persecuting them for being sick. For instance, in the early days of the epidemic when the majority of those contracting HIV in the United States were homosexual, the government did next to nothing to slow the spread of the "gay plague." There were few public health warnings, little push for increased education or funding, and almost no discussion from politicians. In fact, the first time that President Reagan even mentioned the word "AIDS" in public was on September 17, 1985, over four years after the epidemic had begun.[29] By then, 37,000 people (mostly homosexuals) had been diagnosed with AIDS and over 16,000 had died from it (including Reagan's friend Rock Hudson). As if the deafening silence from the president was not bad enough, several senior members of the Reagan administration, including Press Secretary Larry Speakes and Secretary of State George Shultz, often joked about homosexuals and AIDS during interviews.[30] When health officials suggested that more funding and protections were needed for those at risk of contracting the disease, Reagan and his New Right supporters fought against it every chance they could get. Their agenda against homosexuality essentially became an agenda against AIDS support. This reached a low point on June 23, 1986, when the Reagan administration (via the Justice Department) passed down a ruling that employers could legally fire employees who were either HIV-positive or suspected of being so. It was a shameful decision by the federal government at a time when a large number of marginalized and dying people needed their support. As one AIDS activist named Michael Cover once said, "In the history of the AIDS epidemic, President Reagan's legacy is one of silence. It is the silence of tens of thousands who died alone and unacknowledged, stigmatized by our government under his administration."[31]

Unfortunately, the horrific early response of the U.S. government is not unique. Nearly every developed nation in the world has at some point established laws that permitted discrimination against those with HIV or criminalized activities associated with HIV transmission. These include laws that forced disclosure of one's HIV status to employers, laws that blocked HIV-positive people from traveling internationally, and laws that permitted denial of social services.[32] Although most of those laws have been repealed in favor of ones that protect against discrimination, there are still as many as 60 countries that explicitly allow authorities to prosecute people living with HIV for not disclosing their status to their partners. In some cases, legal action was taken against those who exposed others to HIV through unprotected sex even when the other person did not actually contract the virus. Similarly, HIV-positive people have been prosecuted for spitting in public, biting, and for even practicing safe sex.

Many countries also have laws against behaviors commonly associated with HIV transmission.[33] For instance, 76 countries still criminalize same-sex relationships, with several threatening homosexuals with the death penalty. In many places, IV drug users and prostitutes are given overly harsh, punitive sentences rather than being offered rehabilitation or access to social services. This creates an atmosphere of fear that reduces the likelihood that someone with HIV will get tested or seek out treatment from public health authorities. In other words, people who fear being incarcerated are much less likely to reach out for help, which ultimately hinders public efforts to control the epidemic. For this reason, the Global Commission on HIV and the Law recently issued recommendations to nations that have criminalized HIV transmission in some way and asked them to review their counterproductive laws. Since 2010, several nations like Fiji, Senegal, Guyana, and Togo have done just that and removed those laws from their books.

Medical Privacy

Although issues of patient confidentiality have been brought to the forefront as a result of the Digital Revolution and rise of the Internet, the idea has actually been around for several thousand years. One of the earliest known references to medical privacy can be found in the large collection of ancient Greek medical texts commonly attributed to the physician Hippocrates. This

70-volume work, known as the Hippocratic Corpus, was written between the fifth and third centuries BCE by Hippocrates, his students, and his many followers. One of the most enduring parts of the Corpus is the Hippocratic Oath, which is a statement of ethics that is often recited by new physicians before they begin practicing medicine. An excerpt from the original Hippocratic Oath (translated) reads, "And whatsoever I shall see or hear in the course of my profession, as well as outside my profession in my intercourse with men, if it be what should not be published abroad, I will never divulge, holding such things to be holy secrets."[34] It was a bold proclamation—he would protect confidential patient information as if it were something sacred that was entrusted to him. The text went on to elaborate that such secrecy was necessary because without it, patient confidence in the physician would erode along with their trust in the treatment that was prescribed. In other words, a physician, much like a priest or mental health counselor, cannot do their job effectively if the people they are charged with helping do not trust them. It was therefore beneficial to both parties to keep all aspects of their relationship confidential.

The Hippocratic concept of ethics did allow for exceptions to be made if the physician deemed disclosure to be in the best interests of the patient or society or both. For instance, if the physician felt the patient was engaging in behaviors that were destructive to their own health, they often broke confidentiality and spoke with the patient's loved ones. Similarly, when a patient's health endangered the lives of those around them, as in times of epidemics, physicians were typically required by the state to disclose the names and other identifying information to local health boards. This was done so that officials could take the appropriate steps to quarantine any sick individuals and warn those around them to stay away. As mentioned in the chapter on polio (chapter 10), this could involve placing conspicuous signs on the homes of afflicted individuals or even publishing their health information in local newspapers. Such breaches of patient confidentiality were seen as normal and necessary at times when infectious diseases were threatening the broader population. Physicians were no longer bound by their "sacred duty," and patients were expected and even required to sacrifice their right to privacy for the greater good. Confidentiality was therefore situational in that it could be taken away from the patient in times of emergency. With few calls for reform, this remained the standard of medical privacy from the times of Hippocrates until the late 20th century.

And then came HIV and the AIDS pandemic, a disease that was unlike any others that came before it. What is most unique about AIDS is that it has an unusually long asymptomatic period for an epidemic disease. Individuals could silently harbor the virus for years and either not know that they have it or purposely hide it from others. As awful as diseases like smallpox, plague, polio, and yellow fever were, people could see who were infected and take action to avoid them. This was not the case with HIV. Everyone was a suspected carrier, and everyone was potentially dangerous. People were particularly frightened by the possibility of healthy-looking, HIV-positive individuals unknowingly spreading the virus to their family, friends, coworkers, and neighbors by simply being around them. This fear of the unknown permeated the population, leading many to embark on witch hunts that were eerily similar to McCarthyism of the 1950s. Every cough or rash was looked upon with suspicion, especially among groups identified by the CDC as being at a high risk for carrying the virus (e.g., the "4-H Club"). In many communities, concerned citizens organized into local watchdog groups whose mission was to identify those who were carrying HIV and force them out of their schools, workplaces, and neighborhoods. It was the oftentimes shocking actions of these mini HIV "gestapos" that ultimately led the public to demand greater protections of private medical information.

One of the most publicized cases of an HIV witch hunt centered around an Indiana teenager named Ryan White, who contracted the virus as a result of a blood transfusion he received to treat his hemophilia.[35] White was diagnosed in December 1984 following a prolonged battle with pneumonia. His health had been deteriorating rapidly and his T cell counts were so low that doctors only gave him six months to live. By early spring of 1985, his illness had progressed to the point that he was forced to withdraw from school. When all looked lost for the White family, the young teen began to make an unexpected recovery. His health improved so much over the next several months that he started making plans to return to school in the fall. Unfortunately, when members of his Russiaville, Indiana, community found out that a boy with AIDS was trying to enroll in school with their children, they started a petition to prevent him from doing so. One of the leaders of the opposition group, Mitzie Johnson, was quoted as saying, "The big doctors and the government officials don't give a damn about our children. I don't want that boy hurt any more than he has been, but my daughter is never going to school with someone I know has AIDS."[36] Over 50 teachers and 117 parents signed the petition and presented it to the superintendent of the Western School Corporation.

Despite overwhelming evidence that proved it was nearly impossible to contract HIV through casual contact, the school principal and superintendent gave in to the mounting pressure and banned White from returning to school. What followed was a drawn-out, nine-month ordeal filled with lawsuits, trials, injunctions, threats, and intimidation. Every time White won the right to go back to school, the opposition group launched a fresh round of litigation to stop him (using money raised from local bake sales and auctions). This continued until April 10, 1986, when a circuit court judge overruled all previous lower court decisions and determined that White had the legal right to attend school. It was a monumental victory for the White family and for all who had been discriminated against for their HIV status.

The end of the bitter legal battle did not earn them acceptance in their community. The White family continued to face protests and threats on almost a daily basis. They patiently endured the hardship until someone finally shot a bullet through their living room window. Thankfully, no one was home at the time; however, the escalation in violence rattled the family so much that they decided to move to a new city about 30 miles away. Despite being forced out of his school and now his home, Ryan White continued to speak out courageously against discrimination of those with AIDS. He gave frequent interviews to news agencies and spoke in schools around the country in hopes of educating young people about HIV and AIDS. In 1989, a made-for-TV movie based on his life aired on ABC and was watched by an estimated 15 million people. The fame that resulted from it thrust Ryan into the national spotlight as the *de facto* face of the AIDS epidemic in the United States. It was a role that he came to embrace and use to help many others just like himself. Sadly, he would not live long enough to see the full impact of all of his hard work. Ryan White died on April 8, 1990, at the age of 18.

Around the same time that the Ryan White case was being broadcast regularly on the nightly news, a similar case arose in the small city of Arcadia, Florida.[37] Three hemophiliac brothers named Ricky, Robert, and Randy Ray had all contracted HIV through blood transfusions in the early 1980s (diagnosed in 1986). Similar to Ryan White, they were subsequently prevented from attending school once their HIV status became widely known throughout their community. Hate groups like Citizens Against AIDS in Schools mobilized and filed lawsuits to block them from being readmitted. After a lengthy court battle, the boys finally won their right to go back to school on August 5, 1987. The Arcadia community responded by boycotting the elementary school, threatening the Ray family with violence, and setting their home on fire. Fearing for their safety, the family moved to Sarasota in the following year and attempted to start their lives over. Unfortunately, Citizens Against AIDS in Schools followed them there and continued to harass them for several more years.

The Ryan White and Ray cases were a major turning point in the fight against AIDS discrimination. Before 1986, the public largely perceived AIDS to be a disease of drug addicts, racial minorities (Haitians), and homosexuals. It was something that people contracted because they lived immoral lives and made bad decisions that unnecessarily put their health at risk. In other words, there was a pervasive attitude that people with AIDS were themselves at fault for their own condition. As a result, many tended to emotionally look the other way when they saw those with AIDS being relentlessly harassed and discriminated against in their communities. It was a trend that persisted until people began reading stories about innocent, HIV-positive children like

Ryan White being terrorized by irrational mobs at their schools and in their homes. People who formerly did not think much about the AIDS epidemic now expressed outrage over the unjust treatment of these vulnerable kids. They demanded that state and federal authorities provide some level of protection for both kids and adults directly affected by AIDS.

In particular, they fought for the disease to be covered by the ADA, which would in effect make HIV discrimination illegal, and for new laws that would prevent the sharing of someone's HIV status without their permission. These protections would not only improve the quality of life for those already living with HIV, they would also provide peace of mind to those who are considering being tested for the virus. Health officials often had a difficult time convincing at-risk people to get tested because of the fear that they would be "outed" and subsequently ostracized by their community. Many saw the lives of their friends destroyed when blood test results were publicized to their employers, families, and landlords. To some, it was better to live without knowing than to be subjected to constant harassment. This was a major problem for epidemiologists who knew that the key to controlling the AIDS epidemic was to first identify who had HIV so that they can be treated and take measures to not spread it to others. With legal assurances in place that their HIV status will be kept absolutely confidential, health officials hoped that greater numbers of people would agree to be tested, which would lower the rate of transmission in the population.

Early attempts at passing HIV legislation in the United States (e.g., HOPE Act of 1988) were met with significant pushback from lawmakers who felt that the antidiscrimination measures did not allow public health authorities to properly track who had the disease.[38] Instead of anonymity and confidentiality, they wanted state agencies to have a list of names and medical information for every person who tested positive for HIV. AIDS advocates and members of the homosexual community were fervently against such a database because they believed that the government could use it to prosecute them for crimes like IV drug use or sodomy, which was still illegal in many states. Many homosexuals even worried that the government would use it one day to round them up in the same way the Nazis did during the Holocaust. It was fears like these that fueled lawmakers like U.S. Representative Henry Waxman of California to continue fighting for full confidentiality for HIV patients. Their hard work eventually paid off when, on August 18, 1990, President George H. W. Bush signed the Ryan White Comprehensive AIDS Resources Emergency (CARE) Act into law.[39]

In addition to providing millions of dollars in yearly funding for improved HIV care in underserved communities, the law included provisions that granted much greater levels of patient confidentiality in the early phases of medical intervention. Clinics now had to offer counseling to those being tested and inform them exactly how the results of their tests would be disseminated. Furthermore, the CARE Act allowed for clinics to offer anonymous HIV testing. Although it was a significant improvement over the Hippocratic concept of privacy, there were still some serious issues that came up during its implementation. For instance, in some towns, those being tested or treated for HIV had to visit clinics or medical vans that had the word AIDS written on the outside. Anyone seeing them in the vicinity of such places would automatically know intimate details of their medical history. Other more subtle issues of confidentiality arose in the years that followed, indicating that a more comprehensive law was required.

Just about six years after the Ryan White CARE Act established some protections for the HIV community, the federal government passed the Health Insurance Portability and Accountability Act (HIPAA) in an effort to expand privacy rights to all receiving medical care.[40] Title II of the new law established a strict set of guidelines by which personally identifiable medical information (medical records, payment information, etc.) is to be stored and disseminated. It requires that all protected health information (PHI) be kept absolutely confidential by anyone having access to it. PHI cannot be shared with employers, friends, or law enforcement agencies unless the patient waives their legal right to privacy, a court order is issued, abuse of a minor is suspected, or when it is needed to locate a fugitive or missing person. In cases when a person or agency does breach confidentiality, HIPAA empowers the government to impose stiff fines and allows the complainant to file a civil lawsuit. Such protections and punishments were significant because they established medical privacy as a basic right of the individual that superseded the opinions of healthcare providers. Doctors and nurses were no longer permitted to make judgment calls about whether or not disclose patient information. They now had to carefully monitor what they said, wrote, or even insinuated. It was a major victory for the AIDS community because it finally gave them some measure of security. For the first time, they could quietly manage their infection without fear that they would be accidentally or purposely "outed" by the very people they were supposed to trust with their lives.

The AIDS epidemic forever changed how we approach medical privacy in the United States and Europe because it graphically exposed the flaws of the Hippocratic concept. It showed that providing irrational and ignorant people with private medical information about their neighbors created a recipe for violence. Seemingly normal citizens transformed into mobs that shot at and burned the homes of children simply because they were afraid of their disease. Such heinous acts were broadcast all over the country, which started a national dialogue about the need to have laws in place to protect the confidentiality of those who were most vulnerable. That dialogue eventually reached Capitol Hill and the White House. Thankfully, lawmakers saw the inherent weakness in the Hippocratic concept of medical privacy and had the foresight to include all medical conditions and information in the Privacy Rule of HIPAA in 1996. It was a revolutionary change to patient care that has positively impacted not only the AIDS community but also all who fear that their medical information will be used against them in some way.

End of the Sexual Revolution

The Sexual Revolution was a radical, mainstream social movement of the 1960s and 1970s that forever changed how the Western world viewed sexuality and gender roles. It began as a challenge to the perceived oppression of traditional, Victorian concepts of morality that still dominated much of Western culture at the time. Ever since the end of World War I and the cultural transformation of the "Roaring Twenties," young people had become increasingly more independent and less bound by conservative values and roles. For instance, record numbers of women enrolled in colleges and universities in the 1920s, with many choosing to enter into the workforce rather than becoming homemakers after graduation. Women also began exercising greater freedoms in how they dressed and conducted themselves in public. Some cut their hair short, wore short dresses that exposed their legs, and wore lots of makeup. This new breed of self-confident and flamboyant young women, commonly referred to as flappers, proudly enjoyed life and did so without regard for the social inhibitions that had burdened women for centuries. They had no qualms about drinking alcohol or smoking cigarettes in public like their male counterparts or did they shy away from partaking in "petting" (make-out) parties. Stigmas related to sex also started to fade away as more young adults engaged in premarital sex and homosexuality became somewhat less taboo. Such transitions help set the stage for an even more widespread sexual revolution, one that came to completely redefine how we view sex and sexuality.

The Sexual Revolution of the 1960s and 1970s began as outgrowth of other transformative social and scientific movements that were occurring at the time.[41] One of the most influential of these movements was the reemergence of feminism and its push for women to have greater freedom from the traditional roles imposed upon them during the conservative 1940s and 1950s. Most point to the 1963 publication of Betty Friedan's *The Feminine Mystique* as a key rallying cry for a new generation of women activists to organize and renew the fight for equal rights, protection from discrimination and harassment, and control of their own bodies. One of the early battles of the movement centered around the first oral contraceptive pill Enovid and its availability to the female population. At the time of its release in 1960–1961, many states still had old laws on the books that restricted either the distribution or possession of birth control. While such Comstock laws were usually ignored by local officials, their selective enforcement in more conservative areas often posed a significant hurdle to making birth control available to women irrespective of their age or marital status. The feminist movement mounted a unified attack on these outdated laws and eventually overturned them with the help of several Supreme Court cases (e.g., Griswold v. Connecticut [1965], Eisenstadt v. Baird [1972]). As expected, their legal successes resulted in a huge increase in the number women on some form of contraception. For instance, within just five years of its introduction, over 6 million American women were already on the birth control pill.

The full legalization of female birth control was a watershed moment for the feminist movement because it gave women the power to control when and with whom they would have children. They no longer had to worry about unintended pregnancies and the possibility of having to sacrifice their future college education or career goals as a result of them. Women could now more freely have sex and do so with the same autonomy that men have enjoyed for centuries. To many women, the sex act thus became more about experiencing pleasure and less about reproduction. It was a major shift in perception that paved the way for an even greater loosening of sexual standards as the Sexual Revolution continued on.

Complementing the second wave of feminism and increased use of contraception was another important social movement—the Gay Rights Movement. The concerted push for gay rights began in earnest following the Stonewall Riots in 1969. On the night of June 28, police raided a gay bar located at the Stonewall Inn in Greenwich Village and began arresting people indiscriminately.[42] When some patrons were seen being dragged out of the bar and beaten on the streets, hundreds of homosexuals in the area converged on the bar to resist what they felt was police brutality. Before long, that crowd grew into a mob and began to overturn vehicles, set fires, and throw bricks at police. The violence continued to escalate until the New York Police Department brought in their Tactical Patrol Force to suppress the riot. Although the police were eventually successful in clearing the streets of demonstrators, the violent protests resumed over the next several nights.

The Stonewall Riots were crystalizing moment for the gay liberation movement because it marked the first time that the homosexual community had stood up to police harassment as a unified group. It empowered many of them to come out of the shadows and begin fighting for greater civil rights. Organizations like the Gay Activists Alliance and Gay Liberation Front formed in the months that followed the riots, and the first Gay Pride March took place in 1970.[43] Homosexuality gradually became more accepted over time as laws forbidding sodomy and other homosexual acts were removed from the law books, and homosexuality as a mental illness was removed from the American Psychiatric Association (APA) *Diagnostic and Statistical Manual*. Such changes helped foster in a new era of expanded freedom for homosexuals. They could now openly be in homosexual relationships and not fear that the government would imprison them for what they did in the privacy of their bedrooms.

The rise of the Beat and hippie counterculture movements in the 1960s also affected popular views about sex and sexuality.[44] Both groups were composed of mostly young people who broadly embraced liberal, antiestablishment principles such as opposition to the Vietnam War, open drug use, and natural (organic) living. They also sought to throw off many of society's inhibitions related to sex, believing that it was meant to be enjoyed by all without restriction. Their idea of "free love" not only promoted greater levels of sexual experimentation, it also rejected traditional marriage in favor of more open, casual sexual relationships. Sex, to the hippie, was just another form of pleasure that should be explored without intrusion from the government or religious organizations. Although the number of people fully ascribing to the countercultural lifestyle was small in comparison to the population as a whole, their liberal views of sex did gradually permeate much of the rest of society. During the height of the movement, rates of premarital sex among young people skyrocketed as did the prevalence and acceptance of pornography, coed housing at colleges, and greater sexual content in books and on television. It was a time of unprecedented sexual freedom that fundamentally changed our perception as to what is considered to be normal and acceptable sexual behavior.

The Sexual Revolution did not come without some costs.[45] In addition to triggering significant increases in teen pregnancy, divorce, and children raised without a father, the rise in sexual activity in the 1960s led to the uncontrolled spread of many different sexually transmitted diseases (STDs). For instance, the number of reported cases of gonorrhea increased by 165 percent during the 1960s, matching similar trends for syphilis, chlamydia, herpes, and genital warts. Younger generations experienced even steeper increases due to their preference for oral contraception (or no contraception) over condom use. While one may think that such a drastic rise in STD prevalence may have led to more cautious sexual behaviors, data show that it actually had relatively little effect. This is due to the fact that most STDs at the time were readily treatable with antibiotics. Penicillin not only eliminated the risk of dying from neurosyphilis, it could also clear up infections of gonorrhea and chlamydia in a matter of days. Although viral STDs like herpes and genital warts continued to be a nuisance, they did little to dissuade people from having sex. Antibiotics, together with oral contraception, had in effect removed the fear that had been associated with sex for centuries. People no longer saw any real significant long-term consequences of having sex because most mistakes could be corrected with a pill or procedure. Unfortunately, as the AIDS epidemic would later show, their sense of security turned out to be nothing more than an illusion. Sex was still as dangerous as it always had been and maybe even more so.

Most consider the beginning of the HIV/AIDS epidemic to be the *de facto* end of the 1960s Sexual Revolution. AIDS was unlike any other STD that existed in the early 1980s in that it was incurable and almost universally fatal in the early years of the epidemic. The idea that sex could indirectly kill you was terrifying to people, including many who had been strong proponents of the "free love" movement. Every sexual partner was seen as a possible carrier, and every sexual encounter was potentially dangerous. It was a fear that only intensified as the death toll from AIDS continued to rise throughout the decade. The ever-present shadow cast by the epidemic resulted in a gradual shift in how society fundamentally thought about sex. Caution and safety began to take precedence over freedom and pleasure. To many, sex became a very serious life-and-death decision that required great consideration and, in some cases, a blood test. By forcing us to think before we have sex, AIDS essentially ended the era of "do whatever feels good at the time."

Beyond affecting attitudes toward sex, the AIDS epidemic had major impacts on how it was actually practiced. Condom usage increased significantly in 1980s and 1990s as a result of widespread campaigns that promoted "safe sex."[46] First mentioned in a 1982 pamphlet entitled *How to Have Sex in an Epidemic*, the idea of using condoms as a means of protecting oneself from HIV was initially circulated in gay communities in the New York and San Francisco areas. AIDS activists not only handed out free condoms at places like gay bars and health clinics, they educated people in the community about the risks of having unprotected sex. The success of these grassroots public health efforts eventually piqued the interest of the medical community. Before long, safe sex slogans and condom ads became commonplace on television, billboards, posters, and in magazines. Despite pushback from certain religious groups, safe sex practices even made it into the curriculum of public school health classes. Although there were worries that sex education and increased condom availability in schools would lead to higher levels of premarital teenage sex, a number of large studies conducted at the time determined that this was in fact not the case.

By the early 1990s, sex education and safe sex campaigns had become permanent fixtures in schools and public health departments all throughout the world. The results of such interventions have been dramatic. Increased condom use has been found to be positively correlated with lower rates of HIV transmission and decreased levels of other STDs like syphilis, gonorrhea, and herpes. Furthermore, the recent implementation of sex education programs in secondary schools in Africa has led to some changes in behaviors that increase the risk of HIV transmission. It is a trend that is desperately needed as Africa continues to suffer through one of the most serious public health emergencies in its history.

Another Tragedy in Africa

In just over 35 years since being identified, HIV/AIDS has claimed the lives of over 20 million people in Africa and left 15 million of its children as orphans. The death of so many in such a short period of time contributed to lowering the life expectancy of most sub-Saharan African countries by 20–25 years during the height of the epidemic.[47] In fact, some of the hardest hit countries in the southern part of the continent saw their average life expectancies plummet to below 40 years. Although the increased use of antiretroviral drugs and condoms over the last decade has helped slow that trend, HIV continues to infect 1.5 million new people in Africa every year. As of 2015, there were still an estimated 25.5 million people in sub-Saharan Africa who were living with HIV.[48] This is a staggering number considering that Africa accounts for 70 percent of the HIV cases in the world despite having only 16 percent of the total population. In countries like Lesotho, Swaziland, and Botswana, HIV prevalence among adults has continued to skyrocket to over 20 percent (Swaziland currently has a prevalence of 29%). This means that one in five of all adults in those countries are harboring the deadly virus. In terms of total numbers, South Africa currently has the worst HIV epidemic of any country in the world, with 7 million people infected and 380,000 new cases in 2015. While statistics like these clearly show the enormity of the epidemic in Africa, they fail to adequately illustrate the absolute devastation it has inflicted upon the economic, educational, technological, social, and political development of a continent still reeling from hundreds of years of slavery and colonialism.

One of the most significant and lasting effects that the AIDS epidemic has had on Africa is the widespread stagnation of its economy.[49] Studies conducted in the late 1990s and early 2000s found that this economic downturn was caused in large part by a profound reduction in the size and productivity of the skilled labor force. The death and chronic hospitalization of so many young people from AIDS created a void in the workforce that led to lower profits for many private businesses and lower taxes for already strained governments. Lowered outputs also caused a sharp decline in total national exports for several African countries. For instance, the South African mining industry, which accounts for about 7 percent of the nation's total gross domestic product (GDP), was decimated by the spread of HIV among its workers during the 1990s.[50] With nearly 25 percent of its workforce infected with HIV, mining companies saw their profits take a major hit as healthcare costs skyrocketed and outputs declined. The end result of this and other similar industry declines was that economic growth rates declined annually by 2–4 percent across Africa during the peak of the epidemic. That was a huge economic shortfall considering that many of these countries were already having to divert large proportions of their budget to directly combating the epidemic. Instead of investing extra capital into building infrastructure and developing new technologies, these countries were forced to spend billions of dollars every year on domestic programs for the prevention, testing, and treatment of HIV. It was a burden that threw many African economies into a downward spiral that they have yet to recover from.

The effect of AIDS on national economies pales in comparison to the impacts it has had on individuals and families already living in abject poverty. The poor working classes in Africa contract HIV and die of AIDS at much higher rates than those who have stronger incomes and better access to education, condoms, and antiretroviral therapies. Since the poor have very limited means of earning income, the loss or debilitation of a single member of a household can send the entire family into a vicious cycle of unending poverty. Such enormous losses have led to deleterious shifts in household roles as those left behind scramble to survive. For instance, orphaned children commonly forgo their education and enter the workforce as child laborers in order to help support their families. Similarly, widows left with nothing are often forced into working jobs where they are severely underpaid and put at risk for being abused. Elderly relatives are also significantly impacted as they are thrust back into the role of caregiver of their terminally ill children and orphaned grandchildren. A 2002 WHO study that focused on the impact of AIDS on older people in Zimbabwe found that "older people in most African societies are a vulnerable group as a result of a lifetime of hardship, malnutrition, poverty and, in older age, high susceptibility to chronic diseases. The AIDS pandemic is now posing an additional burden on them, further increasing their vulnerability."[51] That burden, shared by all those affected by AIDS, has deepened the suffering of millions in sub-Saharan Africa. It has taken nearly everything from the poor and further widened the gap between them and the other socioeconomic classes living in their communities.

In addition to stunting economic growth, AIDS has also worsened the health of people who have little to no access to advanced health care. Besides all of the normal illnesses that accompany AIDS, the epidemic has brought about a resurgence of tuberculosis in Africa. Epidemiologists estimate that people living with HIV are about 25–30 times more likely to contract TB than noninfected individuals of similar socioeconomic backgrounds.[52] The co-infection problem has become increasingly more common over the last decade and now represents about 12 percent of all HIV infections. Why TB/HIV co-infections are so dangerous is that without a fully functioning immune system (due to being HIV-positive), TB is able to spread throughout a person's body without much restriction. In fact, those who are co-infected progress to active (deadly) forms of TB about 15–20 times more often than those who are TB-positive and HIV-negative. For this reason, TB has become the single largest cause of death in people who have HIV. The co-infection crisis is so extensive in Africa that many epidemiologists now speak of the two diseases in the context of a dual epidemic. It is an important distinction because co-infection has helped give rise to a new and even deadlier menace—multidrug-resistant (MDR) and extensively drug resistant (XDR) TB.

People who are co-infected with HIV and TB represent a perfect breeding ground for antibiotic-resistant mutants of TB because the weakening of the immune system by HIV lowers the overall efficacy of antibiotics. The underlying reason for this is that antibiotics never fully eliminate pathogenic bacteria from a person's body. They work by inhibiting bacterial growth or lowering counts enough for the host immune system to finish them off. When someone has HIV/AIDS, their immune system is unable to kill the last remaining TB bacteria following antibiotic treatment. As a result, some bacteria survive the onslaught (including possible resistant mutants) and begin to repopulate the person's body. The repeating of this failed antibiotic treatment with different drugs in different people eventually creates super-TB mutants that are resistant to every drug known. Although drug-resistant strains of TB can arise independently of HIV, studies have found that people with HIV harbor MDR and XDR-TB twice as frequently as those who are HIV-negative. It is an incredibly frightening statistic considering the number of people in Africa who are infected with HIV and the number of people who have been killed by TB throughout history.

The social stigma faced by those living with HIV in Africa is, in many ways, as toxic as the disease itself. Similar to what was experienced by homosexuals in the United States in the 1980s, an HIV diagnosis in Africa often results in a great deal of internal shame, social alienation, and targeted discrimination. This is especially true in places of extreme poverty, where people ostracized and rejected for being HIV-positive have little legal recourse or support from public programs. They encounter constant harassment in unimaginably difficult environments that are already plagued with high unemployment, low literacy, and high rates of violent crime. Unfortunately, those with HIV are easy targets in such places.

Future of HIV/AIDS

On April 23, 1984, Margaret Heckler, the Secretary of the Department of Health and Human Services, held a press conference in which she announced that the causative agent of AIDS had been isolated and a diagnostic test had been developed. Standing together with the American scientist Robert Gallo who helped pioneer these early achievements, she went onto predict, "We hope to have a vaccine ready for testing in about two years. Yet another terrible disease is about to yield to patience, persistence and outright genius."[53] It was a bold proclamation filled with American hubris—that we would overcome HIV in the same way in which we had conquered smallpox and were conquering polio. Unfortunately, decades have passed since this statement was made and we are no closer in having an effective HIV vaccine than we were then. Our ability to prevent and treat the disease has no doubt improved exponentially over the last three decades; however, HIV has proven to be a worthy adversary against "our patience, persistence and outright genius." The virus has proven to be relatively impervious to vaccine development due to its amazing ability to mutate its own outer surface proteins. Vaccination with one strain of HIV does very little to protect against the thousands of other substrains that may exist in a population at any given time. This mutation issue is compounded by several other factors, including the fact that HIV kills the very cells that are needed for the induction of a good immune response, and HIV proteins do not inherently spark a strong immune response.

Despite limitations, several companies have successfully brought an HIV vaccine through into phase II/III clinical trials.[54] This includes the VaxGen AIDSVAX trials in North America and Thailand in 1998–2004, and RV144 trials started in 2003. Unfortunately, all such trials have ended in relative disappointment. Only one, the combination RV144 vaccine, showed any level of protection in human trials (Thailand in 2009). Participants who received repeated injections of the vaccine contracted HIV 31 percent less often than those who did not. Since a weak vaccine is better than no vaccine, scientists have continued to work on RV144 with the hope that it could be modified to be more effective in the future. A new phase III trial with RV144 has recently begun in South Africa and is expected to yield data in the year 2020.

While many scientists were working to create an HIV vaccine, others focused their efforts on synthesizing chemicals that would inhibit the virus in people who already had it. The first group of these anti-HIV (antiretroviral) drugs that were developed targeted a unique viral enzyme called reverse transcriptase (RT).[55] It was chosen primarily because normal human cells do not have RT and HIV absolutely requires it to replicate its genome. Therefore, inhibition of RT can severely impair the replication of HIV while having no significant effect on the natural processes of the cell. The first reverse transcriptase inhibitor to reach the market was a drug by the name of azidothymidine or AZT. Studies conducted in the late 1980s found that AZT, when given in high doses every day, was very effective at inhibiting HIV in the short term. However, when HIV-positive patients remained on the drug for extended periods of time, the virus started to mutate and become resistant to the new drug. After about a year of treatment, most patients saw HIV levels and T cell counts go back to what they were before they took the drug. Also, early formulations of AZT were toxic to those taking it every day. Side effects included anemia, low neutrophil counts, vomiting, and a degeneration of muscle tissue.

This forced people with HIV to make a difficult decision—face certain death by not getting treatment or go on a drug that significantly lowered the quality of their remaining life. Most chose to take AZT with the idea that it would buy them some time for scientists to develop safer and more effective drugs. By 1993, three new (but similar) RT inhibitors had hit the market.[56] While they were somewhat less toxic than AZT, they suffered from the same problem of viral resistance after extended usage. Other RT inhibitors followed in the next few years with much of the same result. Given alone, all these RT inhibitors ultimately failed to keep HIV suppressed in the long term.

A new era of HIV therapeutics began with the idea of using multiple drugs in combination and with the development of new drugs that targeted HIV enzymes other than RT. Combination therapy relied on the concept of synergy, that drugs will complement one another and have a greater total effect than the sum of their individual effects. Giving patients two or three drugs together could create a cocktail that would attack the virus from different angles and reduce the possibility that resistant HIV mutants would arise. When it was actually tested using multiple RT inhibitors, the results indicated that combination therapy was measurably more effective in both the short and long term. However, resistant HIV mutants still continued to appear in some patients due to the fact that the drugs being used all targeted the same viral protein (RT).

Combination therapy took a major leap forward when scientists announced they had discovered a new HIV inhibitor that targets the viral protease (PR) enzyme.[57] Protease inhibitors block HIV replication at a totally different step in its life cycle than do RT inhibitors. When they were given to patients in combination with two RT inhibitors, the result was a groundbreaking drug cocktail that all but eliminated HIV from the person's body. The large-scale reduction in viral load corresponded with an increase in T cell counts and an elimination of immunosuppression. Termed highly active antiretroviral therapy (HAART), this type of mixed combination therapy has grown to include newer, safer, and more effective drugs, including those that target the viral integrase enzyme. Although it does not actually eliminate all HIV virus particles from the body, it keeps their levels so low that a person can now live with HIV for several decades without ever progressing into AIDS. In other words, HAART allows us to manage HIV in much of the same way we manage diabetes with insulin or hemophilia with injectable blood clotting proteins. HAART has helped transform HIV from a death sentence to a chronic disease that can be controlled for long periods of time.

While HAART has helped to significantly reduce HIV pathogenesis, transmission, and mortality in developed countries, it has not been quite as effective in Africa and other impoverished areas. Examination of potential causes for this disparity revealed that the primary issue lies in the inability of poverty-stricken communities/countries to afford and properly distribute HAART medications. In the United States, the average cost for the HAART regimen is between $1,000 and $3,000 per month for the rest of a person's life. Since few people can afford such exorbitant out-of-pocket costs, most rely on health insurance, government programs like the Ryan White CARE Act, or nonprofit groups to provide the necessary financing. Unfortunately, communities in Africa hit hardest by the epidemic rarely have these types of resources available to them. Not only do they struggle to pay for the medications, many of these communities lack the basic healthcare infrastructure to ensure that people are following the HAART regimen properly.

Realizing that rising costs represented a major hindrance in the worldwide fight against HIV, a global consortium consisting of five UN organizations (e.g., WHO and UNAIDS) and five large pharmaceutical companies launched an initiative designed to provide low-cost antiretroviral drugs to people living in impoverished nations.[58] Beginning in 2000, this Accelerating Access Initiative (AAI) worked with local governments to identify those most in need of antiretroviral therapy and provided it to them at only 10 percent of the commercial price (with funding help from the UN). People who would have never had access to HAART were now living longer, healthier lives and transmitting the virus at much lower rates. When the program began, only about 2.5 percent of the 28.6 million HIV-positive people in the world were receiving antiretroviral therapy on a regular basis. By June 2016, that number had grown to almost 50 percent, or 18.2 million of the 36.7 million infected individuals. Although there is still a long way to go to achieve the ultimate goal of providing HAART to all people infected with HIV, the treatment campaign spearheaded by the AAI has succeeded in slowing the spread of the HIV throughout the world. The rates of new infections and deaths have both dropped by over 40 percent since antiretroviral drugs started being mass distributed to the poor. It is an amazing trend considering these drugs do not actually cure those already infected (like antibiotics) nor do they protect the uninfected (like vaccines).

Another breakthrough in our understanding of how to prevent and treat HIV came from studies that identified numerous individuals who had been repeatedly exposed to HIV but never contracted it. These people hailed from different locations and had different ethnic backgrounds and sexual activities. Included in the studies were homosexual men that engaged in high-risk sex, long-time heterosexual partners of HIV-positive individuals, and female prostitutes from Gambia.

In an effort to ascertain why some individuals were seemingly protected against HIV, scientists isolated their immune cells and began looking for some shared genetic mutation or biochemical property that could explain their innate resistance. In 1996, researchers from Rockefeller University reported that they had identified the specific mutation that caused this unique trait. The mutation was found in a gene that codes for a receptor called CCR5. This protein, which is located on the surface of many different types of host immune cells (including T cells and macrophages), naturally functions during the inflammation process when immune cells are moving between different tissues. As was discovered during this time, CCR5 is also used by HIV as a receptor when the virus first attaches to macrophage cells following its entry into the body. Without CCR5 and the ability to attach, the virus is unable to infect macrophages, which drastically hinders its eventual spread to T cells. Thus, people harboring this mutation (called CCR5Δ32) can be exposed to HIV a thousand times and never become infected since the virus never makes it into the cells that it needs to replicate itself.

The discovery of CCR5Δ32 was an amazing leap forward in HIV research because it opened up new possibilities for therapeutic drugs and other treatments. For instance, if we could somehow artificially block the CCR5 protein in people who do not have the mutation, it may be possible to mimic the resistance trait in those who are already living with HIV. Such an idea sparked a search for synthetic compounds that could act as potential CCR5 blockers (antagonists). In 2007, a novel CCR5 antagonist drug called maraviroc was approved for use in the treatment of HIV.[59] It was found to be both safe and effective at blocking HIV attachment, which has led many physicians to now include it as an additive to the standard HAART treatment regimen.

Another approach for using the CCR5Δ32 mutation as a means of treating HIV centers around the idea of taking bone marrow cells from an person who has the CCR5Δ32 mutation and transplanting them into someone who has the normal CCR5 receptors. Doing so would essentially swap out the person's immune system since the bone marrow is what gives rise to all of the T cells, B cells, and macrophages in the body. If a person receiving this type of treatment were HIV-positive, the virus should in theory be unable to infect any new (mutant) immune cells produced in that recipient because their new bone marrow harbors the CCR5Δ32 mutation.

The proof of principle test case for this approach took place in a Berlin hospital in 2008. It was there that patient by the name of Timothy Ray Brown learned that he had recently developed a deadly form of cancer called adult myeloid leukemia and would need a bone marrow transplant in order to survive. Knowing that Brown was also HIV-positive, doctors saw an opportunity to test their theory. They first found several bone marrow samples that were a match for Brown and determined which also carried the CCR5Δ32 mutation. After identifying an appropriate donor, they proceeded to destroy Brown's existing bone marrow with radiation in order to kill off the defective, cancer-causing cells. Bone marrow from the healthy, CCR5Δ32 donor was then injected directly into several of Brown's long bones. After a short period of time, these new bone marrow cells began to replicate and produce fresh populations of T cells, macrophages, and every other immune cell. Since these new cells all had CCR5Δ32 mutation, the HIV particles that were in his blood could not infect them efficiently. As a result, his viral loads began to drop precipitously, and his T cell counts skyrocketed in just a matter of weeks. His health improved so much that his doctors took him off of all antiretroviral drugs. Now eight years later, Brown still has undetectable levels of HIV throughout his body despite not taking any HIV medications. It thus appears that the CCR5Δ32 transplant procedure functionally cured him of his HIV.

While the Brown case represents an amazing breakthrough in our pursuit of an effective cure for HIV, it has several major issues that prevent it from being implemented on a broader level. First, the procedure requires that an appropriate bone marrow match be found for the person who has HIV. Of all the people in the United States who currently need bone marrow to treat some blood disorder, about 70 percent of them must rely on finding a random stranger that had donated to the national registry. Since only about 2 percent of Americans belong to that registry, it is common for people (especially minorities) to wait for extended periods of time until a matching donor is located. Sadly, about 3,000 people die every year while waiting. These statistics illustrate the near impossibility of finding a bone marrow match for every one of the 36.7 million people in the world that have HIV. Second, the average cost of a bone marrow transplant in developed nations like the

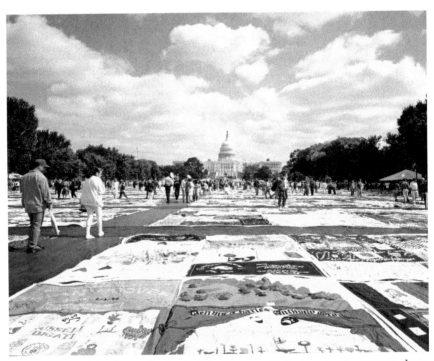

AIDS Memorial Quilt on display in Washington, D.C., to raise awareness about HIV and AIDS. (Carol M. Highsmith Archive, Library of Congress, Prints and Photographs Division)

United States is roughly $500,000–$800,000. Considering that most people living with HIV make less than a dollar a day and are unable to afford basic necessities, it is unlikely that costly bone marrow transplants could be applied on such a global scale. Third, bone marrow transplants are extremely dangerous and can have a mortality rate as high as 35 percent. For this reason, they are usually considered to be a last resort treatment for patients who have fatal blood disorders. Providing them to people with HIV would thus likely kill as many people as they would save. Finally, the CCR5Δ32 mutation is largely found only in Caucasians of Northern European descent and in some Asians and Northern Africans. While about 16 percent of all Northern Europeans have CCR5Δ32 in their genome, people from sub-Saharan Africa and most of Asia rarely do.[60] This is a troubling distribution considering most of the HIV-positive people in the world live in those two locations. As a result, even if they could find ethnically matched bone marrow donors for all people with HIV, chances are that few of them would actually harbor the beneficial CCR5Δ32 mutation.

When looking back on all that has been accomplished over the past 35 years since AIDS was first described, it becomes clear that the future of HIV and AIDS is not as bleak as it was two decades ago. Our collective "patience, persistence, and outright genius" has led to the development a numerous treatments, better preventative measures, and more effective education for those at risk. Infection rates are dropping and people are living with the disease 20–30 years longer than they had previously. Developed nations and global relief agencies have spent billions of dollars to provide lifesaving medications and preventative measures to some of the poorest people in the world. If such investments continue, we may finally see mankind get control of the AIDS epidemic in the same way that it eventually conquered nearly every other epidemic disease it has faced.

CHAPTER TWELVE

The Future of Epidemic Disease

Have we, as a species, progressed technologically to the point that we are no longer susceptible to being wiped out or even largely impacted by new epidemic diseases? It is an interesting question considering that diseases have collectively killed and disfigured billions of people and have been a significant driving force in shaping who we are as human beings. These diseases have toppled our empires, triggered major social changes, altered our genome, inspired revolutionary technological innovations, and influenced many wars. However, over the last 150 years, they have become increasingly less impactful due to the rise of Germ Theory and the introduction of sanitary measures, antibiotics, and vaccines. In fact, of the top 10 causes of mortality in the world, infectious diseases currently account for only 3 of them. It is now more common to hear people speaking about the dangers of heart disease and cancer than about the deadly impacts of tuberculosis and malaria. Rarely do emerging infectious diseases cause widespread panic or develop into new epidemics anymore due to our improved ability to contain them. While such trends seem to indicate that we are, on the whole, winning our battle against these microscopic killers, history has shown us that we are always just one epidemic away from global catastrophe.

What does the future hold for epidemic diseases? Will we ever be able to free ourselves from the grip of old killers like tuberculosis and malaria? Are there any new diseases on the horizon that have the potential to develop into a deadly epidemic? The answers to each of these questions obviously depend on a number of different factors. The first, and arguably most important, is whether we are willing to invest the necessary resources into eliminating infectious diseases in the developing world. Nearly every epidemic disease discussed in this book (and countless more not mentioned) still flourish among the poor. Millions die needlessly every year from diseases that can be treated with antibiotics or prevented with vaccines or basic sanitation.

As both the Smallpox and Polio Eradication Programs have shown, we have the potential to completely eliminate many of these deadly diseases if we are just willing to commit to it. Until that happens, we will continue to be plagued by our oldest pathogens and at risk for brand new ones. There will always be the potential for another "HIV" to be developing somewhere in the jungles of Africa, and there will always be another "cholera" establishing itself in the warm waters of Asia. The seeds of disease will remain until we finally become proactive and fight epidemics where they do the most damage.

Another important factor that may influence our future relationship with epidemic diseases is the manner in which we utilize our weapons against them. Two of the most powerful weapons, antibiotics and vaccines, have been used to save the lives of hundreds of millions of people worldwide over the last century. Like any good weapon, however, their success and safety rely heavily on whether they are used properly by trained professionals. Put a gun into the hands of a police officer and it will be used responsibly to save lives. Put that same weapon in hands of a child or someone who is mentally disturbed and it will cause destruction. The latter situation has arisen over the last 20 years, as the chronic misuse of antibiotics by the general public and pseudoscientific propaganda against vaccines have led us to the brink of a global medical disaster. In that time, we have seen a dangerous increase in antibiotic-resistant bacterial strains and a reemergence of epidemic diseases that were once under control. Although they may not be as trendy as Ebola, Zika, or West Nile, antibiotic resistance and vaccine misinformation represent a more significant threat to the long-term health of the entire population. For this reason, I have chosen to discuss each in greater depth in the sections below.

Antibiotic Resistance—Potential for Catastrophe

The discovery of penicillin in 1928 is widely viewed as being one of the most significant moments in the history of medicine. We gained a new weapon in the fight against deadly epidemic diseases like plague and typhus, and we no longer had to fear dying from minor infections acquired during childbirth, in surgery, or on the battlefield. People on the brink of death from systemic bacterial infections could be brought back to life after just a few days of antibiotic treatment. It was an amazing, almost miraculous, improvement that had some proclaiming we had finally won our centuries-long battle against bacterial diseases.

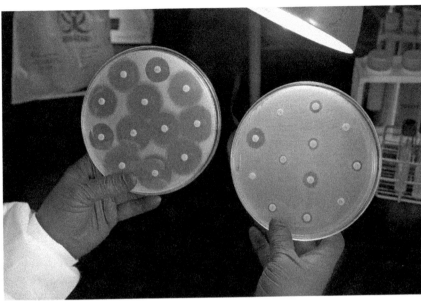

Antibiotic resistant bacteria (on the right) growing very close to paper disks that were soaked with various antibiotics. (Centers for Disease Control and Prevention)

Unfortunately, such optimism faded quickly as reports of antibiotic-resistant strains of Staph, Strep, and other pathogens began appearing all over the world.[1] In some cases, these resistant strains emerged after only one to two years following the release of the antibiotic into the population. For instance, methicillin-resistant *Staph aureus* (MRSA) was first observed in a clinic in Great Britain in 1962, only two years after methicillin began being prescribed for Staph infections. The situation has only grown worse over time as some bacterial strains have become increasingly resistant to multiple antibiotics. In fact, a 2011 survey of infectious disease physicians revealed that over 60 percent of them had seen patients in the previous year with infections that were resistant to all known antibiotics.[2] Such pandrug resistant (PDR) strains are completely impervious to every weapon modern medicine has created over the past 80 years. It is an absolutely frightening development that has public health officials all over the world scrambling for answers. As Dr. Keiji Fukuda, assistant director-general of the World Health Organization, once stated, "Without urgent, coordinated action by many stakeholders, the world is headed for a post-antibiotic era, in which common infections and minor injuries which have been treatable for decades can once again kill."[3]

Antibiotic-resistant bacteria are responsible for several million infections and over 50,000 deaths every year in the United States and Europe alone.[4] That is more people than die from AIDS, Parkinson's, and homicides combined (in the United States). While the most significant resistant pathogens are MRSA and XDR TB, drug-resistant forms of *Pseudomonas*, Enterococci, and *Streptococcus Pneumoniae* also claim lives of thousands. With the prevalence of these resistant strains rising every year, the number of mortalities is sure to increase. A recent study that modeled antibiotic resistance in the future predicted that by 2050, more than 10 million people will die every year from resistant infections.[5] It is a staggering theoretical statistic that is supported by trends that have been seen over the last 20 years. Besides death, the economic burden of having to treat antibiotic-resistant disease is also predicted to be catastrophic. The current yearly cost of treating these infections in the United States is about $20 billion, with another $35 billion being lost in worker productivity. If that trend continues, it is estimated that resistant bacteria will cost the United States over $60 trillion and the world $100 trillion over the next 35 years. The impact of losing so much of the world's combined GDP would be disastrous for the global economy. Many believe that we are on the verge of perhaps the most influential epidemic in history, and few people even know about it because antibiotic resistance is not as newsworthy as other, more visibly shocking diseases like Ebola or Zika. Without immediate and significant changes to how we utilize antibiotics, this epidemic will likely return us to the dark ages of medicine within the next several decades.

The current crisis only exists because of our large-scale unwillingness to responsibly use antibiotics. For instance, one of the most significant causes of increased resistance is the chronic misuse of antibiotics by the general population. Antibiotics are designed to be given at a certain dosage for some defined length of time in order to ensure that all of the pathogenic bacteria are killed by a combination of the drug and patient's immune system. Anything that interferes with that total killing increases the risk that surviving bacteria will develop resistance mutations or acquire resistance genes from other bacteria. For instance, many patients will stop taking their antibiotics after only a few days because they are feeling better. Shortening the treatment regimen in this way is extremely dangerous because it lowers the antibiotic concentration in the blood before the bacteria are fully cleared. Similarly, people will often take old, leftover antibiotics that are sitting around in their medicine cabinets when they start to feel under the weather. Older antibiotics are partially degraded, which means they contain suboptimal amounts of antibiotic needed to inhibit or kill bacteria. In both cases, bacteria are able to survive the antibiotic onslaught and live to fight another day.

A second cause of the growing resistance epidemic is the overuse of antibiotics by the population. Studies done in the United States have found that antibiotics are incorrectly prescribed as much as 30–50 percent of the time.[6] Every sniffle, scrape, and sore throat is now preemptively treated with antibiotics. They are given to patients who are not even sick or who have viral infections (viruses are not affected by antibiotics). Additionally, it has become increasingly common to prescribe broad-spectrum antibiotics like azithromycin (Z-pack) to patients without actually knowing what type of bacterial infection they have. Blindly prescribing antibiotics in this way is dangerous because not all bacteria are equally sensitive to the same drug. As a result, one may be unnecessarily exposed to an antibiotic that is not effective against the specific bacteria that they are infected with. This problem is even more pronounced in developing nations, where antibiotics are commonly available to the population at local drug stores. With no regulation by physicians or nurses, people simply purchase and take random antibiotics any time that they are feeling ill. Overexposure like this is one of the key factors that drive the formation of new resistant strains.

An often overlooked cause of the resistance crisis is the abuse of antibiotics in the agricultural industry. Over 80 percent of all the antibiotics sold in the United States are used to promote growth in livestock. Cows, pigs, and chickens are routinely injected with or fed antibiotics to keep them healthy so that they yield higher quantities of meats and other products. Rather than waiting for animals to get sick before treating them, they are prophylactically given antibiotics on a daily basis to prevent the illness from occurring in the first place. While this may seem like a perfectly reasonable measure to take to maximize profits, the continued use of antibiotics causes the bacteria living on those animals to develop extreme resistance to them. If humans consume meat, eggs, or milk from those animals and fail to prepare the food properly, they can be exposed to deadly, resistant strains of bacteria. Furthermore, since about 90 percent of the antibiotics given to livestock are excreted into the soil and water through their urine, those antibiotics can cause resistant strains to develop in the broader ecosystem. Farmers growing plant crops have also misused antibiotics to maximize profits. For instance, farmers who grow fruit trees often spray antibiotics onto their fields in order to prevent bacterial disease from wiping out their crop. All of the excess antibiotic ends up soaking into the soil and leaching into local water sources. Bacterial populations in those locations, in being continuously exposed to diluted forms of the antibiotics, are at a great risk for developing resistance to them.

Health officials all over the world are attempting to come up with solutions to the growing threat of antibiotic resistance. In the past, this problem was primarily addressed by discovering or synthesizing new antibiotics. As one antibiotic became less effective, a new one was quickly introduced into the market to take its place. Unfortunately, so many antibiotics became obsolete by resistant bacteria that companies began shifting their research and development resources away from new antibiotic discovery. In 1980–1984, there were 19 new antibiotics that were approved for human use by the federal government.[7] Just 20 years later, that number was down to only four new antibiotics (2000–2004). Antibiotic discovery has become unprofitable because of resistance, so only a few companies are still actively searching.

With the prospect of finding better antibiotics fading, many have begun trying to convince physicians, farmers, and the general public to be more cautious when using antibiotics. Physicians are being taught about the extreme dangers of antibiotic resistance earlier in their careers with the hope that they will be more selective in handing out antibiotics. Some countries in Europe have begun requiring physicians to fully diagnose infections before prescribing antibiotics and others have taken certain antibiotics off the market altogether to allow resistant strains to gradually die out. This has been complemented by the rise of the organic movement in food production, which has encouraged farmers to use more natural methods of raising their livestock that do not involve antibiotics or growth hormones. Together with educating the general public about proper antibiotic usage, these interventions will hopefully reverse some of the frightening trends that we have seen and help us avert another deadly pandemic.

The Power of Bad Science

In February 1998, a British surgeon by the name of Andrew Wakefield published a research article in *Lancet* that outlined his belief that the measles, mumps, and rubella (MMR) vaccine predisposes children to intestinal dysfunction and autism-spectrum disorders.[8] His study followed 12 children who had been referred to a pediatric gastroenterology unit following the onset of severe colitis and behavioral symptoms characteristic of autism. Dr. Wakefield and his colleagues took detailed histories of each child and performed extensive neurological and histological testing to see if they could identify any obvious cause for their "sudden" behavioral regression. Upon doing so, it was found that each child started exhibiting the early symptoms of autism just days or weeks after receiving the MMR vaccine. Wakefield used this data to make his case that MMR vaccination was in fact triggering the development of autism. Despite stating "we did not prove an association between measles, mumps, and rubella vaccine and the syndrome described,"[9] the tone and implications inherent to the rest of the article clearly suggest he believed that there was a causal link between the two.

The publication of the Wakefield article set off an absolute firestorm in the medical community. Parents of young children who once celebrated the life-saving miracle of vaccination now refused to vaccinate their children against any childhood disease. They summarily dismissed hundreds of years of epidemiological and immunological evidence that prove vaccines work and save lives and instead began trusting in poorly conducted, anecdotal studies that suggested they do not. Included in the anti-vaccination propaganda were claims that vaccine preservatives (e.g., thimerosal) are toxic to developing brains, receiving too many vaccines at once can cause inflammation in the brain, and vaccines are unnecessary because sanitation had already lowered infectious disease transmission. Many parents even started circulating conspiracy theories that drug companies were colluding with the U.S. government to knowingly inject harmful vaccines into their children just to make bigger profits. Suddenly, everyone was an infectious disease expert because they had read a secondhand account of a study on a blog or website. It was an explosion of ignorance that left many pediatricians having to now convince parents to protect their children from infectious disease. They were having to convince them despite the fact that vaccines have saved at estimated 732,000 American lives in just the 20-year period between 1994 and 2014.

The growing concern for vaccine safety prompted scientists from all over the world to begin looking into possible links between vaccination and autism. Experts from the United States, England, Canada, Finland, and Denmark independently examined several thousand children looking for evidence to support Wakefield's claim. Study after study came to the same conclusion: there was absolutely no link found between the MMR vaccine—or any other vaccine for that matter—and the development of autism. Subsequent follow-up studies by the Centers for Disease Control and Prevention (CDC) in 2011 and 2013 (again involving thousands of children) had identical results.[10] Complementing this mountain of epidemiological evidence, researchers who study brain development in those with autism recently found that biological signs of autism are readily apparent while children are developing *in utero*.[11] In other words, the abnormal brain development that causes the clinical signs of autism begins before birth, long before they are exposed to any vaccine.

A final nail in the "vaccines cause autism" coffin came in 2011, when it was revealed that Wakefield had purposely altered medical histories in his original study in order to get the findings that he wanted.[12] A reassessment of the 12 children in his study found that 3 never had autism and 5 showed autistic symptoms before ever receiving the MMR vaccine. He had also failed to disclose that he had been paid over $600,000 by a law firm that was preparing to sue vaccine manufacturers before he published his article. Such blatant fraud led *The Lancet* to retract his original article and caused Wakefield to lose his license to practice medicine in Great Britain.

In addition to wasting millions of dollars and thousands of research hours that could have used to study other diseases, the autism scare has led to a reemergence of several epidemic diseases that had been previously controlled through vaccination. The most significant of these is measles. Prior to the development of the MMR vaccine in 1963, measles was one of the deadliest diseases in the world, killing over a million people every year. However, as more of the population gained access to the vaccine, the total number of measles cases and deaths began to drop sharply. By the start of the 1990s, measles was exceedingly rare in most developed nations. The United States, which was a leader in the measles vaccination effort, had officially eradicated the disease within its borders by the year 2000.

It was a victory that was short lived, however, as new cases were reported in the following year as a result of people refusing the MMR vaccine.[13] More widespread outbreaks began appearing in 2008, and since then thousands have contracted the deadly disease in the United States alone. For instance, a North Texas megachurch experienced an outbreak in 2013 after the pastor publicly expressed concerns over the safety of vaccines. The United States had 23 separate measles outbreaks in 2014, which resulted in 667 infections. In 2015, a multistate outbreak occurred after an infected traveler brought the disease from overseas to a California amusement park. Over 80 percent of the people infected in that outbreak had refused the MMR vaccine in part because they believed it to be unsafe.

Other vaccine-preventable diseases that have gained a second life due to anti-vaccination efforts include mumps, rubella, whooping cough (pertussis), and diphtheria. These are diseases that had been under control and declining for decades as a result of mandatory vaccination for children starting school. However, with the advent of policies in some states that allow parents to opt out of vaccinations, more unvaccinated children have been flooding playgrounds, camps, and other public areas over the last several years. The results have been alarming in the United States—9,200 new cases of whooping cough in California in 2010, 6,500 cases of mumps in 2006, and the reappearance of congenital rubella after almost a decade of being eradicated. It is a frightening trend that has left public health officials scrambling for solutions.

The spread of misinformation about vaccines is a serious threat to our safety because it allows epidemic diseases that have collectively killed hundreds of millions of people to persist in the population. Most of the diseases described above were declining to levels that people began to speak about them being eradicated on a global level. Mass vaccination campaigns were working and deadly childhood diseases were fading away from our collective memory. Unfortunately, this changed as we started to weaken our most effective weapon against them. By letting epidemic diseases stick around, we are giving them time and opportunity to potentially evolve into something we cannot so easily prevent or treat. We are playing with fire and will only have ourselves to blame if any of these diseases reemerge as full epidemics.

Additionally, willful ignorance about vaccines endangers future vaccination efforts. For instance, if we are eventually successful in generating an effective vaccine against HIV, anti-vaccine activism could impede public acceptance and ultimately lengthen the epidemic. This exact situation has recently arisen following the release of vaccines against the human papillomavirus (HPV). These vaccines, Gardasil and Cervarix, have been studied extensively by the CDC, Food and Drug Administration, and National Cancer Institute and found to be both safe and effective. They prevent infection with cancer-causing strains of HPV and protect the female population from deadly cervical cancer. In fact, several studies have found that rates of HPV transmission have dropped by over 60 percent in locations where the vaccines are available.[14] Furthermore, there has never been a proven case where either vaccine has caused any serious side effects. Despite its success, "anti-vaxxers" are still using pseudoscience and fear mongering to scare people into not vaccinating their children. It is a decision that is actively putting lives at risk.

Notes

Chapter 2

1. Agnolo Di Tura del Grasso, "The Black Death in Siena," in *The Medieval Reader*, ed. Norman F. Cantor (New York: Harper Perennial, 1994), 281.

2. M. Achtman et al., "*Yersinia pestis*, the Cause of Plague, Is a Recently Emerged Clone of *Yersinia pseudotuberculosis*," *Proceedings of the National Academy of Sciences USA* 96, no. 24 (1999): 14043–14048.

3. "Plague Manual: Epidemiology, Distribution, Surveillance and Control," accessed April 1, 2014, http://www.who.int/csr/resources/publications/plague/whocdscsredc992a.pdf.

4. Michaela Harbeck et al., "*Yersinia pestis* DNA from Skeletal Remains from the 6th Century AD Reveals Insights into Justinianic Plague," *PLOS Pathogens* 9, no. 5 (2013): e1003349; William Rosen, *Justinian's Flea: The First Great Plague and the End of the Roman Empire* (New York: Viking Penguin, 2007).

5. Alexander Kazhdan, ed., "Constantinople," in *The Oxford Dictionary of Byzantium* (Oxford: Oxford University Press, 1991), 508.

6. John Frith, "The History of Plague—Part 1. The Three Great Pandemics," *Journal of Military and Veterans Health* 20, no. 2 (2012): 11–16.

7. "Roman Empire," accessed April 1, 2014, https://www.britannica.com/place/Roman-Empire.

8. Guy Halsall, *Barbarian Migrations and the Roman West, 376–568* (Cambridge, UK: Cambridge University Press, 2008), 499–512.

9. Rosen, *Justinian's Flea*.

10. Halsall, *Barbarian Migrations*.

11. John Kelly, *The Great Mortality: An Intimate History of the Black Death, the Most Devastating Plague of All Time* (New York: HarperCollins, 2005).

12. Giovanni Boccaccio, *The Decameron*, trans. and ed. G. H. McWilliam (London: Penguin Classics, 2003).

13. Arnold Pacey, *Technology in World Civilization: A Thousand-Year History* (Cambridge, MA: The MIT Press, 1990), 53–54.

14. Mark Wheelis, "Biological Warfare at the 1346 Siege of Caffa," *Emerging Infectious Diseases* 8, no. 9 (2002): 971–975.

15. Ibid.

16. Ibid.

17. Jeanne Guillemin, "Scientists and the History of Biological Weapons: A Brief Historical Overview of the Development of Biological Weapons in the Twentieth Century," *EMBO Reports* 7, special issue (2006): S45–S49.

18. Ian Kershaw, "The Great Famine and Agrarian Crisis in England 1315–1322," *Past and Present* 59, no. 1 (1973): 3–50.

19. Dorothy Crawford, *Deadly Companions: How Microbes Shaped Our History* (Oxford: Oxford University Press, 2007), 105–106.

20. Alastair Dunn, *The Great Rising of 1381: The Peasants' Revolt and England's Failed Revolution* (Stroud, UK: Tempus, 2002); Christopher Dyer, *Making a Living in the Middle Ages: The People of Britain 850–1520* (New Haven, CT: Yale University Press, 2009).

21. Wheelis, "Biological Warfare."

22. Philip Ziegler, *The Black Death* (New York: HarperCollins, 2009), 84–109.

23. G. G. Coulton, *The Black Death* (London: Ernest Benn, 1929), 59–60.

24. William Langland, *Piers Plowman: The C Version*, trans. George Economou (Philadelphia: University of Pennsylvania Press, 1996), 100–101.

25. Ziegler, *Black Death*.

26. Marc Saperstein and Jacob Rader Marcus, *The Jews in Christian Europe: A Source Book, 315–1791* (Pittsburgh, PA: University of Pittsburgh Press, 2015).

27. Ziegler, *Black Death*.

28. John Aberth, *The Black Death: The Great Mortality of 1348–1350: A Brief History with Documents* (Boston, MA: Bedford/St. Martin's, 2005), 158–159.

29. Marchione di Coppo Stefani, *Cronaca fiorentina. Rerum Italicarum Scriptores*, ed. Niccolo Rodolico, vol. 30 (Florence: Citta di Castello, 1903).

30. J. Matovinovic, "A Short History of Quarantine (Victor C. Vaughan)," *University of Michigan Medical Center Journal* 35, no. 4 (1969): 224–228.

31. Vern Bullough, *The Development of Medicine as a Profession: The Contribution of the Medieval University to Modern Medicine* (New York: Hafner, 1966), 104–110.

32. Anna Montgomery Campbell, *The Black Death and Men of Learning* (New York: Columbia University Press, 1931), 146–180.

33. Millard Meiss, *Painting in Florence and Siena After the Black Death* (Princeton, NJ: Princeton University Press, 1951), 67–74.

34. Christine Boeckl, "The Pisan Triumph of Death and the Papal Constitution Benedictus Deus," *Artibus et Historiae* 18, no. 36 (1997): 55–60.

35. James Snyder, *Northern Renaissance Art: Paintings, Sculpture, the Graphic Arts from 1350 to 1575* (New York: Harry N. Abrams, 1985), 264–265.

36. The Limbourg Brothers, "Procession of Flagellants," in *Belles Heures of Jean de France, duc de Berry* (New York: The Cloisters Collection, 1954).

37. Sophie Oosterwijk, "Of Corpses, Constables, and Kings: The Danse Macabre in Late Medieval and Renaissance Culture," *Journal of the British Archaeological Association* 157 (2004): 66–67.

38. Hafid Laayouni et al., "Convergent Evolution in European and Rroma Populations Reveals Pressure Exerted by Plague on Toll-Like Receptors," *Proceedings of the National Academy of Sciences USA* 111, no. 7 (2014): 2668–2673.

39. S. K. Cohn Jr. and L. T. Weaver, "The Black Death and AIDS: CCR5-Delta32 in Genetics and History," *QJM* 99, no. 8 (2006): 497–503.

40. C. Tollenaere et al., "CCR5 Polymorphism and Plague Resistance in Natural Populations of the Black Rat in Madagascar," *Infection, Genetics and Evolution* 8, no. 6 (2008): 891–897; K. L. Styer et al., "Study of the Role of CCR5 in a Mouse Model of Intranasal Challenge with *Yersinia pestis*," *Microbes and Infection* 9, no. 9 (2007): 1135–1138.

41. T. Butler, "Plague History: Yersin's Discovery of the Causative Bacterium in 1894 Enabled, in the Subsequent Century, Scientific Progress in Understanding the Disease and the Development of Treatments and Vaccines," *Clinical Microbiology and Infection* 20, no. 3 (2014): 202–209.

42. Myron Echenberg, *Plague Ports: The Global Urban Impact of Bubonic Plague, 1894–1901* (New York: New York University Press, 2007), 66–68.

43. Ibid.

Chapter 3

1. John Rhodes, *The End of Plagues: The Global Battle against Infectious Disease* (New York: St. Martin's Press, 2013), 10.

2. N. Barquet and P. Domingo, "Smallpox: The Triumph Over the Most Terrible of the Ministers of Death," *Annals of Internal Medicine* 127, no. 8 (pt. 1) (1997): 635–642.

3. Abbas Behbehani, "The Smallpox Story: Life and Death of an Old Disease," *Microbiological Reviews* 47, no. 4 (1983): 455–509.

4. Ibid.

5. Donald Hopkins, *The Greatest Killer: Smallpox in History* (Chicago, IL: University of Chicago Press, 2002), 104.

6. Cheston Cunha and Burke Cunha, "Great Plagues of the Past and Remaining Questions," in *Paleomicrobiology: Past Human Infections*, ed. D. Raoult and M. Drancourt (Berlin Heidelberg: Springer-Verlag, 2008).

7. Ibid.

8. R. J. Littman and M. L. Littman, "Galen and the Antonine Plague," *American Journal of Philology* 94, no. 3 (1973): 243–255.

9. Cunha and Cunha, "Great Plagues of the Past."

10. J. R. Fears, "The Plague Under Marcus Aurelius and the Decline and Fall of the Roman Empire," *Infectious Disease Clinics of North America* 18, no. 1 (2004): 65–77.

11. Ibid.

12. Rodney Stark, *The Rise of Christianity: How the Obscure, Marginal Jesus Movement Became the Dominant Religious Force in the Western World in a Few Centuries* (San Francisco, CA: Harper, 1996), 73–94.

13. Ibid.

14. Paul Johnson, *A History of Christianity* (New York: Antheneum, 1976).

15. Stark, *Rise of Christianity*.

16. Caroline Finkel, *Osman's Dream: The History of the Ottoman Empire* (New York: Basic Books, 2006), 115–151.

17. Bailey Diffie and George Winius, *Foundations of the Portuguese Empire, 1415–1580*, vol. I (St. Paul: University of Minnesota Press, 1977), 57–95.

18. F. Fenner et al., *Smallpox and Its Eradication* (Geneva, CH: World Health Organization, 1988), 233–240.

19. Ibid.

20. Douglas Wheeler, "A Note on Smallpox in Angola, 1670–1875," *Studia* 13/14 (1964): 351–362.

21. Fenner et al., *Smallpox*.

22. David Henige, "When Did Smallpox Reach the New World (and Why Does It Matter)?," in *Africans in Bondage: Studies in Slavery and the Slave Trade*, ed. Philip Curtin and Paul Lovejoy (Madison: University of Wisconsin-Madison Press, 1986), 11–26.

23. Hopkins, *Greatest Killer*, 205.

24. Ibid.

25. William Prescott, *History of the Conquest of Mexico* (New York: Modern Library, 2001), 157–169.

26. Ibid.

27. Ibid., 170–193.

28. Ibid., 194–220.

29. Ibid., 505–527.

30. Francis Borgia Steck, *Motolinia's History of the Indians of New Spain* (Oceanside, CA: Academy of American Franciscan History, 1951).

31. Prescott, *Conquest of Mexico*, 796–828.

32. Juan de Betanzos, *Narrative of the Incas*, trans. and ed. Roland Hamilton and Dana Buchanon (Austin: University of Texas Press, 1996), 182–302.

33. Ibid.

34. Hopkins, *Greatest Killer*, 214–215.

35. A. W. Crosby, "Virgin Soil Epidemics as a Factor in the Aboriginal Depopulation in America," *William and Mary Quarterly* 33 (1976): 289–299.

36. Increase Mather, *Early History of New England: Being a Relation of Hostile Passages between the Indians and European Voyagers and First Settlers: and a Full Narrative of Hostilities, to the Close of the War with the Pequots, in the Year 1637: Also a Detailed Account of the Origin of the War with King Philip* (Albany, NY: J. Munsell, 1864), 110.

37. Fenner et al., *Smallpox*.

38. J. L. Cumpston, *The History of Smallpox in Australia, 1788–1908* (Melbourne: Government of Australia Printer, 1914).

39. Ibid.

40. Donald Hopkins, *Princes and Peasants: Smallpox in History* (Chicago, IL: University of Chicago Press, 1983).

41. James Carrick Moore, *The History of the Smallpox* (Charleston, SC: Nabu Press, 2010), 96.

42. Hopkins, *Princes and Peasants*.

43. Ibid.

44. Behbehani, "Smallpox Story."

45. Ibid.

46. J. M. Eyler, "Smallpox in History: The Birth, Death, and Impact of a Dread Disease," *Journal of Laboratory and Clinical Medicine* 142, no. 4 (2003): 216–220.

47. Thomas Cone Jr., "Benjamin Franklin's Account of Inoculation (Variolation) in Boston," *Pediatrics* 54, no. 5 (1974): 586.

48. Elizabeth Fenn, *Pox Americana: The Great Smallpox Epidemic of 1775–82* (New York: Hill and Wang, 2001).

49. "Letter from John Adams to Abigail Adams, 26 June 1776," accessed December 14, 2014, https://www.masshist.org/digitaladams/archive/doc?id=L17760626ja.

50. Fenn, *Pox Americana*.

51. Ibid.

52. Ibid.

53. Edward Jenner, "An Inquiry into the Causes and Effects of the Variolae Vaccinae, a Disease Discovered in Some of the Western Counties of England, Particularly Gloucestershire, and Known by the Name of the Cow Pox," in *Classics of Medicine and Surgery*, ed. C. N. B. Camac (New York: Dover, 1959), 213–240.

54. Ibid.

55. Gary Nabel, "Designing Tomorrow's Vaccines," *New England Journal of Medicine* 386, no. 6 (2013): 551–560.

56. Fenner et al., *Smallpox*, 322–418.

57. Ibid.; Donald Henderson, "Smallpox Eradication—A Cold War Victory," *World Health Forum* 19 (1998): 113–119.

58. Ibid.

59. Henderson, "Smallpox Eradication."

60. David Koplow, "Deliberate Extinction: Whether to Destroy the Last Smallpox Virus," *Suffolk University Law Review* 37, no. 1 (2004): 1–50.

61. Ibid.

62. Ken Alibek, *Biohazard: The Chilling True Story of the Largest Covert Biological Weapons Program in the World—Told from Inside by the Man Who Ran It* (Crystal Lake, IL: Delta Publishing, 2000).

63. Richard Preston, "The Demon in the Freezer: How Smallpox, a Disease of Officially Eradicated Twenty Years Ago, Became the Biggest Bioterrorist Threat We Now Face," *New Yorker*, July 12, 1999, 44–61.

64. Ibid.

Chapter 4

1. "Fact Sheet: World Malaria Report 2016," accessed December 30, 2016, http://www.who.int/malaria/media/world-malaria-report-2016/en/.

2. E. Worrall, S. Basu, and K. Hanson, "Is Malaria a Disease of Poverty? A Review of the Literature," *Tropical Medicine and International Health* 10, no. 10 (2005): 1047–1059.

3. A. S. Aly, A. M. Vaughan, and S. H. Kappe, "Malaria Parasite Development in the Mosquito and Infection of the Mammalian Host," *Annual Review of Microbiology* 63 (2009): 195–221.

4. Ibid.

5. Ibid.

6. David J. Conway, Caterina Fanello, Jennifer M. Lloyd et al., "Origin of *Plasmodium falciparum* Malaria Is Traced by Mitochondrial DNA," *Molecular and Biochemical Parasitology* 111 (2000): 163–171.

7. Richard Carter and Kamini Mendis, "Evolutionary and Historical Aspects of the Burden of Malaria," *Clinical Microbiology Reviews* 15, no. 4 (2002): 564–594.

8. Ibid.

9. Ibid.

10. Hippocrates, *Airs, Waters, and Places*, trans. W. H. S. Jones (New York: Putnam, 1923).

11. Ernst Hempelmann and Kristine Krafts, "Bad Air, Amulets and Mosquitoes: 2,000 Years of Changing Perspectives on Malaria," *Malaria Journal* 12 (2013): 232.

12. Robert Sallares, *Malaria and Rome: A History of Malaria in Ancient Italy* (Oxford: Oxford University Press, 2002), 43–114.

13. Pliny the Elder, *Natural History: A Selection*, trans. J. F. Healy (New York: Penguin, 1991), 355–356.

14. Robert Sallares, *Malaria and Rome: A History of Malaria in Ancient Italy* (Oxford: Oxford University Press, 2002), 168–191.

15. J. H. Robinson, *Readings in European History* (Boston, MA: Ginn, 1905), 49–51.

16. B. A. Cunha, "The Death of Alexander the Great: Malaria or Typhoid Fever?," *Infectious Disease Clinics of North America* 18, no. 1 (2004): 53–63.

17. Karen Masterson, *The Malaria Project: The U.S. Government's Secret Mission to Find a Miracle Cure* (New York: Penguin, 2014), 11.

18. Thomas Pakenham, *The Scramble for Africa: White Man's Conquest of the Dark Continent from 1876 to 1912* (New York: Avon Books, 1991), 1–140.

19. Philip Curtin, "The End of the 'White Man's Grave'? Nineteenth-Century Mortality in West Africa," *Journal of Interdisciplinary History* 21, no. 1 (1990): 63–88.

20. Fiammetta Rocco, *The Miraculous Fever-Tree: Malaria, Medicine and the Cure That Changed the World* (London: HarperCollins, 2003).

21. Marie Louise Duran-Reynals, *The Fever Bark Tree: The Pageant of Quinine* (Garden City, NY: Doubleday, 1946).

22. Rocco, *Miraculous Fever-Tree*; Benjamin Blass, *Basic Principles of Drug Discovery and Development* (Cambridge, MA: Academic Press, 2015), 38.

23. Francisco Medina Rodríguez, "Precisions on the History of Quinine," *Reumatología Clínica* 3, no. 4 (2007): 194–196.

24. Saul Jarcho, *Quinine's Predecessor: Francesco Torti and the Early History of Cinchona* (Baltimore, MD: Johns Hopkins University Press, 1993), 14–16.

25. Duran-Reynals, *The Fever Bark Tree*.

26. Mark Honigsbaum, *The Fever Trail: Malaria, the Mosquito and the Quest for Quinine* (London: Macmillan, 2001).

27. R. Kyle and M. Shampe, "Discoverers of Quinine," *Journal of the American Medical Association* 229, no. 4 (1974): 462.

28. Jane Achan et al., "Quinine, an Old Anti-malarial Drug in a Modern World: Role in the Treatment of Malaria," *Malaria Journal* 10 (2011): 144.

29. Bob Whitfield, *Germany, 1848–1914* (Portsmouth, NH: Heinemann, 2000), 127–142.

30. John Davis, ed., *Italy in the Nineteenth Century: 1796–1900* (London: Oxford University Press, 2000), 154–180.

31. Matthew Craven, "Between Law and History: The Berlin Conference of 1884–1885 and the Logic of Free Trade," *London Review of International Law* 3, no. 1 (2015): 31–59.

32. John Luke Gallup and Jeffrey Sachs, "The Economic Burden of Malaria," *American Journal of Tropical Medicine and Hygiene* 64, no. 1 (2001): 85–96; "Economic Costs of Malaria," accessed November 25, 2015, http://www.rollbackmalaria.org/files/files/toolbox/RBM%20Economic%20Costs%20of%20Malaria.pdf.

33. Rustam Aminov, "A Brief History of the Antibiotic Era: Lessons Learned and Challenges for the Future," *Frontiers in Microbiology* 1, no. 134 (2010): 1–7.

34. David McCullough, *The Path between the Seas: The Creation of the Panama Canal, 1870–1914* (New York: Simon and Schuster, 1977), 101–152.

35. Ibid., 153–203.

36. Ibid., 101–152.

37. Ibid., 153–203.

38. Ibid., 243–402.

39. Ibid., 403–489.

40. Ibid., 403–489.

41. Ibid., 101–152.

42. Ronald Ross, "In Exile, Reply—What Ails the Solitude" (1897), in Luke A. Baton and Lisa C. Ranford-Cartwright, "Spreading the Seeds of Million-Murdering Death: Metamorphoses of Malaria in the Mosquito," *Trends in Parasitology* 21, no. 12 (2005): 573–580.

43. McCullough, *Path between the Seas*, 403–489.

44. Ibid., 403–489.

45. C. H. Melville, "The Prevention of Malaria in War," in *The Prevention of Malaria*, ed. Ronald Ross (London: John Murray, 1910), 577–599.

46. J. R. McNeill, "Malarial Mosquitoes Helped Defeat British in Battle That Ended Revolutionary War," *Washington Post*, October 18, 2010.

47. Bernard Brabin, "Malaria's Contribution to World War One—The Unexpected Adversary," *Malaria Journal* 13 (2014): 497.

48. Paul Russell, Luther West, and Reginald Manwell, *Practical Malariology* (Philadelphia, PA: W. B. Saunders, 1946).

49. Vassiliki Smocovitis, "Desperately Seeking Quinine: The Malaria Threat Drove the Allies' WWII Cinchona Mission," *Modern Drug Discovery* 6, no. 5 (2003): 57–58.

50. Ibid.

51. C. W. Hays, "The United States Army and Malaria Control in World War II," *Parassitologia* 42, no. 1–2 (2000): 47–52.

52. Elizabeth Etheridge, *Sentinel for Health: A History of the Centers for Disease Control* (Berkeley: University of California Press, 1992).

53. Hays, "United States Army."

54. J. Richardson, A. Roy, S. L. Shalat et al., "Elevated Serum Pesticide Levels and Risk for Alzheimer Disease," *Journal of the American Medical Association Neurology* 71, no. 3 (2014): 284–290.

55. Carter and Mendis, "Evolutionary and Historical Aspects."

56. Ibid.

57. Ibid.

58. Ibid.

59. Ibid.

Chapter 5

1. Frank Ryan, *Tuberculosis: The Greatest Story Never Told—The Search for the Cure and the New Global Threat* (Sheffield, UK: Swift, 1992), 10.

2. Bruce Rothschild et al., "*Mycobacterium tuberculosis* Complex DNA from an Extinct Bison Dated 17,000 Years Before the Present," *Clinical Infectious Diseases* 33, no. 3 (2001): 305–311.

3. H. D. Chalke, "The Impact of Tuberculosis on History, Literature and Art," *Medical History* 6, no. 4 (1962): 301–318.

4. Friedrich Engels, *The Condition of the Working Class in England in 1844* (Oxford: Oxford University Press, 2009), 29.

5. "Contagion: Historical Views of Diseases and Epidemics—Tuberculosis in Europe and North America, 1800–1922," Harvard University Library Open Collections Program, accessed June 12, 2015, http://ocp.hul.harvard.edu/contagion/tuberculosis.html.

6. David Wagner, *The Poorhouse: America's Forgotten Institution* (Lanham, MD: Rowman and Littlefield, 2005), 1–58.

7. Robert Koch, "An Address on the Fight against Tuberculosis in the Light of the Experience That Has Been Gained in the Successful Combat of Other Infectious Diseases," *British Medical Journal* 2, no. 2117 (1901): 187–193.

8. P. S. Sledzik and N. Bellantoni, "Brief Communication: Bioarcheological and Biocultural Evidence for the New England Vampire Folk Belief," *American Journal of Physical Anthropology* 94, no. 2 (1994): 269–274.

9. Theophilus Thompson, "Hints on Some Relations of Morals and Medicine, with Special Reference to Pulmonary Consumption," *London Journal of Medicine* 3, no. 29 (1851): 403–405.

10. René Jules Dubos and Jean Dubos, *The White Plague: Tuberculosis, Man, and Society* (New Brunswick, NJ: Rutgers University Press, 1952), 44–68; Chalke, "Impact of Tuberculosis."

11. Mark Caldwell, *The Last Crusade: The War on Consumption, 1862–1954* (New York: Atheneum, 1988).

12. Dubos and Dubos, *White Plague*; Chalke, "Impact of Tuberculosis."

13. Peter Warren, "The Evolution of the Sanatorium: The First Half-Century, 1854–1904," *Canadian Bulletin of Medical History* 23, no. 2 (2006): 457–476.

14. George Bodington, *An Essay on the Treatment and Cure of Pulmonary Consumption* (London: Longman, 1840).

15. Warren, "Evolution of the Sanatorium."

16. Richard Sucre, "The Great White Plague: The Culture of Death and the Tuberculosis Sanatorium," accessed March 15, 2015, http://www.faculty.virginia.edu/blueridgesanatorium/death.htm.

17. T. N. Kelynack, "The Tuberculosis Problem," *British Journal of Tuberculosis* 1, no. 1 (1907): 3.

18. Warren, "Evolution of the Sanatorium."

19. Tuberculosis Chemotherapy Centre, "A Concurrent Comparison of Home and Sanatorium Treatment of Pulmonary Tuberculosis in South India," *Bulletin of the World Health Organization* 21, no. 1 (1959): 51–144.

20. Steve Blevins and Michael Bronze, "Robert Koch and the 'Golden Age' of Bacteriology," *International Journal of Infectious Diseases* 14 (2010): e744–e751.

21. "The Postulates of Robert Koch," *Journal of the American Medical Association* 175, no. 11 (1961): 1003–1005.

22. "Robert Koch and Tuberculosis: Koch's Famous Lecture," accessed June 10, 2015, https://www.nobelprize.org/educational/medicine/tuberculosis/readmore.html.

23. Ibid.

24. Blevins and Bronze, "Robert Koch."

25. Ibid.

26. Ibid.

27. Venita Jay, "The Legacy of Carl Weigert," *Journal of Histotechnology* 22, no. 1 (1999): 59–60.

28. V. H. Holsinger, K. T. Rajkowski, and J. R. Stabel, "Milk Pasteurisation and Safety: A Brief History and Update," *Scientific and Technical Review of the Office International des Epizooties* 16, no. 2 (1997): 441–451.

29. Simona Luca and Traian Mihaescu, "History of BCG Vaccine," *Maedica (Buchar)* 8, no. 1 (2013): 53–58.

30. P. E. Fine, "Variation in Protection by BCG: Implications of and for Heterologous Immunity," *Lancet* 346, no. 8986 (1995): 1339–1345.

31. Ariel Roguin, "Rene Theophile Hyacinthe Laënnec (1781–1826): The Man Behind the Stethoscope," *Clinical Medicine and Research* 4, no. 3 (2006): 230–235.

32. Christoph Gradmann, "Robert Koch and the White Death: From Tuberculosis to Tuberculin," *Microbes and Infection* 8 (2006): 294–301.

33. C. von Pirquet, "Frequency of Tuberculosis in Childhood," *Journal of the American Medical Association* 52 (1909): 675–678.

34. C. Mantoux, "L'intradermo-reaction a la tuberculine," *La Presse medicale* 2 (1910): 10–13.

35. Francis Williams, "The Use of X-Ray Examinations in Pulmonary Tuberculosis," *Boston Medical and Surgical Journal* 157 (1907): 850–853.

36. Thomas Mann, *Magic Mountain* (New York: Alfred A. Knopf, 1995), 216.

37. Stefan Kaufmann, "Paul Ehrlich: Founder of Chemotherapy," *Nature Reviews Drug Discovery* 7 (2008): 373.

38. M. Wainwright, "Streptomycin: Discovery and Resultant Controversy," *History and Philosophy of the Life Sciences* 13, no. 1 (1991): 97–124.

39. Ibid.

40. William Rosen, *Miracle Cure: The Creation of Antibiotics and the Birth of Modern Medicine* (New York: Viking, 2017), 204.

41. Wainwright, "Streptomycin."

42. J. Murray, D. E. Schraufnagel, and P. C. Hopewell, "Treatment of Tuberculosis: A Historical Perspective," *Annals of the American Thoracic Society* 12, no. 12 (2015): 1749–1759.

43. W. Fox et al., "The Prevalence of Drug-Resistant Tubercle Bacilli in Untreated Patients with Pulmonary Tuberculosis: A National Survey, 1955–56," *Tubercle* 38 (1957): 71–84.

44. M. D. Iseman, "Tuberculosis Therapy: Past, Present and Future," *European Respiratory Journal* suppl. 36 (2002): 87S–94S.

45. "Global Tuberculosis Report 2014," World Health Organization, accessed July 15, 2015, http://apps.who.int/iris/bitstream/10665/137094/1/9789241564809 _eng.pdf.

46. Kristin Cummings, "Tuberculosis Control: Challenges of an Ancient and Ongoing Epidemic," *Public Health Reports* 122, no. 5 (2007): 683–692.

47. Cesar Bonilla and Jaime Bayona, "Building Political Commitment in Peru for TB Control through Expansion of the DOTS Strategy," *Bulletin of the World Health Organization* 85, no. 5 (2007): 402.

Chapter 6

1. Hans Zinsser, *Rats, Lice, and History* (Abingdon, UK: Routledge, 1935), 153.

2. J. N. Hays, *Epidemics and Pandemics: Their Impacts on Human History* (Santa Barbara, CA: ABC-CLIO, 2005), 1–8.

3. Thucydides, *The Peloponnesian War*, bk. II, trans. "Crawley," rev. ed. T. E. Wick (New York: Modern Library, 1982).

4. Washington Irving, *Chronicle of the Conquest of Granada: From the Mss. of Fray Antonio Agapida* (New York: G. P. Putnam and Son, 1869).

5. Ibid.

6. Zinsser, *Rats*, 243.

7. Angus Konstam, *Pavia 1525: The Climax of the Italian Wars* (Oxford: Osprey Publishing, 1996).

8. André Chastel and Beth Archer, trans., *The Sack of Rome, 1527* (Princeton, NJ: Princeton University Press, 1983).

9. Zinsser, *Rats*, 250–254.

10. Giles Tremlett, *Catherine of Aragon: The Spanish Queen of Henry VIII* (London: Walker Books, 2010).

11. Ibid.

12. Dennis Bratcher, ed., "The Edict of Worms (1521)," accessed August 15, 2015, http://www.crivoice.org/creededictworms.html.

13. Daniel Nexon, *The Struggle for Power in Early Modern Europe: Religious Conflict, Dynastic Empires, and International Change* (Princeton, NJ: Princeton University Press, 2009), 1–2.

14. George Kohn, *Encyclopedia of Plague and Pestilence: From Ancient Times to the Present* (New York: Facts on File, 2007), 69.

15. Peter Wilson, *The Thirty Years War: Europe's Tragedy* (Cambridge, MA: Belknap Press, 2009), 41–48.

16. Ibid., 269–313.

17. Ibid.

18. R. Hare, *Pomp and Pestilence* (New York: Philosophical Library, 1955), 95–152.

19. Zinsser, *Rats*, 272.

20. David Chandler, *The Campaigns of Napoleon* (New York: Simon and Schuster, 1973), 572–592.

21. Owen Connelly, *Blundering to Glory: Napoleon's Military Campaigns* (Wilmington, DE: Scholarly Resources, 2006), 163–190.

22. Antony Brett-James, *1812: Eyewitness Accounts of Napoleon's Defeat in Russia* (New York: Macmillan, 1966).

23. Connelly, *Blundering to Glory*.

24. Brett-James, *1812*.

25. Ibid.

26. David Chandler, *The Campaigns of Napoleon* (New York: Simon and Schuster, 1973), 804–810.

27. Ibid.

28. Leo Tolstoy, *War and Peace* (1869; repr., New York: Vintage, 2008), 1008.

29. Chandler, *Campaigns of Napoleon*.

30. Ibid.

31. Christine Kinealy, *This Great Calamity: The Irish Famine 1845–52* (New York: Gill and Macmillan, 1994).

32. Ibid.

33. George Kohn, *Encyclopedia of Plague and Pestilence: From Ancient Times to the Present* (New York: Facts on File, 2007), 192.

34. Edward Laxton, *The Famine Ships: The Irish Exodus to America* (New York: Henry Holt, 1997).

35. Robert Whyte and James Mangan, eds., *Robert Whyte's 1847 Famine Ship Diary: The Journey of an Irish Coffin Ship* (London: Irish American Book Co., 1994), 95.

36. Cecil Woodham-Smith, *The Great Hunger—Ireland 1845–1849* (London: Penguin Books, 1991), 217–227.

37. Ibid.; Whyte and Mangan, *Robert Whyte's 1847*; Michael Quigley, "Grosse Ile: Canada's Irish Famine Memorial," *Labour/Le Travail* 39 (1997): 195–214.

38. Richard Gabriel, *Man and Wound in the Ancient World: A History of Military Medicine from Sumer to the Fall of Constantinople* (Lincoln, NE: Potomac Books, 2011), 27.

39. V. Soubbotitch, "A Pandemic of Typhus in Serbia in 1914 and 1915," *Proceedings of the Royal Society of Medicine* 11 (1918): 31–39.

40. D. W. Tschanz, "Typhus Fever on the Eastern Front in World War I," accessed January 18, 2016, http://www.montana.edu/historybug/wwi-tef.html.

41. R. L. Atenstaedt, "Trench Fever: The British Medical Response in the Great War," *Journal of the Royal Society of Medicine* 99, no. 11 (2006): 564–568.

42. Dominic Lieven, *The End of Tsarist Russia: The March to World War I and Revolution* (New York: Viking, 2015).

43. Ibid.

44. Ibid.

45. Michael Kort, *The Soviet Colossus: History and Aftermath* (Abingdon, UK: Routledge, 1990), 131.

46. K. David Patterson, "Typhus and Its Control in Russia, 1870–1940," *Medical History* 37 (1993): 361–381.

47. Ibid.

48. C. Nicolle, C. Comte, and L. Conseil, "Transmission expérimentale du typhus exanthématique par le pou du corps," *Comptes Rendus Hebdomadaires des Séances de l'Académie des Sciences* 149 (1909): 486–489.

49. Arthur Allen, *The Fantastic Laboratory of Dr. Weigl: How Two Brave Scientists Battled Typhus and Sabotaged the Nazis* (New York: W. W. Norton, 2015).

50. J. Rutten, *La Mortalite des missionnaires avant et apres l'emploi du vaccine de Weigl. Dossiers de la commission synodale* (Beijing: Peking, 1936), 183–191.

51. Allen, *Fantastic Laboratory*.

52. Ibid.

53. "Jewish Mortality Mounts in Warsaw Ghetto as Nazis Refuse to Check Typhus There," *Jewish Telegraphic Agency*, January 22, 1942.

54. Irma Sonnenberg Menkel, "I Saw Anne Frank Die," *Newsweek*, July 21, 1997.

55. Naomi Baumslag, *Murderous Medicine: Nazi Doctors, Human Experimentation, and Typhus* (Santa Barbara, CA: Praeger, 2005), 117–118.

56. G. G. Otto, *Der Jude als Weltparasit* (Munich, DE: Eher Verlag, 1943), accessed from http://research.calvin.edu/german-propaganda-archive/weltparasit.htm.

57. Paul Weindling, *Epidemics and Genocide in Eastern Europe, 1890–1945* (Oxford: Oxford University Press, 2000), 296.

Chapter 7

1. W. Parkinson, *This Gilded African: Toussaint L'Ouverture* (London: Quartet Books, 1978).

2. "Angola Grapples with Worst Yellow Fever Outbreak in 30 Years," accessed April 1, 2016, http://www.who.int/features/2016/angola-worst-yellow-fever/en/.

3. J. E. Bryant, E. C. Holmes, and A. T. Barrett, "Out of Africa: A Molecular Perspective on the Introduction of Yellow Fever Virus into the Americas," *PLOS Pathogens* 3, no. 5 (2007): 668–673.

4. Leonard Rogers, *Fevers in the Tropics, Their Clinical and Microscopical Differentiation Including the Milroy Lecture* (Charleston, SC: BiblioLife, 2009), 266.

5. H. R. Carter, *Yellow Fever: An Epidemiological and Historical Study of Its Place of Origin* (Baltimore, MD: Williams and Wilkins, 1931).

6. Charles Creighton, *A History of Epidemics in Britain from A.D. 864 to the Extinction of Plague*, vol. 1 (Cambridge, UK: Cambridge University Press, 1891), 621.

7. Pedro Nogueira, "The Early History of Yellow Fever," accessed April 10, 2016, http://jdc.jefferson.edu/yellow_fever_symposium/10.

8. Mulford Stough, "The Yellow Fever in Philadelphia 1793," *Pennsylvania History: A Journal of Mid-Atlantic Studies* 6, no. 1 (1939): 6–13.

9. Benjamin Rush, *An Account of the Bilious Remitting Yellow Fever, as It Appeared in the City of Philadelphia, in the Year 1793* (Charleston, SC: Nabu Press, 2011).

10. "To James Madison from Thomas Jefferson, 1 September 1793," accessed April 20, 2016, https://founders.archives.gov/documents/Madison/01-15-02-0063.

11. Gary Nash, *Forging Freedom: The Formation of Philadelphia's Free Black Community 1760–1820* (Cambridge, MA: Harvard University Press, 1988).

12. "Benjamin Rush to Richard Allen, Mss. Correspondence of Dr. Benjamin Rush, Yellow Fever," pt. IV, 38 (1793).

13. Ibid.

14. Absalom Jones, Richard Allen, and Matthew Clarkson, *A Narrative of the Proceedings of the Black People, During the Late Awful Calamity in Philadelphia, in the Year 1793: and a Refutation of Some Censures, Thrown upon Them in Some Late Publications* (1794; repr., Philadelphia, PA: Rhistoric, 1969).

15. "Benjamin Rush (Philadelphia) Letter to Julia Stockton Rush, 1793 September 18," accessed June 24, 2016, https://repository.duke.edu/dc/rushbenjaminandjulia/brpst016018.

16. "Benjamin Rush to Richard Allen."

17. Mathew Carey, *A Short Account of the Malignant Fever Which Prevailed in Philadelphia, 1793* (Philadelphia, 1793), 13–28, 65–68, 83–92.

18. Jones et al., *Narrative*.

19. Ibid.

20. Benjamin Henry Latrobe, *Journal of Latrobe: The Notes and Sketches of an Architect, Naturalist and Traveler in the United States from 1796 to 1820* (Carlisle, MA: Applewood Books, 2007), 97.

21. Jim Byrne, "The Philadelphia Lazaretto: A Most Unloved Institution," accessed April 27, 2016, http://pabook2.libraries.psu.edu/palitmap/Lazaretto.html.

22. Bill Marshall, *France and the Americas: Culture, Politics, and History* (Santa Barbara, CA: ABC-CLIO, 2005), 17–26.

23. Fred Anderson, *The War That Made America: A Short History of the French and Indian War* (New York: Viking, 2005).

24. Clarence Munford and Michael Zeuske, "Black Slavery, Class Struggle, Fear and Revolution in St. Domingue and Cuba, 1785–1795," *Journal of Negro History* 73, no. 1/4 (1988): 12–32.

25. Philip Curtin, "The Declaration of the Rights of Man in Saint-Domingue, 1788–1791," *Hispanic American Historical Review* 30, no. 2 (1950): 157–175.

26. "Declaration of the Rights of Man—1789," accessed May 1, 2016, http://avalon.law.yale.edu/18th_century/rightsof.asp.

27. C. L. R. James, *The Black Jacobins: Toussaint L'Ouverture and the San Domingo Revolution* (London: PenguinVintage, 1989).

28. Junius Rodriguez, *Encyclopedia of Emancipation and Abolition in the Transatlantic World* (Abingdon, UK: Routledge, 2007), 283; D. Geggus, "Yellow Fever in the 1790s: The British Army in Occupied Saint Domingue," *Medical History* 23 (1979): 38–58.

29. Geggus, "Yellow Fever"; J. R. McNeill, *Mosquito Empires: Ecology and War in the Greater Caribbean, 1620–1914* (Cambridge, UK: Cambridge University Press, 2010).

30. McNeill, *Mosquito Empires*.

31. H. Meziere, *Le General Leclerc et l'expedition de Saint-Domingue* (Paris: Bibliotheque Napoleonienne Tallandier, 1990).

32. John Marr and John Cathey, "The 1802 Saint-Domingue Yellow Fever Epidemic and the Louisiana Purchase," *Journal of Public Health Management Practice* 19, no. 1 (2013): 77–82.

33. John Miller and Mark Molesky, *Our Oldest Enemy: A History of America's Disastrous Relationship with France* (New York: Doubleday, 2004), 104.

34. Lester King, "Sword of Pestilence: The New Orleans Yellow Fever Epidemic of 1853," *Journal of the American Medical Association* 197, no. 6 (1966): 517–518.

35. Molly Crosby, *The American Plague: The Untold Story of Yellow Fever, the Epidemic That Shaped Our History* (New York: Berkley Books, 2007).

36. Glenn Robins, *The Bishop of the Old South: The Ministry and Civil War Legacy of Leonidas Polk* (Macon, GA: Mercer University Press, 2006), 63.

37. Mariola Espinosa, "The Question of Racial Immunity to Yellow Fever in History and Historiography," *Social Science History* 38 (2014): 437–453.

38. Crosby, *American Plague*.

39. Ibid.

40. Jerrold Michael, "The National Board of Health: 1879–1883," *Public Health Reports* 126, no. 1 (2011): 123–129.

41. *Congressional Record: Proceedings and Debates of the 45th Congress* (Washington, DC: U.S. Government Printing Office, 1879), 2264.

42. *Transactions of the Medical Association of the State of Alabama: The Report of the State Board of Health* (Mobile, AL: Journal of the Medical Association of the State of Alabama, 1879), 65.

43. Michael, "National Board of Health."

44. Cassandra Copeland, Curtis Jolly, and Henry Thompson, "The History and Potential of Trade between Cuba and the US," *Journal of Business and Economics* 2, no. 3 (2011): 163–174.

45. Louis Perez, *The War of 1898: The United States and Cuba in History and Historiography* (Chapel Hill: University of North Carolina Press, 1998).

46. John Stevens, *Sensationalism and the New York Press* (New York: Columbia University Press, 1991), 91–102.

47. Michael Richman, "A 'Splendid Little War' Built America's Empire," *Washington Post*, April 8, 1998.

48. Annie Riley Hale, *Excerpts from Rooseveltian Fact and Fable* (New York: Broadway Publishing, 1908).

49. A. Agramonte, "A Review of Research in Yellow Fever," *Annals of Internal Medicine* 2 (1928–1929): 138–154.

50. Enrique Chaves-Carballo, "Carlos Finlay and Yellow Fever: Triumph Over Adversity," *Military Medicine* 170, no. 10 (2005): 881.

51. C. E. Finlay, *Carlos Finlay and Yellow Fever* (New York: Oxford University Press, 1940).

52. Chaves-Carballo, "Carlos Finlay."

53. Howard Atwood Kelly, *Walter Reed and Yellow Fever* (Baltimore, MD: Medical Standard Book Co., 1906).

54. James Carroll, "A Brief Review of the Etiology of Yellow Fever," *New York Medical Journal* 79 (1904): 211–245.

55. Ibid.

56. Ibid.

57. Laura Cutter, "Walter Reed, Yellow Fever, and Informed Consent," *Military Medicine* 181, no. 1 (2016): 90–91.

58. Walter Reed, James Carroll, and Aristides Agramonte, "The Etiology of Yellow Fever: An Additional Note," *Journal of the American Medical Association* 36 (1901): 431–440.

59. Max Theiler, "Susceptibility of White Mice to the Virus of Yellow Fever," *Science* 71 (1930): 367.

60. M. Theiler and L. Whitman, "The Danger with Vaccination with Neurotropic Yellow Fever Virus Alone," *Bulletin Mensuel de l'Office International d'hygiene Publique* 27 (1935): 1342–1347.

61. M. Theiler and L. Whitman, "Quantitative Studies of the Virus and Immune Serum Used in Vaccination against Yellow Fever," *American Journal of Tropical Medicine* 15 (1935): 347–356.

62. W. A. Sawyer et al., "Jaundice in Army Personnel in the Western Region of the United States and Its Relation to Vaccination against Yellow Fever," *American Journal of Hygiene* 39 (1944): 337–430.

63. M. Theiler and H. H. Smith, "The Use of Yellow Fever Modified by *In Vitro* Cultivation for Human Immunization," *Journal of Experimental Medicine* 65 (1937): 787–800.

64. Erling Norrby, "Yellow Fever and Max Theiler: The Only Nobel Prize for a Virus Vaccine," *Journal of Experimental Medicine* 204, no. 12 (2007): 2779–2784.

Chapter 8

1. George Wood, *A Treatise on the Practice of Medicine*, vol. 1 (Philadelphia, PA: J.B. Lippincott, 1858), 715.

2. A. A. Kousoulis, "Etymology of Cholera," *Emerging Infectious Diseases* 18, no. 3 (2012): 540.

3. R. Pollitzer, "Cholera Studies," *Bulletin of the World Health Organization* 10 (1954): 421–461.

4. R. S. Bray, *Armies of Pestilence: The Impact of Disease on History* (Cambridge, UK: James Clarke, 1996), 159.

5. C. Macnamara, *A History of Asiatic Cholera* (London: Macmillan, 1876).

6. Pollitzer, "Cholera Studies."

7. J. N. Hays, *Epidemics and Pandemics: Their Impacts on Human History* (Santa Barbara, CA: ABC-CLIO, 2005), 211–225.

8. John Noble Wilford, "How Epidemics Helped Shape the Modern Metropolis," *New York Times*, April 15, 2008.

9. Yury Bosin, "Russia, Cholera Riots of 1830–1831," in *International Encyclopedia of Revolution and Protest*, ed. Immanuel Ness (Hoboken, NJ: Blackwell, 2009), 2877–2878.

10. Wilford, "How Epidemics Helped Shape."

11. John Pintard, *Letters from John Pintard to His Daughter, Eliza Noel Pintard Davidson, 1816–1833*, vol. 4 (New York: New York Historical Society, 1941).

12. R. E. McGrew, *Russia and the Cholera: 1823–1832* (Madison: University of Wisconsin Press, 1965).

13. Aleksandr Nikitenko, *The Diary of a Russian Censor*, ed. and trans. Helen Jacobson (Amherst: University of Massachusetts Press, 1975), 34–35.

14. Ibid.

15. *Liverpool Mercury*, October 13, 1826.

16. *Liverpool Mercury*, October 26, 1827.

17. B. Bailey, *Burke and Hare: The Year of the Ghouls* (Edinburgh, UK: Mainstream, 2002).

18. Lisa Rosner, *Being the True and Spectacular History of Edinburgh's Notorious Burke and Hare and of the Man of Science Who Abetted Them in the Commission of Their Most Heinous Crimes* (Philadelphia: University of Pennsylvania Press, 2010), 74.

19. A. W. Bates, *The Anatomy of Robert Knox: Murder, Mad Science, and Medical Regulation* (Sussex, UK: Sussex Academic Press, 2010).

20. Geoffrey Gill, Sean Burrell, and Jody Brown, "Fear and Frustration: The Liverpool Cholera Riots of 1832," *Lancet* 358, no. 9277 (2001): 233–237.

21. Ibid.

22. Ibid.

23. Ibid.

24. Dean Kirby, *Angel Meadow: Victorian Britain's Most Savage Slum* (Barnsley, UK: Pen and Sword, 2016), 37–38.

25. Theodore Friedgut, "Labor Violence and Regime Brutality in Tsarist Russia: The Iuzovka Cholera Riots of 1892," *Slavic Review* 46, no. 2 (1987): 245–265.

26. James Harvey Robinson, *Readings in European History: From the Opening of the Protestant Revolt to the Present Day* (Charleston, SC: Nabu Press, 2010), 333–334.

27. Anthony Wild, *The East India Company: Trade and Conquest from 1600* (New York: HarperCollins, 2000).

28. Ibid.

29. "Kumbh Mela 2013," accessed July 1, 2016, http://kumbhmelaallahabad .gov.in/english/index.html.

30. Ibid.

31. Norman Howard-Jones, *The Scientific Background of the International Sanitary Conferences 1851–1938* (Geneva. CH: World Health Organization, 1975).

32. Samuel Abbot, trans., *Report to the International Sanitary Conference of a Commission from That Body, to Which Were Referred the Questions Relative to the Origin, Endemicity, Transmissibility and Propagation of Asiatic Cholera* (Boston, MA: International Sanitary Conference, 1867).

33. Ibid.

34. David Arnold, "Cholera and Colonialism in British India," *Past and Present* 113 (1986): 118–151.

35. Ibid.

36. C. Macnamara, *A History of Asiatic Cholera* (London: Macmillan, 1876), 91–92.

37. David Long, *The Hajj Today: A Survey of the Contemporary Pilgrimage to Makkah* (Albany: State University of New York Press, 1979), 69–73.

38. Achille Proust, *Essai sur l'hygiéne, avec une carte indiquant la marche des épidémies de choléra par les routes de terre et la voie maritime* (Paris: G. Masson, 1873).

39. Howard-Jones, *Scientific Background*.

40. Ibid.

41. Valeska Huber, "The Unification of the Globe by Disease? The International Sanitary Conferences on Cholera, 1851–1894," *Historical Journal* 49, no. 2 (2006): 453–476.

42. M. French Sheldon, *Sultan to Sultan: Adventures Among the Masai and Other Tribes of East Africa* (Norman, OK: Saxon, 1892), 29.

43. "BMJ Readers Choose the 'Sanitary Revolution' as Greatest Medical Advance Since 1840," *British Medical Journal* 334 (2007): 111.

44. Friedrich Engels, *The Condition of the Working Class in England in 1844* (Oxford: Oxford University Press, 2009).

45. *London Gazette*, October 21, 1831.

46. A. Susan Williams, *The Rich Man and the Diseased Poor in Early Victorian Literature* (London: Macmillan, 1987), 9.

47. Michael Brown, "From Foetid Air to Filth: The Cultural Transformation of British Epidemiological Thought, ca. 1780–1848," *Bulletin of the History of Medicine* 82 (2008): 515–544.

48. Southwood Smith, "Contagion and Sanitary Laws," *Westminster Review* 3 (1825): 142.

49. Ibid., 522.

50. Brown, "Foetid Air to Filth."

51. Edwin Chadwick, *Report on the Sanitary Condition of the Labouring Population and on the Means of Its Improvement* (London, 1842).

52. Elizabeth Fee and Theodore Brown, "The Public Health Act of 1848," *Bulletin of the World Health Organization* 83, no. 11 (2005): 866–867.

53. K. Calman, "The 1848 Public Health Act and Its Relevance to Improving Public Health in England Now," *British Medical Journal* 317, no. 7158 (1998): 596–598.

54. Christopher Hamlin and Sally Sheard, "Revolutions in Public Health: 1848, and 1998?," *British Medical Journal* 317, no. 7158 (1998): 587–591.

55. Ibid.

56. Stephen Halliday, *The Great Stink of London: Sir Joseph Bazalgette and the Cleansing of the Victorian Metropolis* (Stroud, UK: The History Press, 2001).

57. N. Howard-Jones, "Cholera Treatment in the Nineteenth Century," *Journal of the History of Medicine* 27 (1982): 373–395.

58. W. B. O'Shaughnessy, "Experiments on Blood in Cholera," *Lancet* 17, no. 435 (1831): 490.

59. W. B. O'Shaughnessy, *Report on the Chemical Pathology of the Malignant Cholera* (London: Highley, 1832).

60. Ibid.

61. T. Latta, "Malignant Cholera. Documents Communicated by the Central Board of Health, London, Relative to the Treatment of Cholera by the Copious Injection of Aqueous and Saline Fluids into the Veins," *Lancet* 18, no. 457 (1832): 274–280.

62. B. A. Foëx, "How the Cholera Epidemic of 1831 Resulted in a New Technique for Fluid Resuscitation," *Emergency Medicine Journal* 20 (2003): 316–318.

63. *Lancet* 18, no. 457 (1832): 284.

64. Michael Ramsay, "John Snow, MD: Anaesthetist to the Queen of England and Pioneer Epidemiologist," *Baylor University Medical Center Proceedings* 19 (2006): 24–28.

65. Ibid.

66. John Snow, *On the Mode of Communication of Cholera* (London: Churchill, 1849): 6–9.

67. John Snow, "The Cholera Near Golden-Square, and at Deptford," *Medical Times and Gazette* 209 (1854): 321–322.

68. Ibid.

69. Edwin Lankester, *Cholera: What Is It? And How to Prevent It* (Abingdon, UK: Gary Routledge and Sons, 1866), 34–35.

70. John Snow, *On the Mode of Communication of Cholera*, 2nd ed. (London: Churchill, 1855).

71. Ibid.

72. John Eyler, "The Changing Assessments of John Snow's and William Farr's Cholera Studies," *Sozial- und Präventivmedizin* 46 (2001): 225–232.

73. Ibid.

74. James Wakley, ed., "Dr. Farr's Cholera Report," *Lancet* 92, no. 2346 (1868): 223.

75. D. Lippi and E. Gotuzzo, "The Greatest Steps towards the Discovery of *Vibrio cholera*," *Clinical Microbiology and Infection* 20, no. 3 (2014): 191–195.

76. Filippo Pacini, "Osservazioni microscopiche e deduzioni patologiche sul cholera asiatico," *Gazzetta Medica Italiana Toscana* 6 (1854): 397–405.

77. Ibid.

78. Robert Koch, "Fünfter Bericht der Leiters der deutschen wissenshaftlichen Commission zur Erforschung der Cholera," *Deutsche Medizinische Wochenschrift* 10 (1884): 111–112.

79. "Drinking-Water," accessed August 1, 2016, http://www.who.int/mediacentre /factsheets/fs391/en/.

80. "International Notes Cholera—Peru, 1991," *MMWR Weekly* 40, no. 6 (1991): 108–110.

81. "Cholera Outbreak among Rwandan Refugees—Democratic Republic of Congo, April 1997," *MMWR Weekly* 47, no. 19 (1997): 389–391.

82. Guy Dinmore, "Rwandans Flee Big Rebel Push," *Reuters World Service*, July 11, 1994.

83. "Cholera Outbreak."

84. I. Chirisa et al., "The 2008/2009 Cholera Outbreak in Harare, Zimbabwe: Case of Failure in Urban Environmental Health and Planning," *Review of Environmental Health* 30, no. 2 (2015): 117–124.

85. Renaud Piarroux et al., "Understanding the Cholera Epidemic, Haiti," *Emerging Infectious Diseases* 17, no. 7 (2011): 1161–1168.

86. Ibid.

87. Jonathan Katzaug, "U.N. Admits Role in Cholera Epidemic in Haiti," *New York Times*, August 17, 2016.

Chapter 9

1. S. L. Knobler et al., eds., *The Threat of Pandemic Influenza: Are We Ready?* (Washington, DC: National Academies Press, 2005).

2. Sandra Opdycke, *The Flu Epidemic of 1918: America's Experience in the Global Health Crisis (Critical Moments in American History)* (Abingdon, UK: Routledge, 2014), 168.

3. T. M. Tumpey et al., "Characterization of the Reconstructed 1918 Spanish Influenza Pandemic Virus," *Science* 310 (2005): 77–80.

4. Bogumiła Kempińska-Mirosławska and Agnieszka Woźniak-Kosek, "The Influenza Epidemic of 1889–90 in Selected European Cities—A Picture Based on the Reports of Two Poznań Daily Newspapers from the Second Half of the Nineteenth Century," *Medical Science Monitor* 19 (2013): 1131–1141.

5. Ibid.

6. Claire Jackson, "History Lessons: The Asian Flu Pandemic," *British Journal of General Practice* 59, no. 565 (2009): 622–623.

7. J. Corbett McDonald, "Between Ourselves," *RCGP Archives* ACE G3–4 (December 1957).

8. Nancy Tomes, "'Destroyer and Teacher': Managing the Masses during the 1918–1919 Influenza Pandemic," *Public Health Reports* suppl. 3, no. 125 (2010): 48–62.

9. Ibid.

10. "Epidemic Lessons against Next Time," *New York Times*, November 17, 1918.

11. Tomes, "'Destroyer and Teacher.'"

12. R. J. Hatchett, C. E. Mecher, and M. Lipsitch, "Public Health Interventions and Epidemic Intensity during the 1918 Influenza Pandemic," *Proceedings of the National Academy of Sciences USA* 104, no. 18 (2007): 7582–7587; M. C. J. Bootsma and N. M. Ferguson, "The Effect of Public Health Measures on the 1918 Influenza Epidemic in U.S. Cities," *Proceedings of the National Academy of Sciences USA* 104, no. 18 (2007): 7588–7593.

13. "Influenza Spread Causes Mayor to Declare City in Quarantine," *Charlotte Observer*, October 5, 1918, 7.

14. R. D. Fleischmann et al., "Whole-Genome Random Sequencing and Assembly of *Haemophilus influenzae* Rd," *Science* 269, no. 5223 (1995): 496–512.

15. J. K. Taubenberger et al., "Initial Genetic Characterization of the 1918 'Spanish' Influenza Virus," *Science* 275, no. 5307 (1997): 1793–1796.

16. J. K. Taubenberger et al., "Characterization of the 1918 Influenza Virus Polymerase Genes," *Nature* 437 (2005): 889–893.

17. Tumpey et al., "Characterization."

18. J. van Aken, "Is It Wise to Resurrect a Deadly Virus?," *Heredity* 98 (2007): 1–2.

19. "Reviving the Virus," accessed August 20, 2016, http://www.pbs.org/wgbh/nova/sciencenow/3318/02-poll-nf.html.

20. R. Pfeiffer, "Aus dem Institut für Infektionskrankheiten. II. Vorläufige Mittheilungen über die Erreger der Influenza" [From the Institute for Infectious Diseases. II. Provisional communication on the cause of influenza], *Deutsche medicinische Wochenschrift* 18 (1892): 28; P. Olitsky and F. Gates, "Experimental Study of the Nasopharyngeal Secretions from Influenza Patients," *Journal of the American Medical Association* 74 (1920): 1497–1499.

21. W. Smith, C. H. Andrewes, and P. P. Laidlaw, "A Virus Obtained from Influenza Patients," *Lancet* 222, no. 5732 (1933): 66–68.

22. A. A. Smorodintsev et al., "Investigation on Volunteers Infected with the Influenza Virus," *American Journal of Medical Science* 194 (1937): 59–70.

23. Thomas Francis Jr., "Vaccination against Influenza," *Bulletin of the World Health Organization* 8, no. 5–6 (1953): 725–741.

24. Ibid.

25. Thomas Francis Jr., "A New Type of Virus from Epidemic Influenza," *Science* 92 (1940): 405–408.

26. Francis, "Vaccination."

27. C. Hannoun, "The Evolving History of Influenza Viruses and Influenza Vaccines," *Expert Review of Vaccines* 12, no. 9 (2013): 1085–1094.

28. "Into the History of Influenza Control . . . ," accessed August 25, 2016, http://www.who.int/influenza/gip-anniversary/en/.

29. Christopher Ambrose and Myron Levin, "The Rationale for Quadrivalent Influenza Vaccines," *Human Vaccines and Immunotherapeutics* 8, no. 1 (2012): 81–88.

Chapter 10

1. Nina Seavey, Paul Wagner, and Jane Smith, *A Paralyzing Fear: The Triumph Over Polio in America* (New York: TV Books, 1998), 19.

2. Michael Underwood, *A Treatise on the Diseases of Children, with General Directions for the Management of Infants from Birth* (London: Printed for J. Mathews, 1789).

3. J. Heine, *Beobachtungen über Lähmungszustände der untern Extremitäten und deren Behandlung* (Stuttgart: Franz Heinrich Köhler, 1840).

4. B. Trevelyan, M. Smallman-Raynor, and A. D. Cliff, "The Spatial Dynamics of Poliomyelitis in the United States: From Epidemic Emergence to Vaccine-Induced Retreat, 1910–1971," *Annals of the Association of American Geographers* 95, no. 2 (2005): 269–293.

5. Richard Rhodes, *A Hole in the World* (Lawrence: University of Kansas Press, 1990), 37.

6. Judith Beatty, "My Polio Story Is an Inconvenient Truth to Those Who Refuse Vaccines," *Huffington Post*, August 15, 2016.

7. A. Yelnik and I. Laffont, "The Psychological Aspects of Polio Survivors through Their Life Experience," *Annals of Physical and Rehabilitation Medicine* 53, no. 1 (2010): 60–67.

8. Neal Nathanson and Olen Kew, "From Emergence to Eradication: The Epidemiology of Poliomyelitis Deconstructed," *American Journal of Epidemiology* 172 (2010): 1213–1229.

9. Ibid.

10. M. Martinez-Bakker, A. A. King, and P. Rohani, "Unraveling the Transmission Ecology of Polio," *PLOS Biology* 13, no. 6 (2015): 1–21.

11. Phillip Drinker and Charles F. McKhann III, "The Use of a New Apparatus for the Prolonged Administration of Artificial Respiration: I. A Fatal Case of Poliomyelitis," *Journal of the American Medical Association* 92, no. 20 (1929): 1658–1660.

12. Ibid.

13. G. S. Bause, "Emerson Respirator or 'Iron Lung,'" *Anesthesiology* 110, no. 4 (2009): 812.

14. Larry Alexander, "Iron Lung and Other Equipment," accessed September 15, 2016, http://amhistory.si.edu/polio/howpolio/ironlung.htm.

15. Fiona Kelly et al., "Intensive Care Medicine Is 60 Years Old: The History and Future of the Intensive Care Unit," *Clinical Medicine* 14, no. 4 (2014): 376–379.

16. Robert Lindsey, "Francis Ford Coppola: Promises to Keep," *New York Times*, July 24, 1988.

17. "Our History," accessed October 1, 2016, http://www.mars.com/global/about -us/history.

18. "Candyland," accessed October 2, 2016, https://www.hasbro.com/common /instruct/Candy_Land_50th_Anniversary_Edition.PDF.

19. Naomi Rogers, *Polio Wars: Sister Kenny and the Golden Age of American Medicine* (Oxford: Oxford University Press, 2013).

20. Elizabeth Kenny and Martha Ostenso, *And They Shall Walk: The Life Story of Sister Elizabeth Kenny* (New York: Dodd, Mead, 1943).

21. Wallace Cole and Miland Knapp, "The Kenny Treatment of Infantile Paralysis: A Preliminary Report," *Journal of the American Medical Association* 116, no. 23 (1941): 2577–2580.

22. J. F. Pohl and E. Kenny, *The Kenny Concept of Infantile Paralysis and Its Treatment* (Minneapolis, MN: Bruce Publishing, 1943).

23. James Tobin, *The Man He Became: How FDR Defied Polio to Win the Presidency* (New York: Simon and Schuster, 2013).

24. Ibid.

25. Ibid.

26. "Birthday Balls: Franklin D. Roosevelt and the March of Dimes," accessed October 15, 2016, http://docs.fdrlibrary.marist.edu/bdtext.html.

27. Franklin D. Roosevelt, "Radio Address on the President's First Birthday Ball for Crippled Children," January 30, 1934, accessed from http://www.presi dency.ucsb.edu/ws/?pid=14728.

28. "Birthday Balls."

29. Ibid.

30. Franklin D. Roosevelt, "Radio Address for the Fifth Birthday Ball for Crippled Children," January 29, 1938, accessed from http://www.presidency.ucsb .edu/ws/?pid=15584.

31. "A History of the March of Dimes," accessed November 1, 2016, http:// www.marchofdimes.org/mission/a-history-of-the-march-of-dimes.aspx.

32. William Barrett, "The Largest U.S. Charities for 2016," *Forbes*, December 14, 2016.

33. Mark O'Brien and Gillian Kendall, *How I Became a Human Being: A Disabled Man's Quest for Independence* (Madison: University of Wisconsin Press, 2003), 3.

34. "Section 504, Rehabilitation Act of 1973," accessed December 16, 2016, https://www.dol.gov/oasam/regs/statutes/sec504.htm.

35. Maria Fleming, ed., *A Place at the Table: Struggles for Equality in America* (Oxford: Oxford University Press, 2001), 114.

36. "Remarks of President George Bush at the Signing of the Americans with Disabilities Act," accessed December 20, 2016, https://www.eeoc.gov/eeoc /history/35th/videos/ada_signing_text.html.

37. Sydney Halpern and Lesser Harms, *The Morality of Risk in Medical Research* (Chicago, IL: University of Chicago Press, 2004), 48–72.

38. Ibid.

39. Susan Lederer, *Subjected to Science: Human Experimentation in America Before the Second World War* (Baltimore, MD: Johns Hopkins University Press, 1995), 108–109.

40. A. Sabin and P. Olitsky, "Cultivation of Poliomyelitis Virus *in vitro* in Human Embryonic Nervous Tissue," *Proceedings of the Society for Experimental Biology and Medicine* 34 (1936): 357–359.

41. J. F. Enders, T. H. Weller, and F. C. Robbins, "Cultivation of the Lansing Strain of Poliomyelitis Virus in Cultures of Various Human Embryonic Tissues," *Science* 109 (1949): 85–87.

42. J. E. Juskewitch, C. J. Tapia, and A. J. Windebank, "Lessons from the Salk Polio Vaccine: Methods for and Risks of Rapid Translation," *Clinical and Translational Science* 3, no. 4 (2010): 182–185.

43. J. E. Salk, "Studies in Human Subjects on Active Immunization against Poliomyelitis. I. A Preliminary Report of Experiments in Progress," *Journal of the American Medical Association* 151 (1953): 1081–1098.

44. J. S. Smith, *Patenting the Sun: Polio and the Salk Vaccine* (New York: William Morrow, 1990).

45. Ibid.

46. Ibid.

47. Juskewitch et al., "Lessons."

48. C. Carroll-Pankhurst et al., "Thirty-five Year Mortality Following Receipt of SV40-Contaminated Polio Vaccine during the Neonatal Period," *British Journal of Cancer* 85, no. 9 (2001): 1295–1297.

49. Ibid.

50. Marguerite Rose Jiménez, "Biographical Memoirs: Albert Sabin 1906–1993," National Academy of Sciences, 2014, accessed from http://www.nasonline.org/publications/biographical-memoirs/memoir-pdfs/sabin-albert.pdf.

51. A. Sabin and R. Ward, "The Natural History of Human Poliomyelitis: I. Distribution of Virus in Nervous and Non-Nervous Tissues," *Journal of Experimental Medicine* 73, no. 6 (1941): 771–793.

52. Jiménez, "Biographical Memoirs."

53. Dorothy Horstmann, "The Sabin Live Poliovirus Vaccination Trials in the USSR, 1959," *Yale Journal of Biology and Medicine* 64 (1991): 499–512.

54. Ibid.

55. Ibid.

56. Ibid.

57. "Polio Eradication," accessed December 30, 2016, http://polioeradication.org/.

Chapter 11

1. Mary Fisher, "A Whisper of AIDS: Address to the Republican National Convention," August 19, 1992, accessed from http://gos.sbc.edu/f/fisher.html.

2. "Pneumocystis Pneumonia—Los Angeles," *MMWR Weekly Report* 30 (1981): 250–252.

3. M. W. Ross, E. J. Essien, and I. Torres, "Conspiracy Beliefs About the Origin of HIV/AIDS in Four Racial/Ethnic Groups," *Journal of Acquired Immune Deficiency Syndromes* 41, no. 3 (2006): 342–344.

4. Thomas Boghardt, "Operation INFEKTION: Soviet Bloc Intelligence and Its AIDS Disinformation Campaign," *Studies in Intelligence* 53, no. 4 (2009): 1–24.

5. Ibid.

6. Alan Cantwell, *AIDS and the Doctors of Death: An Inquiry into the Origin of the AIDS Epidemic* (Los Angeles, CA: Aries Rising Press, 1988).

7. Wolf Szmuness et al., "Hepatitis B Vaccine—Demonstration of Efficacy in a Controlled Clinical Trial in a High-Risk Population in the United States," *New England Journal of Medicine* 303 (1980): 833–841.

8. Ross et al., "Conspiracy Beliefs."

9. M. Worobey et al., "Origin of AIDS: Contaminated Polio Vaccine Theory Refuted," *Nature* 428, no. 6985 (2004): 820.

10. Tuofu Zhu et al., "An African HIV-1 Sequence from 1959 and Implications for the Origin of the Epidemic," *Nature* 391, no. 6667 (1998): 594–597.

11. Paul Sharp and Beatrice Hahn, "Origins of HIV and the AIDS Pandemic," *Cold Spring Harbor Perspectives in Medicine* 1, no. 1 (2011): 1–22.

12. Craig Timberg and Daniel Halperin, *Tinderbox: How the West Sparked the AIDS Epidemic and How the World Can Finally Overcome It* (London: Penguin Press, 2012).

13. Ibid.

14. Paul Volberding, ed., *Global HIV/AIDS Medicine* (Amsterdam: Elsevier, 2008), 758–759.

15. M. Thomas Gilbert et al., "The Emergence of HIV/AIDS in the Americas and Beyond," *Proceedings of the National Academy of Sciences USA* 104, no. 4 (2007): 18566–18570.

16. Ibid.

17. "Current Trends Prevention of Acquired Immune Deficiency Syndrome (AIDS): Report of Inter-Agency Recommendations," *MMWR Weekly Report* 32, no. 8 (1983): 101–103.

18. Paul Farmer, *AIDS and Accusation: Haiti and the Geography of Blame* (Berkeley: University of California Press, 1990).

19. Marlise Simons, "For Haiti's Tourism, the Stigma of AIDS Is Fatal," *New York Times*, November 29, 1983.

20. Bruce Lambert, "Now, No Haitians Can Donate Blood," *New York Times*, March 14, 1990.

21. Nicole Bitette and Corky Siemaszko, "New York Attorney General Probes Help Wanted Ad That States 'No Haitians' Need Apply," *New York Daily News*, October 19, 2015.

22. G. M. Herek and E. K. Glunt, "An Epidemic of Stigma: Public Reactions to AIDS," *American Psychologist* 43, no. 11 (1988): 886–891.

23. Sergio Rueda et al., "Examining the Associations between HIV-Related Stigma and Health Outcomes in People Living with HIV/AIDS: A Series of Meta-Analyses," *British Medical Journal Open* 6, no. 7 (2016): 1–15.

24. L. Li et al., "Impacts of HIV/AIDS Stigma on Family Identity and Interactions in China," *Families, Systems, and Health* 26, no. 4 (2008): 431–442.

25. Deepa Rao et al., "Stigma in the Workplace: Employer Attitudes About People with HIV in Beijing, Hong Kong, and Chicago," *Social Science and Medicine* 67, no. 10 (2008): 1541–1549.

26. G. Green and S. Platt, "Fear and Loathing in Health Care Settings Reported by People with HIV," *Sociology of Health and Illness* 19, no. 1 (1997): 70–92.

27. "HIV/AIDS: Discrimination Reported in Health Care in 60% of European Countries," accessed March 5, 2017, http://www.unric.org/en/latest-un-buzz /30493-hivaids-discrimination-reported-in-health-care-in-60-of-european -countries.

28. "Global Report: UNAIDS Report on the Global AIDS Epidemic 2013," accessed March 10, 2017, http://www.unaids.org/sites/default/files/media_asset /UNAIDS_Global_Report_2013_en_1.pdf.

29. Richard Lawson, "Fatal Inaction: The Reagan Administration's Unearthed Response to the AIDS Crisis Is Chilling," *Vanity Fair*, December 1, 2015.

30. Ibid.

31. Allen White, "Reagan's AIDS Legacy/Silence Equals Death," *SF Gate*, June 8, 2004.

32. UNAIDS, *Criminalisation of HIV Non-Disclosure, Exposure and Transmission: Background and Current Landscape* (Geneva, CH: UNAIDS, September 2011).

33. Ibid.

34. G. L. Higgins, "History of Confidentiality in Medicine: The Physician-Patient Relationship," *Canadian Family Physician* 35 (1989): 921–926.

35. Ryan White and Ann Marie Cunningham, *Ryan White: My Own Story* (London: Penguin Books, 1992).

36. Michael Specter, "AIDS Victim's Right to Attend Public School Tested in Corn Belt," *Washington Post*, September 3, 1985.

37. "Family in AIDS Case Quits Florida Town After House Burns," *New York Times*, August 30, 1987.

38. "Building Trust: Confidentiality and the Ryan White HIV/AIDS Program," accessed March 15, 2017, https://hab.hrsa.gov/livinghistory/issues/Confidential ity.pdf.

39. "Ryan White HIV/AIDS Program Legislation," accessed March 20, 2017, https://hab.hrsa.gov/about-ryan-white-hivaids-program/ryan-white -hivaids-program-legislation.

40. "Health Insurance Portability and Accountability Act of 1996," accessed March 28, 2017, https://www.congress.gov/104/plaws/publ191/PLAW-104publ191 .pdf.

41. Steven Angelides, "The 'Second Sexual Revolution,' Moral Panic, and the Evasion of Teenage Sexual Subjectivity," *Women's History Review* 21, no. 5 (2012): 831–847.

42. David Carter, *Stonewall: The Riots That Sparked the Gay Revolution* (New York: St. Martin's Press, 2004).

43. Ibid.

44. Peter Braunstein and Michael William Doyle, *Imagine Nation: The American Counterculture of the 1960s and '70s* (Abingdon, UK: Routledge, 2002).

45. Brian Alexander, "Free Love: Was There a Price to Pay?," accessed June 1, 2017, http://www.nbcnews.com/id/19053382/ns/health-sexual_health/t/free-love-was-there-price-pay/#.WU5dhNyQzIU.

46. A. Salem, "A Condom Sense Approach to AIDS Prevention: A Historical Perspective," *South Dakota Journal of Medicine* 45, no. 10 (1992): 294–296.

47. S. Mboup et al., "HIV/AIDS," in *Disease and Mortality in Sub-Saharan Africa*, ed. D. T. Jamison et al. (Washington, DC: The International Bank for Reconstruction and Development, 2006), 1–24.

48. "HIV/AIDS," accessed January 15, 2017, http://www.who.int/mediacentre/factsheets/fs360/en/.

49. Simon Dixon, Scott McDonald, and Jennifer Roberts, "The Impact of HIV and AIDS on Africa's Economic Development," *British Medical Journal* 324, no. 7331 (2002): 232–234.

50. Ibid.

51. "Impact of AIDS on Older People in Africa: Zimbabwe Case Study," accessed January 23, 2017, http://apps.who.int/iris/bitstream/10665/67545/1/WHO_NMH_NPH_ALC_02.12.pdf.

52. "Tuberculosis and HIV," accessed January 25, 2017, http://www.who.int/hiv/topics/tb/about_tb/en/.

53. Stephanie Nolen, *28: Stories of AIDS in Africa* (London: Walker Books, 2007), 199.

54. José Esparza, "What Has 30 Years of HIV Vaccine Research Taught Us?," *Vaccines* 1 (2013): 513–526.

55. Stefano Vella et al., "The History of Antiretroviral Therapy and of its Implementation in Resource-Limited Areas of the World," *AIDS* 26 (2012): 1231–1241.

56. Ibid.

57. Ibid.

58. S. Van der Borght et al., "The Accelerating Access Initiative: Experience with a Multinational Workplace Programme in Africa," *Bulletin of the World Health Organization* 87 (2009): 794–798.

59. S. Sayana and H. Khanlou, "Maraviroc: A New CCR5 Antagonist," *Expert Review of Anti-infective Therapy* 7, no. 1 (2009): 9–19.

60. J. Novembre, A. P. Galvani, and M. Slatkin, "The Geographic Spread of the CCR5 Δ32 HIV-Resistance Allele," *PLOS Biology* 3, no. 11 (2005): 1954–1962.

Chapter 12

1. C. Lee Ventola, "The Antibiotic Resistance Crisis: Part 1: Causes and Threats," *Pharmacy and Therapeutics* 40, no. 4 (2015): 277–283.

2. B. Spellberg and D. N. Gilbert, "The Future of Antibiotics and Resistance: A Tribute to a Career of Leadership by John Bartlett," *Clinical Infectious Diseases* 59, suppl. 2 (2014): S71–S75.

3. "WHO's First Global Report on Antibiotic Resistance Reveals Serious, Worldwide Threat to Public Health," accessed February 1, 2017, http://www .who.int/mediacentre/news/releases/2014/amr-report/en/.

4. C. Lee Ventola, "The Antibiotic Resistance Crisis."

5. "Antimicrobial Resistance: Tackling a Crisis for the Health and Wealth of Nations," accessed February 5, 2017, https://amr-review.org/sites/default/files /AMR%20Review%20Paper%20-%20Tackling%20a%20crisis%20for%20 the%20health%20and%20wealth%20of%20nations_1.pdf.

6. C. E. Luyt et al., "Antibiotic Stewardship in the Intensive Care Unit," *Critical Care* 18, no. 5 (2014): 480.

7. J. G. Bartlett, D. N. Gilbert, and B. Spellberg, "Seven Ways to Preserve the Miracle of Antibiotics," *Clinical Infectious Diseases* 56, no. 10 (2013): 1445–1450.

8. A. J. Wakefield et al., "Ileal-Lymphoid-Nodular Hyperplasia, Non-specific Colitis, and Pervasive Developmental Disorder in Children," *Lancet* 351, no. 9103 (1998): 637–641.

9. Ibid.

10. F. DeStefano, C. S. Price, and E. S. Weintraub, "Increasing Exposure to Antibody-Stimulating Proteins and Polysaccharides in Vaccines Is Not Associated with Risk of Autism," *Journal of Pediatrics* 163, no. 2 (2013): 561–567.

11. H. C. Hazlett et al., "Early Brain Development in Infants at High Risk for Autism Spectrum Disorder," *Nature* 542, no. 7641 (2017): 348–351.

12. T. S. Sathyanarayana Rao and Chittaranjan Andrade, "The MMR Vaccine and Autism: Sensation, Refutation, Retraction, and Fraud," *Indian Journal of Psychiatry* 53, no. 2 (2011): 95–96.

13. "Measles Cases and Outbreaks," accessed March 15, 2017, https://www .cdc.gov/measles/cases-outbreaks.html.

14. J. T. Schiller, X. Castellsague, and S. M. Garland, "A Review of Clinical Trials of Human Papillomavirus Prophylactic Vaccines," *Vaccine* 30, suppl. 5 (2012): F123–F138.

Index

About the Author

Joshua S. Loomis, PhD, is a microbiologist and professor at East Strouds-burg University. While earning his doctoral degree at the Pennsylvania State University College of Medicine, he worked on dissecting mechanisms by which viruses assemble during replication. His postdoctoral research at the University of Miami Sylvester Cancer Institute focused on the use of geneti-cally engineered viruses as novel treatments for cancer. In 2005, he accepted a faculty position at Nova Southeastern University and remained there for 10 years. While at NSU, he frequently taught courses in microbiology, genet-ics, immunology, cell biology, and epidemic disease. Dr. Loomis moved to East Stroudsburg University in 2015 and continued his teaching and research in microbiology. He has since become a partner in the Small World Initiative, a global consortium of scientists and students working together in search of novel antibiotics produced by soil microorganisms. Loomis has published his research in numerous scientific journals, including the *Journal of Virology* and *Nature Immunology*. He continues to run an active research program with his undergraduate and graduate students in many different subfields of microbiology, which include virology, biofilm formation, and antibiotic discovery.